The Pediatric Foot and Ankle

Michelle L. Butterworth
John T. Marcoux
Editors

The Pediatric Foot and Ankle

Diagnosis and Management

Springer

Editors
Michelle L. Butterworth, DPM, FACFAS
Williamsburg Regional Hospital
Kingstree, SC
USA

John T. Marcoux, DPM, FACFAS
Steward - St. Elizabeth's Medical Center
Brighton, MA
USA

ISBN 978-3-030-29786-2 ISBN 978-3-030-29788-6 (eBook)
https://doi.org/10.1007/978-3-030-29788-6

This Springer imprint is published by the registered company Springer Nature Switzerland AG
The registered company address is: Gewerbestrasse 11, 6330 Cham, Switzerland

This textbook is dedicated to our educators and training mentors at the Temple University School of Podiatric Medicine, the University of Pennsylvania Health Systems-Presbyterian Medical Center residency program, and the Podiatry Institute. Their professional guidance, motivation, and pursuit of excellence have always driven us to continuously keep raising the bar for the next generation of foot and ankle surgeons. In addition, this textbook is also dedicated to the many residents and students that we have had or will have the privilege to educate during our careers. May they all continue to pay it forward as we have!

Foreword

There are few accomplishments more satisfying for a foot and ankle surgeon than achieving a successful, long-term correction of a disabling and/or painful deformity in a child or adolescent's lower extremity.

Podopediatrics is a growing area of most foot and ankle surgeons' practices. The importance of addressing deformities early in their development has long been recognized for more severe lower limb, ankle, and foot deformities but now is being more fully explored, identified, and treated in many mild-to-moderate conditions. Surgery in the child or adolescent patient is much more than just "surgery on a small adult." The surgeries are often done on a growing lower extremity and foot and require careful planning with considerable attention to detail to achieve a lasting, good, long-term outcome. The timing of the surgery must often be deliberated and can affect the final result. Additionally, if present, neuromuscular disease can affect the treatment options and should be considered. The goal of surgery in the pediatric patient population often cannot entirely resolve a gait abnormality, neuromuscular disease, or pedal condition but should strive for lasting improvement in the quality of life for the juvenile patient.

The editors of this textbook have gathered together an outstanding, accomplished, and experienced group of surgeons who regularly perform foot and ankle surgery in the pediatric patient population. Among these authors are leading surgeons, traumatologists, professors, researchers, and most importantly parents. They clearly understand the trepidation of any parents electing to proceed with foot and ankle surgery on their child. Many of these authors have also given their time to medical mission trips to foreign countries, where surgery on the pediatric and adolescent foot and ankle are among the most common procedures performed.

This textbook has been carefully laid out to highlight the more common procedures done for this juvenile patient population. However, children are like "snowflakes," and no two congenital abnormalities or pediatric traumas are identical, further highlighting the criticality of proper patient and procedural selection. Therefore, this textbook is best used as a foundation for improving one's knowledge base in this continuously evolving and changing area of foot and ankle surgery. The editors and authors of this fine textbook have certainly achieved this goal and have successfully completed their mission.

Michael S. Downey, DPM, FACFAS
Division of Podiatric Surgery
Penn Presbyterian Medical Center
Philadelphia, PA, USA

Department of Surgery
Temple University of Podiatric Medicine
Philadelphia, PA, USA

The Podiatry Institute
Decatur, GA, USA

Preface

It is with great excitement that we present this textbook on the pediatric foot and ankle. We are extremely grateful for our teachers and mentors throughout our education, training, and careers. Without them, we would not have our passion for teaching and our thirst for knowledge to share with students, residents, and our fellow colleagues. It is because of our great educators and role models that we had the ambition and chose to embark on this great endeavor so that we can pay it forward to our profession.

We were very fortunate to have completed a 4-year surgical residency specializing in reconstructive surgery of the foot, ankle, and leg. One aspect of training that our residency initially lacked, however, was the evaluation and management of pediatric foot and ankle deformities. Then, with a stroke of luck and good fortune and a lot of efforts by our attendings, especially Dr. Kieran Mahan, we gained privileges at the Temple Children's Hospital in Philadelphia, PA, and our eyes were opened to a whole new realm of medicine. This amazing opportunity helped us broaden our skills and become well-rounded physicians and surgeons, encompassing all aspects of foot and ankle care.

The pediatric population is a very special patient group, and we have found them to be some of the most rewarding. When these patients endure surgery, it is usually because of significant deformity and/or trauma. And although most of these patients are a true pleasure to treat, their deformities and pathology can be quite challenging. Their physiology and psychology are very different from the adult; therefore, they have to be treated differently than the adult. We do, however, have to deal with adults, as parents and chaperones of these patients, so the problem as a whole can be very complex. It takes a very patient and understanding physician to encompass the entire family, address their concerns, and gain their trust in treating their beloved child. But once that trust is achieved, an incredible relationship is created.

The goal of this textbook is to be all encompassing including normal anatomy and development and evaluation and management of most pediatric foot and ankle entities. The chapters include clinical and radiographic evaluation and treatment options, both conservative and surgical. The most common pediatric problems from digital deformities, neurological abnormalities, clubfoot, flatfoot, sports medicine, and trauma have been included.

This textbook has been a labor of love. It has been a true honor and pleasure to work with such talented authors, we are proud to call our friends and colleagues, as they have shared their areas of expertise for the benefit of us all. It is our hope that this textbook will be a valuable and practical resource and provide you with great knowledge and assist you in evaluating and treating your pediatric patients. To be able to improve a juvenile's lifestyle, keep them mobile, eliminate or at least decrease their pain, and even return them to the athletic field makes a heart happy like no other. We hope you gain as much joy from treating this patient population as we do.

Kingstree, SC, USA Michelle L. Butterworth, DPM, FACFAS
Brighton, MA, USA John T. Marcoux, DPM, FACFAS

The updated online version of this book can be found at
https://doi.org/10.1007/978-3-030-29788-6_15

Acknowledgments

This textbook is the culmination of a journey that could not have been possible without the love, encouragement, support, and at times patience of our families, friends, and colleagues. We are deeply indebted to our contributing authors for their willingness to share their expertise on pediatric foot and ankle pathology. We appreciate the dedication and countless hours that were required to complete each chapter. They are truly experts in the field, and we are honored to have them as a vital part of this very special endeavor. We would also like to extend special thanks to Mr. Kristopher Spring and Prakash Jagannathan at Springer for their persistence and guidance throughout the editorial process.

Contents

Contributors

Patrick Stephen Agnew, DPM, FACFAS Family and Community Medicine, Eastern Virginia Medical School, Norfolk, VA, USA

Irina Bazarov, DPM Department of Podiatry, Kaiser Permanente, San Jose, CA, USA

Michelle L. Butterworth, DPM, FACFAS Williamsburg Regional Hospital, Kingstree, SC, USA

Craig A. Camasta, DPM, FACFAS Pediatric and Adult Reconstructive Foot & Ankle Surgery Fellowship, Atlanta, GA, USA

Department of Surgery, Emory St. Joseph's Hospital, Atlanta, GA, USA

Faculty, The Podiatry Institute, Decatur, GA, USA

Brian B. Carpenter, DPM, FACFAS Department of Orthopaedics, The University of North Texas Health Science Center, Fort Worth, TX, USA

Robert A. Christman, DPM, EdM College of Podiatric Medicine, Western University of Health Sciences, Pomona, CA, USA

Marissa S. David, DPM Podiatric Surgery Resident (PGY-III), Kaiser Permanente Santa Clara and GSAA, Santa Clara, CA, USA

Patrick A. DeHeer, DPM, FACFAP, FACFAS, FASPS, FFPM RCPS (Glasg) St. Vincent Hospital, Indianapolis, IN, USA

Private Practice Hoosier Foot & Ankle, Franklin, IN, USA

Robert Duggan, LAT, DPM, FACFAS Caldwell Foot and Ankle, Caldwell UNC Health Care, University of North Carolina Healthcare, Lenoir, NC, USA

University of Central Florida College of Medicine, Orlando, FL, USA

Timothy A. Graeser, DPM, AACFAS Private Practice, Motio Foot and Ankle Specialists, Winter Springs, FL, USA

Edwin J. Harris, DPM, FACFAS Loyola University Chicago, Stritch School of Medicine, Department of Orthopedics and Rehabilitation, Maywood, IL, USA

Rosiland Franklin University of Health Sciences, Dr. William M. Scholl College of Podiatric Medicine, Department of Podiatric Surgery and Applied Biomechanics, North Chicago, IL, USA

Daniel J. Hatch, DPM, FACFAS Medical Center of the Rockies, Loveland, CO, USA

North Colorado Podiatric Surgical Residency, Greeley, CO, USA

Byron L. Hutchinson, DPM, FACFAS Franciscan Medical Group: CHIFranciscan Foot & Ankle Associates: Highline Clinic, Seattle, WA, USA

Jessica M. Knight, DPM, AACFAS Weil Foot and Ankle Institute, Northwest Community Hospital Medical Group, Arlington Heights, IL, USA

Bradley M. Lamm, DPM, FACFAS Foot and Ankle Deformity Center and Fellowship, Paley Orthopedic and Spine Institute at St. Mary's Medical Center and Palm Beach Childerns Hospital, West Palm Beach, FL, USA

Caitlin Mahan Madden, DPM Private Practice, Podiatry Care Specialists, West Chester, PA, USA

Kieran T. Mahan, DPM Department of Podiatric Surgery, Temple University School of Podiatric Medicine, Philadelphia, PA, USA

Department of Podiatric Medicine and Surgery, Temple University Hospital, Philadelphia, PA, USA

Faculty, The Podiatry Institute, Decatur, GA, USA

College of Physicians of Philadelphia, Philadelphia, PA, USA

John T. Marcoux, DPM, FACFAS Steward – St. Elizabeth's Medical Center, Brighton, MA, USA

Emily D. Pugh, DPM, AACFAS Foot and Ankle Surgeon, Harvard Vanguard Medical Associates, Wellesley, MA, USA

Glenn M. Weinraub, DPM, FACFAS Department of Orthopaedic Surgery, TPMG- GSAA, San Leandro, CA, USA

Midwestern University, Glendale, AZ, USA

Western University, Pomona, CA, USA

Mitzi L. Williams, DPM, FACFAS, FACFAP Kaiser San Francisco Bay Area Foot and Ankle Residency Program, Department of Orthopedics and Podiatric Surgery, Kaiser Permanente, Oakland, CA, USA

Pediatry Institute Faculty Member, American Academy of Foot and Ankle, Osteosynthesis, Oakland, CA, USA

The Pediatric History and Physical Examination

1

Edwin J. Harris

Introduction

The purpose of the pediatric history and physical examination is to collect information. The objectives of the history are to identify and fully understand the chief complaint or complaints and all of their ramifications, acquire pertinent past medical and surgical information relevant to the chief complaints, identify other factors that may influence diagnosis and treatment, and begin the formation of a differential diagnosis. Obtaining the history is not a passive process. The examiner questions the historian, and the historian responds. Answers to the questions lead to new questions and the data base grows. The differential diagnosis is narrowed based on this information. If the history is properly obtained, the physical examination can be focused to support one of the diagnoses or rule several out.

Diagnostic errors can result from misinterpretation of these data but more often result from inattention to detail and failure to appreciate the importance of information obtained in the history.

E. J. Harris (✉)
Loyola University Chicago, Stritch School of Medicine, Department of Orthopedics and Rehabilitation, Maywood, IL, USA

Rosiland Franklin University of Health Sciences, Dr. William M. Scholl College of Podiatric Medicine, Department of Podiatric Surgery and Applied Biomechanics, North Chicago, IL, USA

The Historian

In pediatric practice, the patient is rarely the historian. The child may provide some useful information and the examiner should try to obtain as much information from the child as possible taking the child's age into consideration. Somebody other than the person experiencing the problem is relating the information and may be interjecting his or her own personal experiences and biases complicated by misinformation volunteered by well-meaning friends and relations, medical students, nurses, resident physicians, primary care physicians, referring physicians, and Internet searches. On occasion, the historian may even purposely withhold information because he or she finds it embarrassing or may think that those data are none of the examiner's business.

The historian's command of English may require an interpreter who is versed in translating medical concepts. Professional interpreters make every effort to translate verbatim, but circumstances may arise when an appropriate word may not be available and the interpreter is forced to improvise. Friends and family members, especially children, make very poor interpreters, and their services should not be used.

M. L. Butterworth, J. T. Marcoux (eds.), *The Pediatric Foot and Ankle*,
https://doi.org/10.1007/978-3-030-29788-6_1

The Information

Certain portions of the past medical history take on special significance. Some concerns are developmental in origin and possibly hereditary, adding importance to the developmental and family histories. Gait disturbances may really be movement disorders, prompting the examiner to search for risk factors suggestive of neurological pathology. Some might be the result of past medical conditions that have left permanent anatomical change, while others may be the residual of past trauma.

Organizing the Medical History

The Chief Complaint or Complaints

More diagnostic errors occur at this portion of the workup than anywhere else by failing to fully understand the chief complaint or complaints. There may be communication problems resulting from misunderstanding or the examiner may fail to recognize that there are actually several complaints that may or may not be related. The result is failure to identify the problem or problems correctly, leading to incorrect diagnosis and faulty treatment.

The chief complaint or complaints should be expressed in lay terminology. Medical terms offered by the caregiver should be changed into simple non-medical terms that are easily understood and agreed on by both the historian and the physician because, more often than not, the historian does not really understand the meaning of these terms. Worst-case scenario is that the historian is inadvertently relating incorrect secondhand information obtained from other sources. Mindful that the information is most likely not provided by the child, the historian may superimpose his or her own ideas based on personal experience, interpretation of the situation, or both.

Careful study of the chief complaint may reveal that there are actually several complaints. The inexperienced physician may make the incorrect supposition that all of the complaints are related when they may be separate isolated complaints with different etiologies. Each of these must be carefully explored and prioritized.

The History of the Chief Complaint or Complaints

All complaints have a natural history that aids in their understanding. The age of the patient at the onset of symptoms is important, since many orthopedic abnormalities are clustered in specific age groups. For example, most of the intoeing and outtoeing problems recognized before the child begins to walk are usually found in the foot. Between the ages of 1 and 2, rotational limb abnormalities are most likely in the tibiofibular segment. Past the age of 2, intoeing problems are more likely in the femur.

The history of the chief complaint or complaints should include their manifestations, onset of the symptom, the circumstances in which they developed, and any treatment rendered to date. This includes the location, quality, severity, timing, circumstances producing the symptom, and associated manifestations. Timing should include onset, duration, and frequency. Significant negatives will also help in the differential diagnosis. At this point in the workup, it is acceptable to begin to formulate a list of differential diagnoses that will help guide the remainder of the history and focus the physical examination.

The Past Medical History

The past medical history has two components – the immediate or current medical history and the more remote past medical history. Since many problems encountered in pediatric practice are acute, it is better to start with current events.

Overall Impressions

Asking the parents for their impression of the child's general health may reveal more about the caregiver's impression of the child than the actual medical state. This helps the examiner to better interpret what the caregiver relates. As an example, the caregiver may state that the child's general health is poor but, when questioned in detail, may actually indicate behavioral issues, dietary problems, or social interactions. Conversely, the caregiver may have a very cavalier attitude about more serious issues such as seizures, chronic diseases, and other illnesses.

Medications

All medications past and present should be reviewed. These may have immediate health implications or may suggest diseases that may have been forgotten or deliberately not divulged. Caregivers may be under the impression that only prescription drugs are important, but inquiries about over-the-counter medications, homeopathic remedies, and other alternative medications should be made. Some may be innocuous, but others have unappreciated pharmacological properties. The caregivers may be reluctant to report these medications because they fear that they might meet with physician disapproval. The same can be said for nontraditional medical treatments. As a part of the inquiry on medications, the examiner must specifically explore the effects of these medications both on the disease being treated and on the child in general. This should include the name of the medication, the dose, the response, the course of treatment, and the reason why the medication was used. This is especially important for medications having more than one indication. How far back in time the examiner probes the medication history is dictated by the chief complaint.

Alternative medical care includes massage therapy, acupuncture, chiropractic care, homeopathic medications, herbal medications, and vitamins. Most infants and children take vitamin supplements, but the clinician should be aware that certain vitamin therapies can become excessive and may actually be harmful.

Allergies

Allergic reactions can be caused by medications, foods, and environmental allergen including latex and other contact allergens. The examiner must attempt to determine whether an adverse response to any of these is a true allergy, an idiosyncrasy, or a parental concern not based in fact. As examples, caregivers often relate that the child is allergic to penicillin. Penicillin is a broad term and it should be remembered that native penicillin is rarely used today because of antibiotic resistance. Most exposure is to the semisynthetic penicillins and cephalosporins. In some cases, penicillin-related antibiotics are avoided because another family member supposedly has an allergy to these medications. In this case, there is no documented allergy for that child. In other cases there may be nausea or vomiting following use of a drug that is actually the result of the disease being treated and not the medication. Other adverse responses are clearly allergic in nature. Respiratory difficulty, generalized urticaria, angioedema, and anaphylaxis result from a severe allergic reaction. In some cases, the caregiver will report somnolence or euphoria following ingestion of certain medications. Here, a true allergy is questionable. Similarly, macular rashes on the chest with certain antibiotics may be a nonallergic response. There is a fine line between an allergy and an idiosyncrasy. Placing the child at risk for subsequent adverse response is not justified. However, denying a child an entire class of medications when no true allergy exists is equally problematic. If a true allergy exists, this is an excellent educational opportunity to stress the need for immediate medical attention as soon as symptoms develop and to have injectable epinephrine on hand.

Childhood Illnesses

Childhood diseases for which vaccinations are available include rubella, rubeola, varicella, pertussis, mumps, poliomyelitis, diphtheria, and tetanus. Vaccination programs are highly successful and carry very little risk. As the result, these diseases are uncommon in the community.

Other childhood illnesses include type I diabetes, scarlet fever, rheumatic fever, roseola, fifth disease, hand-foot-mouth disease, asthma, and other forms of reactive airway disease, respiratory syncytial viral infections, Asperger syndrome, autism, and learning and behavioral disorders.

Immunizations

Immunizations protect both the child and the community from the communicable diseases of childhood. These include mumps, measles, pertussis, polio, rubella, varicella, haemophilus infections, hepatitis B, and tetanus. Some parents refuse vaccinations based on religious beliefs or concerns that vaccinations may be harmful to the children. At the current moment, there is no supportive evidence that vaccinations cause autism or any of the group of illnesses purportedly caused by the vaccination programs. The harm of withholding vaccinations exceeds the theoretical risks. Every effort should be made to insure that the child's vaccinations are up to date. It should be kept in mind that some parents choose to decline vaccinations for their children and are unlikely to be persuaded.

Special inquiries about tetanus immunization and last booster injection are critical pieces of information when penetrating trauma is the chief complaint. Recent data suggests that certain vaccinations do not confer lifetime immunity and boosters are necessary.

Surgical History

The surgical history identifies past surgical diseases and responses to anesthesia. Caregivers remember major interventions, such as tonsillectomy, adenoidectomy, appendectomy, intussusception, hernia repair, and similar procedures. They often forget about others such as tympanostomy, dental procedures, and revision of circumcisions or do not consider these surgical even though they require general anesthesia. The same can be said for upper and lower endoscopies, urological imaging procedures, examination under anesthesia, and MRI. Infants and young children require general anesthesia or deep sedation for these procedures. Searching for the reason for these interventions often yields forgotten information regarding general health issues. Responses to anesthesia may help plan further lower extremity procedures and help select the appropriate facility for their performance.

Trauma

Fractures, lacerations, and other injuries should be noted. This includes the nature of the trauma, how it happened, treatment, and the sequel. The examiner should always be aware of repeat or unusual patterns of injury that might suggest non-accidental trauma.

Admissions

The dates and reasons for hospital admissions as well as the treatment rendered should be obtained. If indicated, medical records should be requested. Emergency room and urgent care visits should be identified as well.

Social and Developmental History

The number of siblings, their ages, and the patient's position in the sibship should be determined. This requires compassionate questions about the number of pregnancies and the number of live births and surviving children. Since the causes of sibling demise include stillborns, genetic events, childhood disease, and trauma, if possible, the cause of demise should be identified.

The living situation should also be explored. The number and relationships of other household dwellers should be determined. This may be important when other family members bring the child for examination and treatment. The principal responsible caregiver should be identified. If the principal caregiver is not a parent, the examiner must determine whether that person is empowered legally to give consent for any invasive treatment or even the initial physical examination.

Inquiry should be made about the child's educational status. This includes the academic year; performance in school; interaction with peers; in-school occupational, physical, and speech therapy; and any special educational needs. The examiner should also inquire about sports participation, hobbies, and other avocations.

Certain information including smoking, alcohol consumption, drug, and sexual activity may be difficult to obtain. These are not encountered in the very young children, but may be activities engaged in by preteens or teenagers. The patient would be extremely unlikely to divulge this information in the presence of a parent or other caregiver. Separating the child from the caregiver to obtain this information is a technique employed by the primary care provider or pediatrician, but is usually not an option for a specialist.

The Developmental History

The developmental history is the chronology of the child's progression from fetal state to the current time. The status of the mother's health at the time of conception is important. Medications prescribed for the mother's health during pregnancy (sometimes before pregnancy is recognized) can have adverse effects on the developing fetus. For example, the effects of thalidomide were not recognized for several years. Recreational drug use, alcohol, and tobacco smoking also adversely affect the fetus.

Complications occurring during pregnancy affect fetal development and survival. Premature labor is often a sign of fetopathy. Uterine abnormalities such as bicornuate uterus and fibroids can also influence pregnancy. Placenta previa, placenta abruption, nuchal cord, and malpositioning can influence the survival and development of the fetus and increase the risk of neurological damage during delivery.

Length of gestation has significance. Labor may be premature, spontaneous, or induced. If induced, the examiner should determine the reason. Prolonged labor may be a factor in central nervous system pathology as the result of hypoxia and intracranial bleeding.

Assisted vaginal delivery can result in clavicular fractures and brachial plexopathy. Cesarean section carries its own set of risks and is not the method of choice for most pregnancies. If a cesarean section is required, the examiner should determine the reason.

Breech presentations carry their own sets of risks. Abnormal positioning can be corrected immediately prior to delivery with obstetrical maneuvers, but certain other presentations are not deliverable vaginally. Not only do these require cesarean section, but they carry their own orthopedic morbidities. For instance, frank breech presentation is often associated with the triad of hip dysplasia/dislocation, knee subluxation, and calcaneovalgus foot deformity.

Infant data associated with delivery include length, weight, and Apgar scores [1] (Table 1.1).

Identifying the length of stay after delivery may also give valuable information. A healthy

Table 1.1 Apgar score

Color	
Blue, pale	0
Body pink, extremities blue	1
Completely pink	2
Heart rate	
Absent	0
< 100 beats per minute	1
> 100 beats per minute	2
Response to nasal stimulation	
No response	0
Grimace	1
Sneeze, cough	2
Respiratory effort	
Absent	0
Slow, irregular	1
Crying	2
Muscle tone	
Limp	0
Some extremity flexion	1
Active movement	2

Scores determined at 1 and 5 minutes after birth. Healthy 7–10, mild to moderate depressed 4–6, seriously ill 0–3 neonate is usually discharged home with the mother within 48 hours. If there is significance post-delivery icterus, the length of stay may be increased. Initial difficulties with feeding and respiration and workup for neonatal fever and infection will increase the length of stay. These latter may require blood cultures, special imaging, and spinal tap.

Major motor landmarks include development of head control, rolling from prone to supine and supine to prone, sitting, crawling, standing, cruising, independent walking, speech, development of cerebral dominance, and bowel and bladder training (Table 1.2).

Family History

The examiner should begin by inquiring about the occurrence of the same or similar problems in other family members. Additional questioning searches for anemia, bleeding disorders, diabetes, hypertension, asthma, ischemic heart disease, tuberculosis, hypercholesterolemia, liver disease, cerebral vascular accident, renal disease, hepatic disease, cognitive dysfunction, immune diseases, epilepsy, alcohol and drug abuse, cancer, the various forms of arthritis, and blood dyscrasias. Inquiry about sickle cell trait and disease should be made in patients who are genetically prone. Questions about other family member response to general anesthesia might give information about possible malignant hyperthermia. Giving the caregiver some prompts by systems makes going through a long list unnecessary. The examiner needs to be aware that the historians may withhold information if they feel threatened by its revelation.

Table 1.2 Developmental milestones

Head control
One month moves head from side to side while prone
Two months holds head and neck up begins to push while prone
Three months will control head when supine and lifted by arms
Pushing up well on arms while prone
Rolling over
4–5 months rolling over first prone to supine
5 months rolling over both ways
Sitting
Six months sitting independently
Crawling
Seven months crawling, scooting, army crawling
Standing
Seven to nine months pulls to stand
Cruising
Nine to ten months cruising around objects
Walking
Twelve to thirteen months independent walking
Cerebral dominance
Twenty-four months develops hand preference
Bowel and bladder control
Thirty to forty months bowel and bladder trained

Systems Review

A general review includes both objective and subjective information such as nutritional status, weight stability, weakness, fatigue, unexplained fever, loss of appetite, and information on general well-being.

Information about the head includes such things as headache, dizziness, and history of head injury.

Assessment of the eyes includes the patient's perception of his or her vision, the use of glasses or contact lenses, redness, burning, excessive tearing, loss of vision, glaucoma, and cataracts.

Evaluation of the ears includes loss of hearing, tinnitus, and episodes of otitis.

The review of nose problems includes frequent upper respiratory infections, sinusitis, obstruction, discharge, and epistaxis.

Appraisal of the throat includes status of the dentition, mobility of the tongue, swallowing, throat pain, and hoarseness.

The neck is evaluated for known deformities, pain on range of motion, and general tenderness. Questions about thyroid pathology are also included.

Lymphatic pathology may occur in the neck, axilla, and inguinal and popliteal areas. Questions about local masses and pain will help identify generalized lymphatic pathology. The location of the involved nodes often identifies the remote site of the real pathology.

Pulmonary review includes presence of cough, dyspnea, wheezing, pain on inspiration or expiration, cyanosis, and exposure to chronic pulmonary diseases such as tuberculosis.

Cardiovascular evaluation includes chest pain, rhythm disorders, extremity edema, hypertension, and history of known cardiac disease such as rheumatic fever, murmur, and syncope.

Gastrointestinal review includes dysphagia, pain on swallowing, nausea, vomiting, abnormal bowel patterns, rectal bleeding, icterus, disease of the liver and gallbladder, and hepatitis.

Urinary tract review includes hematuria, dysuria, nocturia, and polyuria, incontinence, and urinary tract infection.

Genital tract review for males includes history of hernia, testicular pain, scrotal masses, and sexually transmitted diseases. For females, age at onset of menarche, history of sexually transmitted diseases, pregnancy, and use of contraceptives are explored.

Musculoskeletal review includes congenital and acquired deformities, joint pain, stiffness, edema, and history of fractures.

Neurological review includes syncope, seizures, muscle weakness, altered sensations, decreased sensation, loss of sensation, paralysis, tremors, and headaches.

Psychiatric review includes anxiety, nightmares, irritability, depression, learning difficulties, and behavioral disorders.

Endocrine review places particular emphasis on disease of the thyroid; adrenals, and diabetes.

Hematologic exploration includes anemia, abnormal bleeding, unexplained ecchymoses, and sickle cell status in the genetically predisposed.

The Physical Examination

Like the history, the physical examination can be tailored to meet the needs of the chief complaint or complaints. Subject to the complaint, the examination may be problem focused or comprehensive. However, all levels of physical examination have basic common components.

The physical examination often has to be modified depending on the child. The comprehensive nature of the examination must be maintained, but the examiner should not feel bound by any particular format. In general, components of the examination requiring patient cooperation should be performed first while the child's focus can be maintained. Portions of the examination based on observation should also be performed early in the encounter. Particularly in the young child, manipulation and position changes should be minimized. As much as possible, it should be performed in one anatomical position. This often means that the sequence of the examination needs to be modified. Unpleasant or painful portions of the examination should be performed last. As a final note, the safest place for an apprehensive or uncooperative child is on the parent's lap.

Vital Signs

Vital signs are considered integral to all physical examinations, and most electronic medical records systems require them with every patient encounter. These include temperature, heart rate, respiratory rate, height, weight, BMI, and pain rating.

Temperature

Temperature can be measured by a number of routes utilizing a variety of instruments. Mercury glass thermometers have been largely replaced with electronic digital thermometers because of the hazards of mercury. Procedures include oral, rectal, axillary, tympanic membrane, forehead skin, and temple artery routes. Tympanic and forehead skin measurements are not reliable. Temporal artery, tympanic membrane, and axillary measurements suffice for screening but lack reliability. Elevated measurements by these routes should be verified by repeating the oral or rectal routes. Current recommendations are the oral route for children 4 years and older and the rectal route for infants, toddlers, and children under 4 years of age. Results can be recorded in degrees Celsius and Fahrenheit (Table 1.3). When sequential temperatures are monitored,

Table 1.3 Temperature equivalents Fahrenheit to Celsius

98.2 °F	36.8 °C
98.4 °F	36.9 °C
98.6 °F	37.0 °C
98.8 °F	37.1 °C
99.0 °F	37.2 °C
99.2 °F	37.3 °C
99.4 °F	37.4 °C
99.6 °F	37.6 °C
99.8 °F	37.7 °C
100.0 °F	37.8 °C
100.2 °F	37.9 °C
100.4 °F	38.0 °C
100.6 °F	38.1 °C
100.8 °F	38.2 °C
101.0 °F	38.3 °C
101.2 °F	38.4 °C
101.4 °F	38.6 °C
101.6 °F	38.7 °C
101.8 °F	38.8 °C
102.0 °F	38.9 °C
102.2 °F	39.0 °C
102.4 °F	39.1 °C
102.8 °F	39.3 °C
103.0 °F	39.4 °C

Table 1.4 Fever thresholds by route

Fever is present if:
Oral temperature is over 99.5 F (37.5 C)
Rectal temperature is over 100.4 F (38.0 C)
Axillary temperature is over 99.0 F (37.2 C)[a]
Tympanic membrane temperature is over 100.4 F (38.0 C)[a]
Temporal artery temperature is over 100.4 F (38.0 C)[a]
Pacifier temperature is over 100.0 F (37.8 C)
Thermocrystal forehead temperature not recommended

[a]Accuracy of axillary, tympanic membrane and temporal artery temperatures is questionable and should be verified by oral or rectal route

all recordings should be determined by the same method – avoiding mixing oral and rectal routes. Fever thresholds by route are listed in Table 1.4.

Heart Rate

Heart rate can be measured by palpating an artery or by auscultating the chest. Radial, dorsalis pedis, posterior tibial, and popliteal arteries are considered peripheral arteries, while carotid, brachial, and femoral arteries are considered central and are the sites preferred for seriously ill children in shock. The rate and rhythm can be verified both by palpating an appropriate artery and by auscultation. The quality of the pulse can only be determined by palpation. The rate is best determined by counting the beats in 30 seconds and multiplying by 2. If there is an obvious unusual rhythm, the rate should be counted over 1 minute.

Blood Pressure

Blood pressure can be measured at any age. Cuff size is the most important factor in accurately determining pressure. Neonate and infant cuffs average 5.5 cm in width in order to appropriately fit the middle of the upper arm. Toddlers and children can be measured utilizing cuff width of 7 cm. A 10 cm width cuff is appropriate for older children and preteens. Past that age, a 14 cm adult cuff will suffice. Systolic and diastolic pressures are recorded along with the pulse pressure. Abnormalities include pulsus paradoxus defined as an abnormal decrease in systolic pressure during inspiration and abnormal pulse pressure reflecting the state of systemic vascular resistance. Occasionally, Korotkoff sounds cannot be heard. It helps to raise the arm above the shoulder before inflating the cuff. Otherwise, systolic pressure is determined by palpation of the radial artery as cuff pressure is lowered. Minimum systolic pressure in children is determined by the formula $P = 70$ mm/hg + age in years × 2.

Respiratory Rate

Determining respiratory rate is problematic because the child often alters the rate and rhythm if he is aware that respiratory rate is being observed. There are two ways of avoiding this error. The first technique is to spend 30 seconds determining pulse rate by radial palpation. Next, the examiner spends 30 seconds measuring respiratory rate by observing chest excursions during respiratory effort while continuing chest auscultation. The second technique is to auscultate the heart and count respirations at the same time.

Height

Height is recorded in inches or centimeters and is usually done with the shoes off. A number of wall charts and similar devices are commercially available. Height can be recorded in conjunction with age to give a percentile rank for the child comparing other children of the same gender.

Weight

Accurate weight is important for maintaining correct vital statistics and for dosing medications. Parents are likely to incorrectly estimate the child's weight, so it is better to place the child on a scale. Weight is recorded in pounds or kilograms. Conversions are as follows: pounds to kilograms multiply pounds by 0.45 and kilograms to pounds multiply kilograms by 2.2.

BMI

The formula for calculating body mass index is the child's weight in kilograms divided by the child's height in centimeters squared. This is rather cumbersome to do manually, and there are a number of available online programs that will calculate based on age, gender, weight in kilograms, and height in centimeters. Many electronic medical records programs calculate this automatically when vital signs are entered.

Pain Estimation

Estimation of the severity of entrance level pain is determined using the Visual Analog Pain Scale. The examiner shows the child a chart of multiple facial expressions ranging from happy smiling to severe distress. Many children will greatly overestimate the severity of the pain on initial evaluation and rate it higher than the examiner's estimation of his affect.

The General Physical Examination

The Head

The head and face are easily examined as a unit for symmetry and shape. The head is examined for microcephaly and macrocephaly. Head circumference is measured and recorded. This can be graphed for determination of percentile rank. Asymmetry of the eyes, plagiocephaly, and other variations of symmetry suggest in utero molding. The fontanels are examined for fullness, flatness, and size. Muscle weakness of the face is easily assessed independent of examination the cranial nerves. Certain facial characteristics such as slanting of the palpebral fissures and thickness of the tongue are diagnostic for conditions such as Down syndrome and are immediately recognized by simple inspection.

The Eyes

The eyes are examined for symmetry of the pupils, roundness, response to light, and accommodation. The extraocular movement patterns are also easily examined. The sclerae are examined for color and presence of icterus. Lids are examined for ptosis and globes for proptosis.

The Ears

Ears are examined for position on the head, patency of the canals, tenderness, evidence of discharge, and the status of the tympanic membranes.

The Nose

The nares are inspected for patency. The septum is evaluated for position and lesions. The mucosa is examined for color. Any discharge is noted.

The Mouth and Throat

The lips are evaluated for color and presence of lesions. The dentition is inspected for carries. Buccal and gingival mucosa are evaluated for color, presence of lesions, and hypertrophy. The tongue is evaluated for lesions, fasciculations, and mobility. The uvula is inspected for position and mobility. The tonsils are inspected for size, color, and the presence of inflammation.

The Neck

The neck is examined for range of motion and the presence of pain. Obvious deformities such as high riding shoulders and torticollis are easily identified. The cervical, submental, and supraclavicular lymph nodes are palpated for size, mobility, and tenderness. The trachea should be in midline. The thyroid should be smooth, symmetrical, and nodule-free. The carotid arteries are usually not palpated in children.

The Chest and Lungs

The chest is inspected for symmetry and obvious deformities such as pectus excavatum and carinatum. Breath sounds over the large airway passages and the periphery are evaluated by auscultation. Percussion and evaluation for fremitus are performed as indicated.

The Heart

The heart is examined for rate and rhythm. S1 and S2 should be easily heard. Other adventitious sounds such as S3 and S4, opening snaps, and ejection clicks should not be heard. Murmurs are occasionally heard and their significance depends on their volume, frequency, and location. Frequently, on inspiration, S2 is split at the base. This is not considered pathological in most cases.

The Abdomen

The abdomen should be inspected visually first. The umbilicus should be midline. The presence of surgical scars and abnormal venous patterns should be noted. Next should come auscultation of bowel sounds, the renal arteries, the aorta, and common iliac arteries. Percussion and palpation should always follow auscultation. Superficial and deep palpation is performed to detect masses and the position of the liver and spleen.

The Spine

The child stands with his back to the examiner. The spine should be straight and the shoulders level. The iliac crests should be level, the natal cleft vertical, and the inferior gluteal folds at the same level. The back is examined for midline lesions such as hair patches, dimples, lipomas, and hemangiomas that might suggest cord pathology. The child is then examined from the side noting the amount of thoracic kyphosis and lumbar lordosis.

The Upper Extremities

The upper extremities should be evaluated for skin and nail lesions, joint tenderness, range of motion, tone, and muscle strength. Obvious skeletal deformities are also noted.

The Neurological Examination

The general neurological examination begins with an assessment of cognitive function. Interaction with the examiner, degree of alertness, and orientation in space and time are all easy observations to make.

The cranial nerve should be grossly tested (Table 1.5).

Gait should be evaluated for the overall pattern (full-flat toe-off, heel to toe, toe to heel,

Table 1.5 Cranial nerves

Cranial nerve I	Olfactory nerve and tract
	Test: sense of smell
Cranial nerve II	Optic nerve and tract
	Test: visual acuity
	Test: Perimetry
Cranial nerves III, IV, Vi	Oculomotor, trochlear, abducens
	Test: finger following for ocular muscle movement
	Test: accommodation
	Test: light reflex
	Test: consensual light reflex
Cranial nerve V	Trigeminal
	Test: sensation
	Test: corneal reflex
	Test: chewing to evaluate masseters
Cranial nerve VII	Facial
	Test: smile, whistle
	Test: taste
	Test: facial symmetry
Cranial nerve VIII	Acoustic
	Test: hearing acuity
	Test: Webber and Rinne tests
	Test: vestibular tests
Cranial nerve IX	Glossopharyngeal
	Test: gag reflex
Cranial nerve X	Vagus
	Test: sensory exam of pharynx
	Test: carotid sinus reflex
Cranial nerve XI	Spinal accessory
	Test: shrug shoulders and rotate head
	Test: observe muscle symmetry
Cranial nerve XII	Hypoglossal
	Test: examine tongue for symmetry, atrophy, tremors

and toe-toe). The direction of the foot to the line of progression should also be noted. Balance, unusual movement patterns, muscle shape, bulk, and strength all round out the general motor portion of the examination.

The sensory examination includes evaluation of sharp dull, two-point, hot/cold, and vibration. Position in space and time and balance using the Romberg test identify posterior column lesions.

Upper and lower deep tendon reflexes and search for pathological reflexes round out the neurological examination. Superficial reflexes are evaluated as indicated (Table 1.6).

Tonic and positional reflex patterns are evaluated as indicated. These are summarized in Table 1.7.

Table 1.6 Superficial reflexes

Corneal	Cranial nerves V and VII
Gag reflex	Cranial nerves IX and X
Upper abdominal	T7, 8, 9, 10
Lower abdominal	T10, 11, 12
Cremasteric	L1
Plantar	S1, 2

Table 1.7 Postural reflexes

Flexor withdrawal
Positioning: Patient supine, head midline, legs extended
Stimulus: Stimulate sole of foot
Abnormal response: Massive flexion of tested extremity
Involution: Age 2 months
Extensor thrust
Positioning: Patient supine, head midline, one extremity extended, the other flexed
Stimulus: Stimulate sole of flexed foot
Response: Extension of stimulated leg
Involution: Age 2 months
Asymmetrical tonic neck
Positioning: Patient supine, head midline, extremities extended
Stimulus: Turn head to one side
Response: Extension of limbs on face side, flexion of limbs on occipital side
Involution: Age 4–6 months
Symmetrical tonic neck
Positioning: Patient prone over examiner's knees
Stimulus: Ventroflex head
Response: Arms flex, legs extend
(opposite response when head is dorsiflexed)
Involution: Age 4–6 months
Supporting reaction
Positioning: Support patient in standing position
Stimulus: Bounce patient on soles of feet
Response: Increased leg extensor tone, plantarflexion of feet
Involution: Age 4 months
Neck righting

Table 1.7 (continued)

Positioning: Patient supine, head midline, extremities extended
Stimulus: Turn head to one side
Response: Total body rotation in direction of head rotation
Involution: Age 6 months
Moro
Positioning: Patient supine, limbs extended
Stimulus: Sudden noise, movement of exam table, head drop from 1–2 inches
Response: Abduction, extension, movement of limbs to midline
Involution: Age 4 months
Stepping reflex
Positioning: Patient suspended
Stimulus: Dorsum of foot touches underside of examining table
Response: Flexion of knee and hip
Involution: Age 4–5 months
Parachute reflex
Positioning: Infant suspended prone
Stimulus: Sudden lowering toward table
Response: Extends arms and legs
Involution: Persists throughout life

The Lower Extremity Examination

The Skin

In the absence of disease, the child's skin is normal in color. Local erythema usually means inflammatory disease such as infection in the form of cellulitis. Any inflammatory disease of the skin and articulations can produce erythema. Other color changes such as rubrocyanosis are signs of vasomotor instability. For instance, unilateral rubor is frequently associated with chronic regional pain syndrome. Generalized pallor may be associated with anemia, blood loss, and impending shock.

Diaphoresis can be seen in otherwise normal children. It is usually symmetrical in both upper and lower extremities. Changes associated with a single extremity suggest vasomotor instability. Excessive perspiration may lead to contact dermatitis and other forms of skin disease. When it occurs in conjunction with verruca, it is often associated with mosaic types that are difficult to manage.

Skin temperature is normally cooler distally becoming warmer moving in a proximal direction and should be comparable from side to side. Unusual gradations in temperature may also be a sign of vasomotor instability.

Superficial veins are commonly seen but should be barely noticeable and not tortuous. Focal aggregates of superficial veins or violaceous skin masses may represent hemangiomas.

Certain skin lesions suggest specific systemic diseases. These include café au lait spots seen in neurofibromatosis, hemangiomas that can be associated with Sturge- Weber syndrome, midline spine lesions associated with various forms of spinal dysraphisms, linear sebaceous nevi, periungual fibromas associated with tuberous sclerosis, and unilateral hemangiomas with overgrowth of the part characteristic of Klippel-Trenaunay syndrome (Fig. 1.1a–c).

Nail changes are particularly difficult to evaluate since so many diseases appear similar. These include thickening of the nails, discoloration of the nail surfaces, mycotic changes, and infections. Onychomycosis is relatively common. However, not every nail that is discolored, furrowed, fragmented and associated with subungual debris is a mycosis. Differential diagnoses include Darier's disease, pachyonychia congenita, nail changes associated with thyroid disease, contact dermatitis, eczema of the nail bed, lichen planus, psoriasis, traumatic nail disease, and yeast infections.

A variety of nevi are seen regularly on the lower extremities. These include compound nevi, junctional nevi, and dysplastic nevi. Size, consistency of color, elevation, and definitions of the margins are critical factors in diagnosis and decision-making. Lesions in inaccessible locations or in areas difficult to monitor should be excised because they may undergo transformation without the patient aware that this is happening.

Peripheral Vascular Examination

With the exception of congenital vascular anomalies, peripheral arterial and venous diseases are extremely rare in childhood. Lymphatic abnormalities are the exception to this rule.

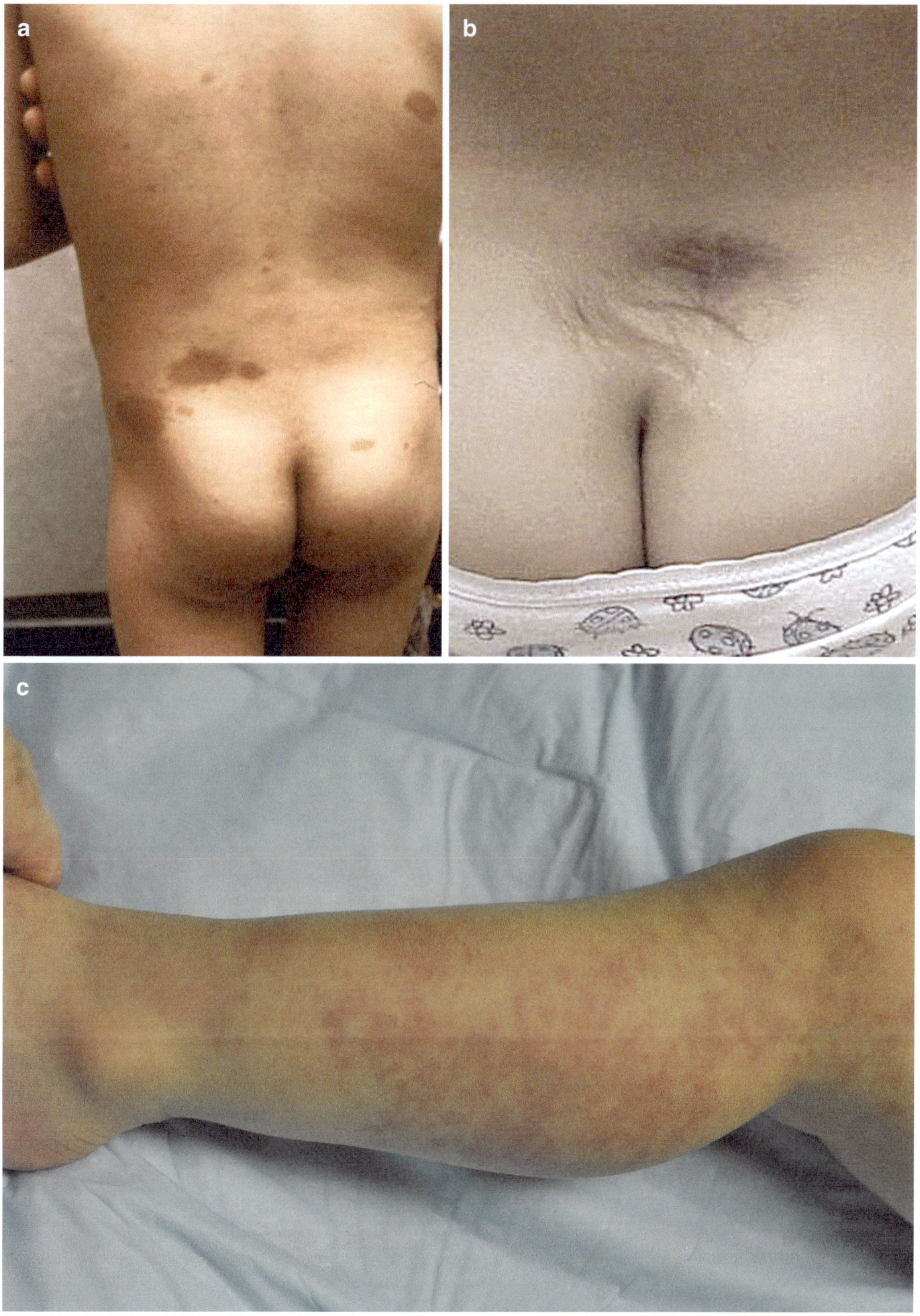

Fig. 1.1 (a–**c**) Certain skin lesions strongly suggest specific systemic diseases. Café-au-lait lesions (**a**) are the cutaneous manifestations of neurofibromatosis. Hair patches (**b**) and other midline spinal lesions suggest underlying neural tube abnormalities. Hemangiomas (**c**) with overgrowth of the part are seen in diseases such as Klippel-Weber-Trenaunay syndrome

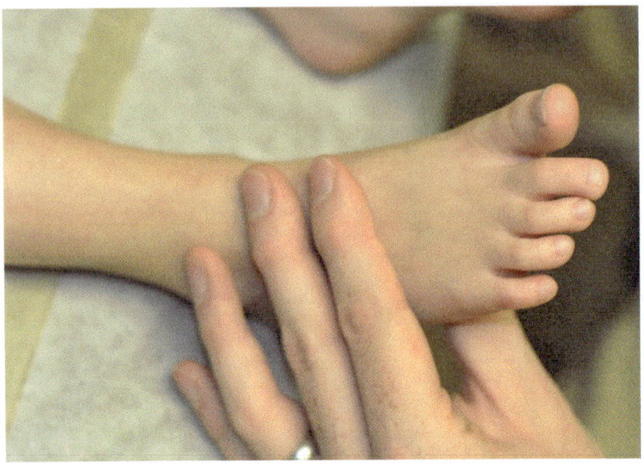

Fig. 1.2 The dorsalis pedis pulse is best palpated using the contralateral hand and placing the tips of the fingers over the course of the artery

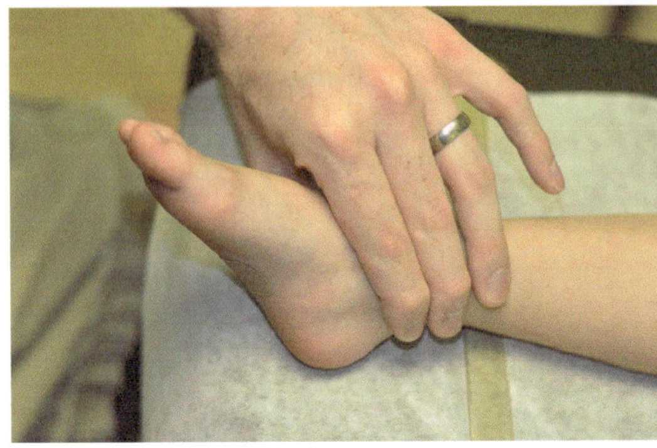

Fig. 1.3 The posterior tibial artery is best palpated using the contralateral hand and placing the tips of the fingers below the medial malleolus. Firm pressure is applied and slowly released until the pulsation is felt

The assessment begins with an evaluation of the skin color, temperature, and status of the skin and appendages. Capillary fill time is measured in seconds. The most important observation is palpation of the arteries.

The Dorsalis Pedis

The dorsalis pedis is usually easily palpable on the dorsal aspect of the foot in infants and children. The examiner palpates the dorsum of the foot with the contralateral hand placing the flats of the finger tips in the area of the artery and then gently compressing the skin until the pulsation is felt (Fig. 1.2).

In some children, the dorsalis pedis does not arise from the anterior tibial artery and may either be palpated as retrograde flow from the plantar or it may come from the perforating peroneal artery. Anterior tibial artery variations occur in approximately 80–90% of patients with idiopathic talipes equinovarus. In some cases, the anterior tibial artery ends above the malleoli, while in others, the anterior tibial artery may be anomalous at any point up to the trifurcation of the popliteal artery [2, 3].

The Posterior Tibial Artery

The posterior tibial artery may be difficult to palpate in young children. This does not infer vascular pathology, and the artery can easily be identified with Doppler. The examiner inspects each foot by using the contralateral hand. The thumb is placed along the lateral and plantar side of the foot, and the fingers extend over the tarsus to allow the tips of the fingers to pass below and proximal to the medial malleolus. Pressure is applied and then slowly relaxed until the pulse is felt (Fig. 1.3).

Posterior tibial artery variations are reported both in talipes equinovarus and congenital convex pes valgus and other congenital deformities [4–7].

The Popliteal Artery

The popliteal artery can be palpated with the child in either the supine or the prone position. In the supine position, the examiner places the thumbs along the patella and the fingertips meet in midline in the popliteal space. Pressure is applied in order to compress the popliteal artery against the posterior femur or the posterior tibia and then slowly released until the pulsation is felt (Fig. 1.4a). Alternately, the patient is placed in the prone position and the knee slightly flexed. The popliteal artery is felt in the popliteal space (Fig. 1.4b).

The Femoral Artery

The femoral artery is palpated in the groin. Since this is regarded as a central rather than

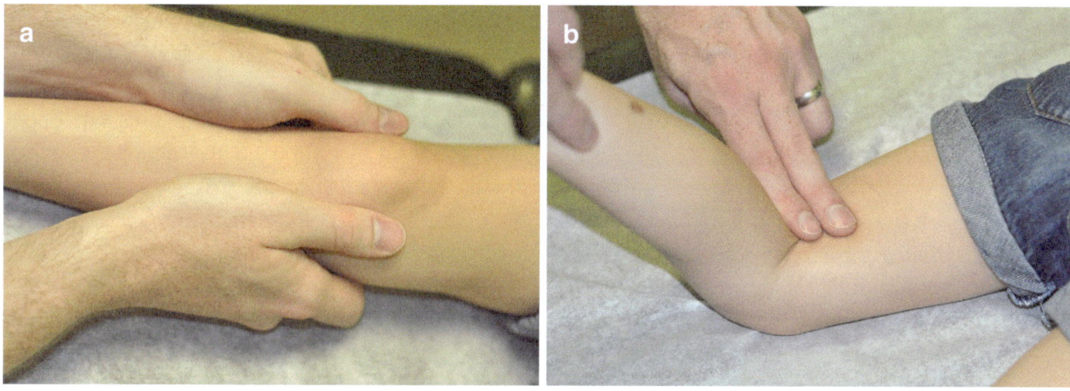

Fig. 1.4 (**a**, **b**) The popliteal artery can be palpated in two ways. The examiner places each thumb along the patella and his fingertips meet in the popliteal space (**a**). The artery is compressed against the posterior surface of the upper tibia until the pulse is felt. Alternately, the child is placed prone (**b**), the knee is flexed slightly, and the examiner's fingers compress the artery deep in the popliteal space. The popliteal lymph nodes are palpated at the same time

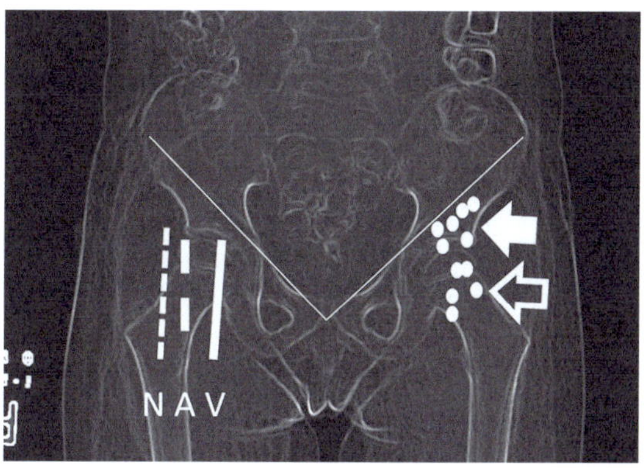

Fig. 1.5 On the left side, the positions of the femoral nerve (N), femoral artery (A), and femoral vein (V) are indicated. On the right side, the solid arrow points to the superficial inguinal lymph nodes and the open arrow to the superficial subinguinal lymph nodes

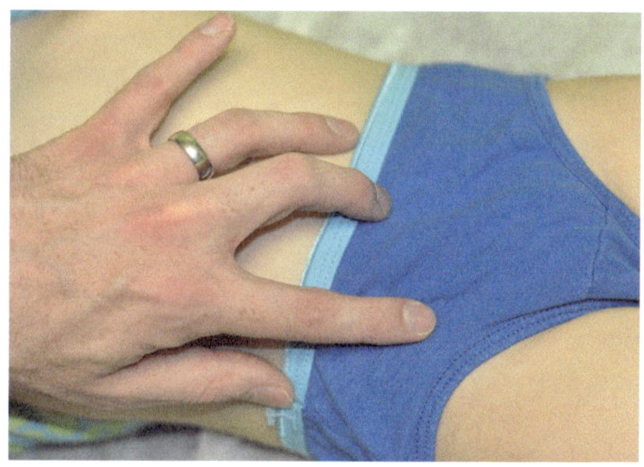

Fig. 1.6 The femoral artery is quickly located by placing the contralateral thumb on the anterior superior iliac spine and the long finger on the symphysis pubis. The index finger drops to the groin and usually is directly on the femoral artery. The procedure is reversed for the opposite side

peripheral artery, it is a vessel of choice in emergency assessment in infants and young children. It is palpated directly below the inguinal ligament. The location of the femoral artery with respect to the nerve and vein should be recalled. The most lateral structure is the femoral nerve. Immediately medial to it is the femoral artery and medial to the artery is the femoral vein (Fig. 1.5). A simple technique for locating the femoral artery is to stand to the lateral of the child. On the right side, the examiner places the thumb of the left hand on the anterior superior iliac spine and the long finger on the symphysis pubis. The index finger drops to the groin and in most cases will be directly on the femoral artery. The procedure is reversed for the left side (Fig. 1.6).

The Lymphatics

The superficial inguinal, superficial subinguinal, and popliteal nodes are the three groups of lymph nodes accessible in the lower extremity. The superficial inguinal nodes lie just distal to the inguinal ligament and drain the perineum, male and female genitalia, buttocks, and abdominal wall below the umbilicus. The superficial subinguinal nodes lie on either side of the proximal portion of the saphenous vein and largely drain the lymphatics of the lower extremity (Fig. 1.5). The popliteal nodes drain the lymphatics following the anterior and posterior tibial arteries.

The superficial inguinal nodes are palpated just below the inguinal ligament close to midline, and the superficial subinguinal nodes are palpated in the femoral triangle. Given the areas of their lymphatic drainage, nodes are often palpable in healthy infants and children. They should be small, freely movable, and painless to palpation. Since the popliteal nodes are in an area of considerable amounts of fat, they are not routinely identified on examination of healthy children.

General Inspection of the Lower Limbs

Visual inspection is performed with emphasis on limb length, muscle size, and anatomical position of the parts. Difference in limb length and transverse diameter may be very obvious and associated with other limb abnormalities. More often, the difference is less obvious and noticeable only when the posterior pelvic landmarks are asymmetrical in stance or with special limb positioning (Allis or Galeazzi tests). Atrophy of the muscle is easily identified by simple visual inspection, although it may be difficult to distinguish mild muscle atrophy from mild muscle hypertrophy. Bowing of the lower extremities can be appreciated by evaluating the relationship of the medial femoral condyles and the malleoli. Tibia varum is identified when the malleoli touch and the medial knees are separated. Genu valgum occurs when the medial knees touch and the malleoli are separated. These can be quantified by measuring the separation in inches or centimeters, or the angle formed by the axes of the femur and tibia can be measured. The position of the patellae and the position of the foot on the lower leg are also easily seen on simple inspection.

Enlargements of a limb can be identified by comparing one side to the other. This could represent simple edema. It may be pitting or brawny. Edema can have inflammatory causes but could also be caused by lymphatic obstruction and hypoplasia. These latter include Milroy's disease and lymphedema praecox. Arteriovenous malformations can also produce edema. Hemihypertrophy and hemiatrophy must also be considered in the differential diagnosis. Comparison of the upper and lower limbs may help determine whether an individual limb is increased in size or the opposite limb is hypoplastic. Hypertrophy of the lower limb can be associated with macrodystrophis lipoidicum, muscular hypertrophy, and other forms of focal or regional gigantism. Hemiatrophy is seen in muscle wasting disease, denervation, and congenital anomalies such as talipes equinovarus, tethered cord, and other issues characterized by denervation (Fig. 1.7).

The Evaluation of Gait

The human walking pattern evolves from toddlers to childhood and depends both on neurological maturation and learned behavior. Toddlers walk with wide ankle separation and external rotation to expand the base of support. The initial gait pattern is full-flat toe-off with exaggerated knee and hip flexion for foot clearance during swing phase. The heel toe pattern develops around age 2 and persists throughout life. The foot progression angle is also evolving, starting out with wide external rotation and becoming less as the child approaches age 2 years. The gait pattern can be modified by neurological dysfunction in the form of movement disorder, static limb abnormalities, or combinations of both.

The gait laboratory may be useful for pinpointing gait abnormalities, but much diagnostic information can be acquired through simple observation in the clinic by viewing the patient walking to and fro and from side to side. The gait evaluation should be performed with the least amount of clothing on the child as conditions allow. Evaluation should be done with and without shoes. The key elements are the position of the foot to the line of progression, malleolar

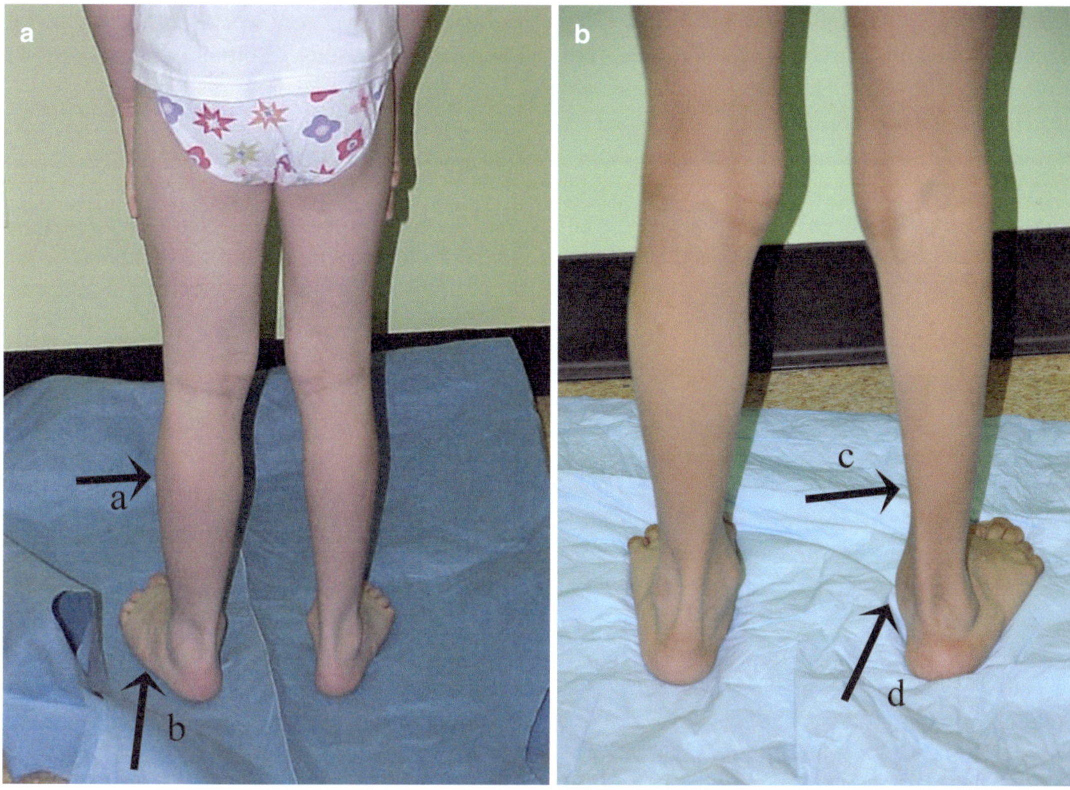

Fig. 1.7 (**a**, **b**) Limb hypertrophy and atrophy can usually be identified by simple inspection. Hypertrophy (**a**) can be seen in the thigh, calf (arrow a), and the foot (arrow b). Atrophy (**b**) in the calf (arrow c) and a small foot (arrow d) is seen in many skeletal conditions such as talipes equinovarus

separation in stance and gait (the angle and base of gait), stability, and the swing-stance patterns.

Foot Progression Angle

With the exception of adduction and abduction deformities in the foot such as pes cavus, metatarsus adductus, and forefoot abduction, abnormal foot progression angles are almost always supramalleolar in origin. Simple inspection identifies foot issues, and they are unlikely causes of intoeing or outtoeing noted while the child is wearing shoes. Further, intrinsic foot abnormalities are usually identified and treated successfully in infancy before the child begins to walk. Abnormalities in tibial torsion and femoral antetorsion (femoral anteversion) account for the majority of intoeing and outtoeing gait abnormalities in late toddlers and children.

Intermalleolar Distance

The amount of malleolar separation is a function of age. Toddlers as they begin to walk have tibia varum, bringing the malleoli close together while the knees are separated. This may be partially hidden by abduction of the limbs in the toddlers in order to provide some degree of additional stability. As the child ages, the tibia varum, which is physiologic in toddlers, gives way to genu valgum. This separates the malleoli when the knees just touch.

Stability in Gait

Stability in gait is a function of neurological maturation. Toddlers just beginning to walk are externally rotated with a wide base of gait. This balances the center of gravity over a larger surface area. Stability requires normal neurological function. As central nervous system myelination progresses, gait becomes more refined and stable. The degree of stability is also influenced by inverter-everter control and hip and trunk stability. As examples, peroneal muscle weakness may result in inappropriate inversion during stance. Weakness of the gluteus medius will result in joint instability and a Trendelenburg gait.

Stance and Swing

The relative ratios of stance and swing phases are easily evaluated. Abbreviated stance phase is almost always the result of pain in the limb and reflects the need to unload the painful limb by shortening stance phase, inappropriate knee extension, and early heel off. This is referred to as the antalgic gait pattern. It may be caused by pathology anywhere in the lower extremity. Children from the toddler stage even up to age 8 or 9 may identify the location of the pain quite some distance away from the actual source (referred pain). As an example, pain originating at the level of the hip is often referred to the medial knee. The examination of the extremity must include at least two joints above the apparent source of the pain.

Toddlers beginning to walk demonstrate exaggerated hip and knee flexion during swing. Stance phase begins with a full flat pattern followed by toe off at the end of stance [8]. As the child approaches age 2, the pattern becomes more mature with a distinct heel contact followed by full flat and toe off resembling adult gait.

There is no period in the development of gait when toe to toe walking is considered developmental and physiologic [8]. Variations from normal include premature heel off, toe to toe pattern, and toe to heel pattern. Premature heel off is often a finding of mild equinus deformity restricting full ankle dorsiflexion. Abnormal pronation is a compensatory mechanism allowing the heel to come closer to the ground during the early part of stance. Toe to toe pattern almost always occurs in association with severe fixed equinus. A toe to heel pattern results from weakness in the anterior compartment muscles resulting in drop foot.

The Lower Extremity Examination

The first part of the examination is visual inspection to identify obvious deformity of the lower extremities. These include abnormal digit position, forefoot adduction or abduction, medial column sag, prominent medial talar head, inverted and everted heel, unusual ankle positions, tibia varum, genu valgum, and difference in limb length. This is followed by measuring the lower extremity ranges of motion for both diagnostic and clinical decision-making.

Palpation for pain and edema are next. Localized edema and erythema associated with pain are the first indicators of local articular disease, joint sepsis, systemic disease, and trauma. Beginning with the distal interphalangeal joints, the entire lower extremity is palpated for local findings and range of motion.

Forefoot Ranges of Motion

Hallux range of motion is measured with the foot both on and off-weight-bearing looking for pain and restricted joint mobility. The procedure is repeated for the lesser digits.

In the absence of ligamentous laxity, there is little midfoot range of motion available, but the examiner may identify dorsiflexion or plantarflexion of the first ray which usually signifies some sagittal plane abnormality of part of the medial column.

Subtalar Range of Motion

Subtalar and ankle ranges of motion are critical to the diagnosis and treatment plans for most of the major foot and ankle deformities.

There are several methods for measuring subtalar range of motion, but the simplest tech-

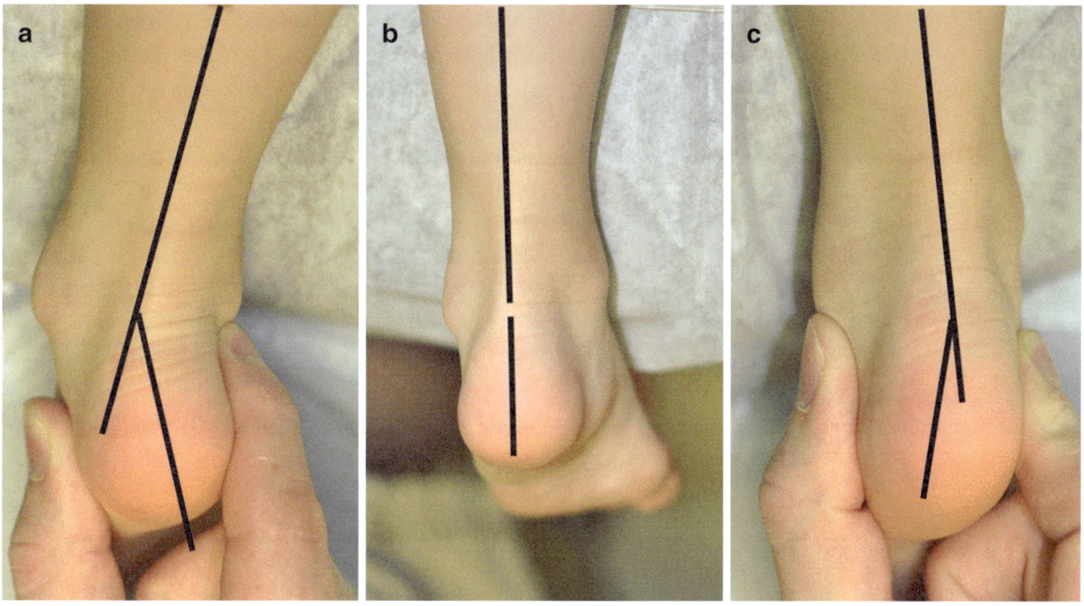

Fig. 1.8 (**a**–**c**) Subtalar range of motion is best measured with the child prone. The axis of the tibia is the proximal reference and the calcaneal bisection the distal reference. Inversion (supination) is measured (**a**), the heel bisection is in the same position as the tibial axis (**b**), and eversion (pronation) is measured (**c**)

nique is to place the child prone and measure the line of the heel bisection against the long axis of the tibia. When the heel bisection is in the same plane as the tibial bisection, this is interpreted as zero. Maximal inversion and eversion from that point are measured and recorded (Fig. 1.8). At the same time, the examiner estimates the amount of plantarflexion and dorsiflexion of the foot that occurs during measurement of subtalar range. This helps determine the orientation of the subtalar joint axis. Greater dorsiflexion and plantarflexion during this portion of the examination suggest a higher than normal position of the subtalar joint axis. More horizontal axes will show little foot dorsiflexion and plantarflexion.

There are many issues with trying to define and determine subtalar joint neutrality. The range of motion is more important. Normal comfortable subtalar function in children seems to occur around the vertical heel. Most symptoms occur when children function near, at, or in some cases slightly beyond the normal range of heel eversion.

Values obtained during measurements are both operator and instrumentation variable. A good rule of thumb for pediatric patients is 30° of inversion and 10° of eversion.

Forefoot to Rearfoot Relationship

Forefoot to rearfoot relationship is evaluated by determining the plane of the forefoot through the first metatarsal and fifth metatarsal heads and comparing it to the bisection of the heel (Fig. 1.9). Varus relationship of the forefoot usually indicates some dorsiflexion in the medial column between the navicular, the cuneiforms, and the first metatarsal base. Plantarflexion of the medial column producing a valgus forefoot-to-rearfoot relationship is usually associated with some degree of cavus deformity.

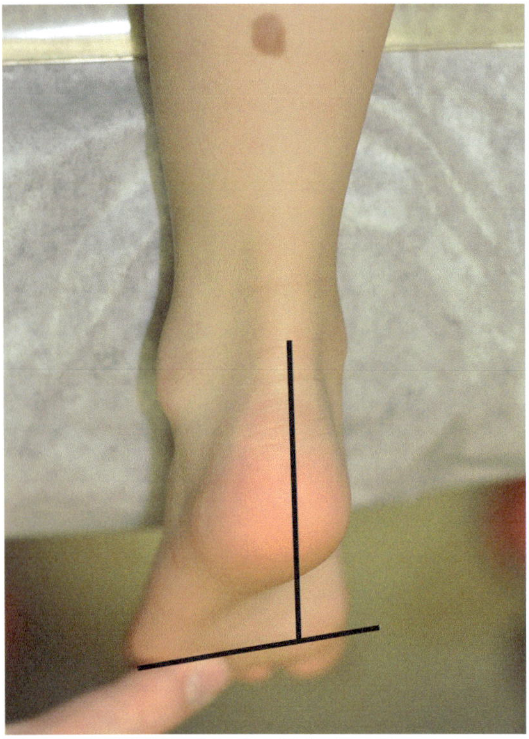

Fig. 1.9 Forefoot varus and valgus are best measured with the child prone. A line passing along the first and fifth metatarsal heads is measured against the calcaneal bisection

Ankle Range of Motion

Abnormal ankle range of motion is a component of many foot deformities. Like subtalar range of motion measurements, the results are both examiner and instrument dependent. Some standardization of the technique is necessary, and it is recommended to follow the physical therapy literature by measuring ankle dorsiflexion and plantarflexion with the heel bisection parallel with the axis of the tibia. Although this is somewhat artificial, any error in the technique will be canceled out, since it is applied to all patients the same way. Dorsiflexion of the ankle in maximal pronation produces more motion because the subtalar joint pronation allows the lateral margin of the foot to dorsiflex. Conversely, measurement with the rearfoot inverted will decrease the range of ankle joint motion.

The technique is best performed with the patient in the prone position. The calcaneal bisection is placed in the same plane as the tibial bisection and ankle dorsiflexion is measured using the lateral margin of the foot and the axis of the fibula as the references. This is performed first with the patient allowing passive range of motion and again with the patient assisting in dorsiflexion. Plantarflexion is measured the same way.

Dorsiflexion range of motion is first measured with the knee in the extended position (Fig. 1.10a) and again in the flexed position (Fig. 1.10b). Since the gastrocnemius takes much of its origin from the posterior condyles of the femur above the level of the knee joint, flexing the knee effectively lengthens the gastrocnemius muscle allowing evaluation of the soleus. This is the basis of the Silfverskiold test to be discussed later.

Dorsiflexion ranges of motion vary from patient to patient, but the examiner should expect at least 10° with the knee in extension and as much as 20° with the knee in flexion. Exaggerated range of motion occurs with ligamentous laxity.

The Silfverskiold test clarifies the anatomical nature of equinus deformity [9]. By evaluating the range of motion at the ankle with the knee in the extended and flexed position, the various components of the triceps mechanism can be evaluated for contracture (Fig. 1.11a–d). Ten degrees of dorsiflexion in knee extension and 20° of knee flexion is a normal range of motion for most children and indicates the absence of ankle joint equinus.

Limitation of ankle dorsiflexion to neutral or below in knee extension followed by additional dorsiflexion to near normal with the knee flexed implicates the gastrocnemius component as the contracted portion. If surgical intervention is indicated, some form of gastrocnemius lengthening is the procedure of choice.

Inadequate ankle dorsiflexion with the knee extended and flexed implicates both the gastrocnemius and the soleus components, but with this test, it is impossible to further isolate the gastrocnemius component.

This interpretation of the Silfverskiold test is only valid for neurologically normal children. Of interest, Silfverskiold's original article dealt with children who were not neurologically normal [9]. The neurologically abnormal child, especially in the presence of spasticity, is interpreted differently. In some cases, the issue is really hypertonicity. Tone is modified by the position of the more proximal joints and decreases distally permitting more motion. The result could be misinterpreted, since flexing the knee might decrease tone enough in the leg to erroneously indicate the need for gastrocnemius lengthening alone.

Other factors can impact ankle range of motion. Cavus deformities restrict ankle joint motion because the plantarflexion of the forefoot against the rear foot raises the talus higher in the ankle mortise. When the range of motion is evaluated, the talar neck abuts against the anterior tibia, producing a "bony block" equinus. Alterations in the talar dome can produce a similar restriction of motion by flattening down the

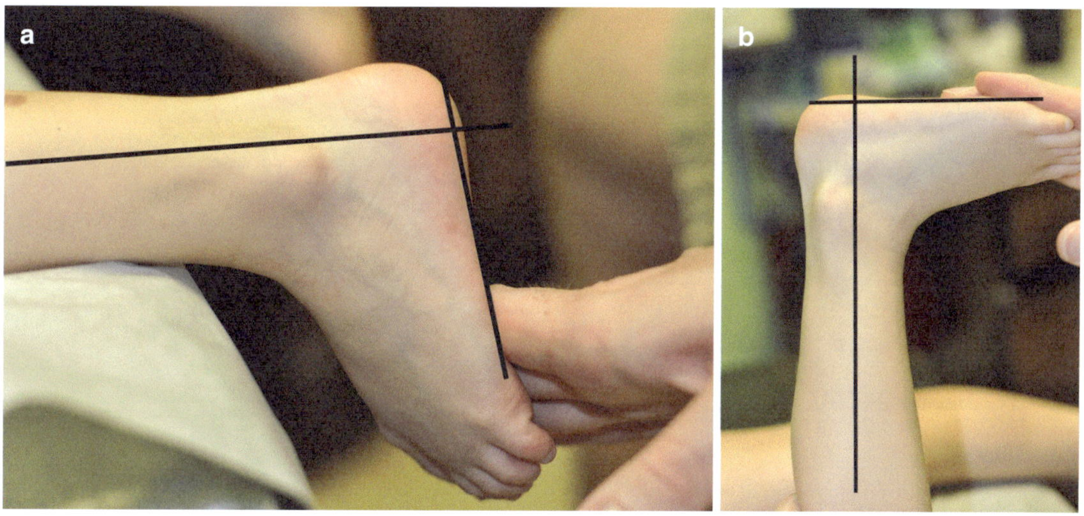

Fig. 1.10 (**a**, **b**) Ankle dorsiflexion is best measured with the child prone and the heel bisection in the same plane as the tibial axis. Ankle dorsiflexion is first measured with the knee extended (**a**) and repeated with the knee flexed (**b**)

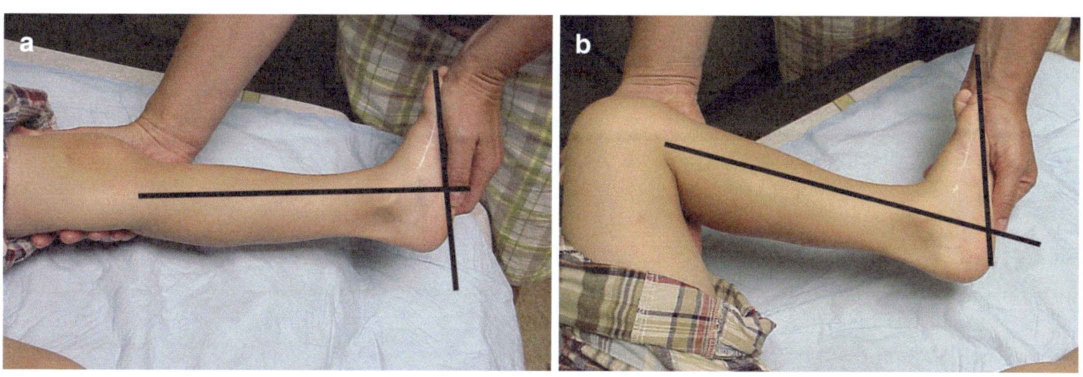

Fig. 1.11 (**a–d**) The Silfverskiold test is used to determine which component of the triceps mechanism contributes most to ankle equinus. Ankle dorsiflexion with the knee first extended and then flexed (**a**, **b**) show limited dorsiflexion in extension but more dorsiflexion with the knee flexed – implicating the gastrocnemius as the cause. Ankle dorsiflexion is abnormal in both positions (**c**, **d**) suggesting the soleus (and possibly also the gastrocnemius) as the cause

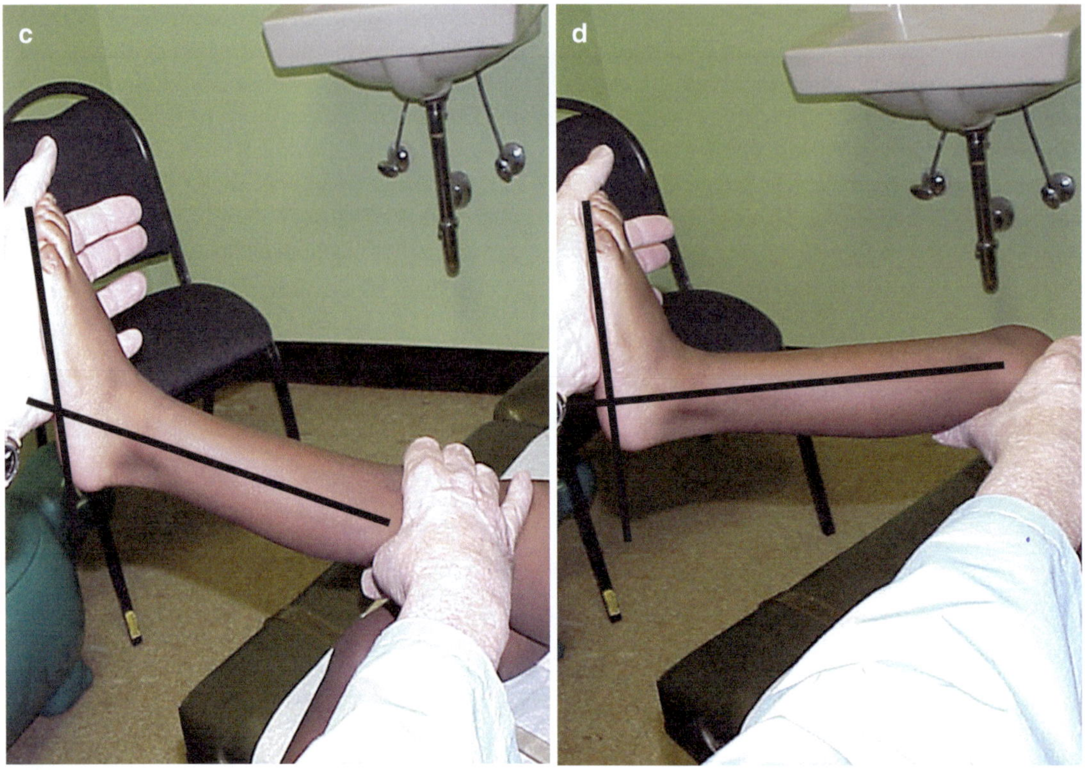

Fig. 1.11 (continued)

talar articular surface. This is a common complication following operative treatment for talipes equinovarus (Fig. 1.12).

The Relationship of the Knee Axis to the Ankle Axis (Tibial Torsion)

Most physicals are performed in the examining room. There is limited equipment available. Consequently, simple cost-efficient techniques are desirable. Although there are sophisticated tools available for measuring tibial torsion, they are impractical for most examinations because of the cost in medical resources [10–23] as well as the amount of radiation involved [24, 25].

In infancy, the ankle axis is internally rotated to the knee axis, which progressively externally rotates with age so that by approximately age 5, the ankle axis should be externally rotated 15–20° to the knee axis. The knee axis is easy to define, and simple flexion and extension of the knee will give the examiner the visual cue needed to establish that reference. The ankle axis, on the other hand, has no regularly occurring anatomical landmarks. Flexion and extension of the ankle does not define the axis. It has become the standard to use a line passing between the tips of the medial and lateral malleoli instead. This line does not correspond to the true ankle joint axis and there is considerable debate about the relationship. However, it will suffice for clinical measurement of tibial torsion.

The relationship between the knee and the ankle axis is determined by placing the child supine on the examining table. The hip is flexed at right angles to the trunk. Knee extension and flexion is ranged, and the femur is moved medially and laterally until the tibia is extending and flexing in the sagittal plane of the body, positioning the knee axis in the plane of the examining table. The tibia is gently externally rotated just to resistance, and a gravity goniometer or any other suitable device is placed on the tips of the medial

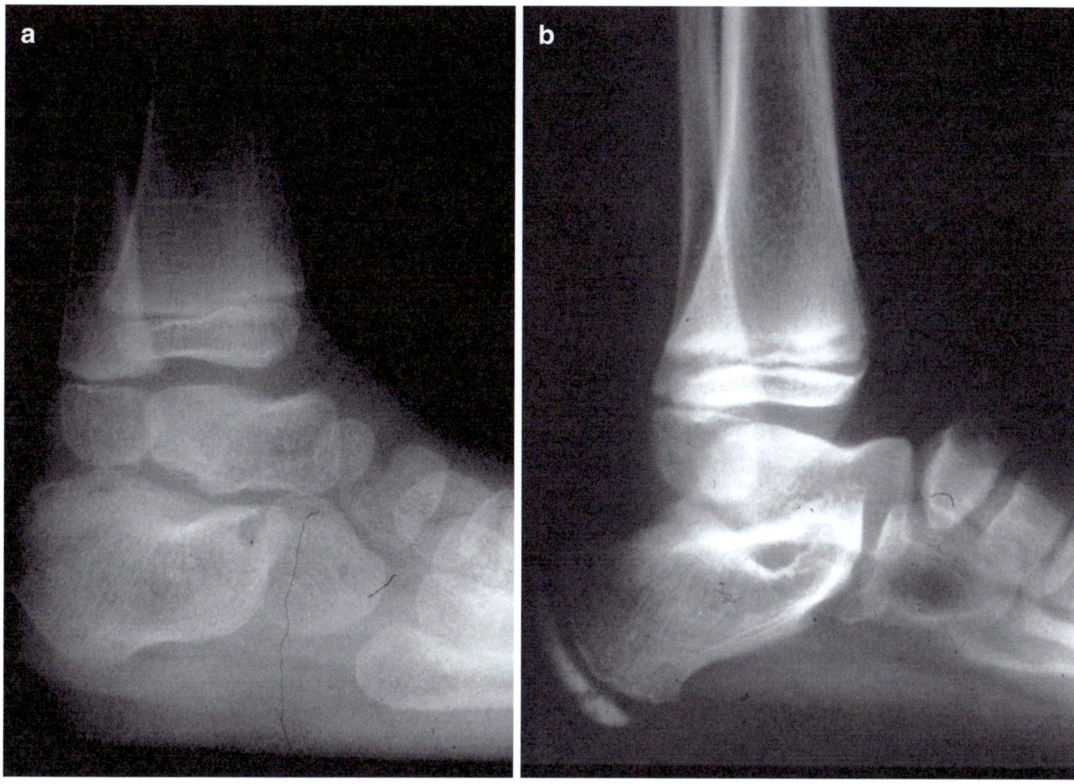

Fig. 1.12 (**a**, **b**) Flattening of the talar dome restricts ankle motion. This may produce anatomical equinus (the heel is off the weight-bearing surface in **a**) or restriction both due to flattening of the talar dome and forefoot equinus or cavus (**b**)

and lateral malleoli. The relationship of the ankle axis to the knee axis is measured directly in degrees (Fig. 1.13).

Flexion and Extension of the Knee

The normal knee hyperextends about 5° and flexes to the limits allowed by the posterior calf pressing against the posterior thigh (Fig. 1.14a, b). When the knee is fully extended, the tibia is locked in external rotation against the femur. When the knee is flexed, there is much more transverse plane rotation within the knee joint itself.

The Popliteal Angle

The popliteal angle is measured with the hip flexed at 90°. The knee is extended as much as possible. The angle formed by the axis of the tibia and the axis of the femur is measured as the acute angle (Fig. 1.15). Many physical therapists report the popliteal angle as the obtuse angle. This could cause some confusion between specialties. This test best identifies hamstring contracture. Large popliteal angles are also seen in conditions such as spondylolisthesis, lumbosacral inflammatory disease, and neuromuscular diseases producing contractures.

Coronal or Frontal Plane Association of the Tibia to the Femur

The normal infant tibiofemoral relationship is usually a varus angle (colloquially referred to as bow legs). The malleoli are in contact, but the medial femoral condyles are separated. As the infant matures, the tibiofemoral relationship reverses so that the medial femoral condyles touch and the malleoli are separated (knock knees in lay terms). In both cases, the limbs should be symmetrical. Assigning numerical values to these two conditions without radiographs is difficult. A rough measurement can be made by deep palpation of the femur and tibia then placing the arms of a goniometer on the two structures (Fig. 1.16). For a more simple reference, the intermalleolar distance or the distance between the femoral condyles can be measured and recorded in centimeters (Fig. 1.17). Unilateral tibia varum should raise the question of Blount's disease. Symmetrical deviations in either direction outside of the normal range are findings associated with rickets. Radiographs of the knees are needed to further define the differential diagnosis between these two.

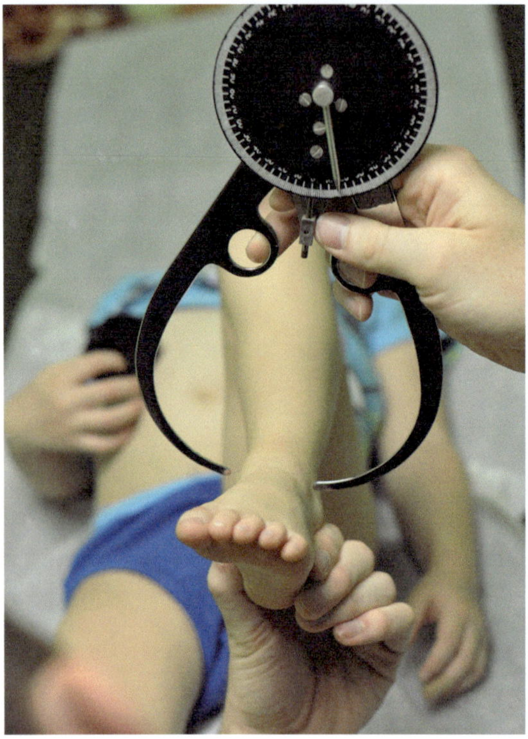

Fig. 1.13 Measuring tibial torsion by the transmalleolar axis technique. The child is placed supine. The knee and hip are flexed to 90°. The femur is placed vertical and the tibia externally rotated just to resistance. The arms of the goniometer are placed on the medial and lateral malleoli and the rotation is measured directly

Ranges of Motion of the Hip

These include internal-external rotation, abduction-abduction, and flexion-extension.

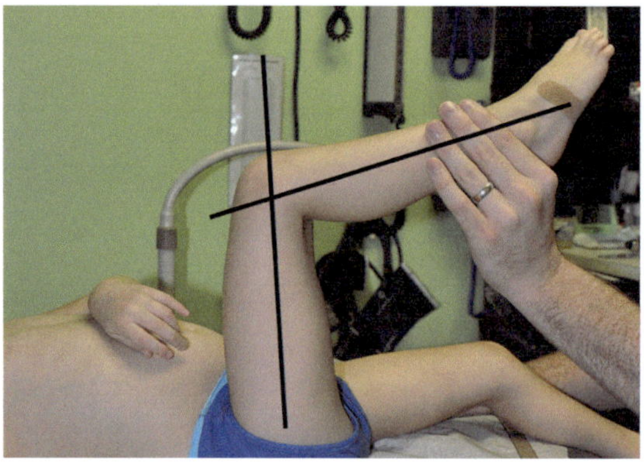

Fig. 1.15 The popliteal angle. The child is placed supine and the knee and hip are flexed to 90°. The knee is gradually extended to resistance and the acute angle made by the axes of the tibia and femur is recorded as the popliteal angle

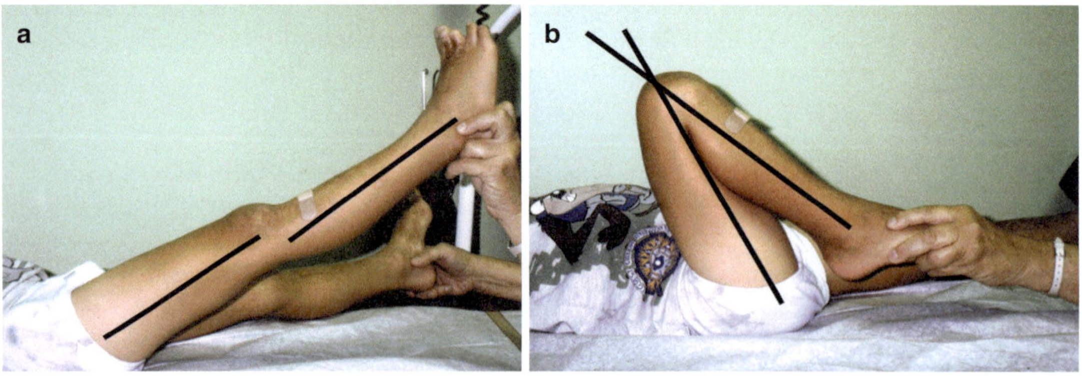

Fig. 1.14 (**a**, **b**) The axes of the tibia and femur are used to measure knee motion in extension (**a**) and flexion (**b**)

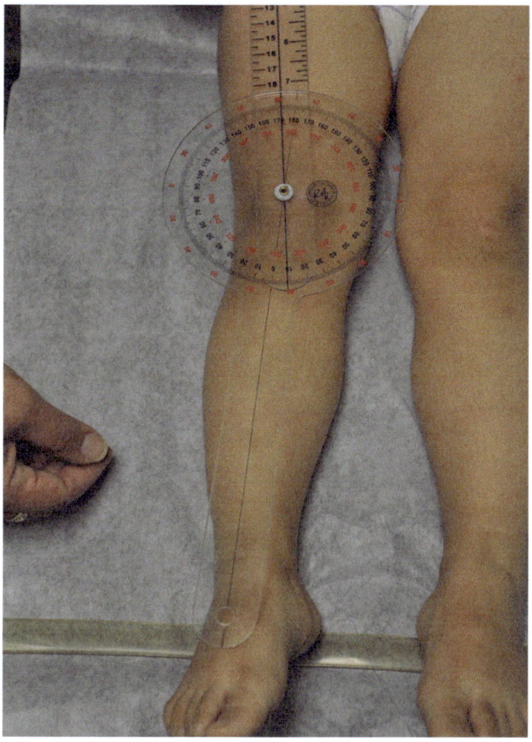

Fig. 1.16 The tibiofemoral angle can be measured by palpating the shafts of the tibia and femur. The arms of a goniometer are placed over them and the angle measured directly in degrees

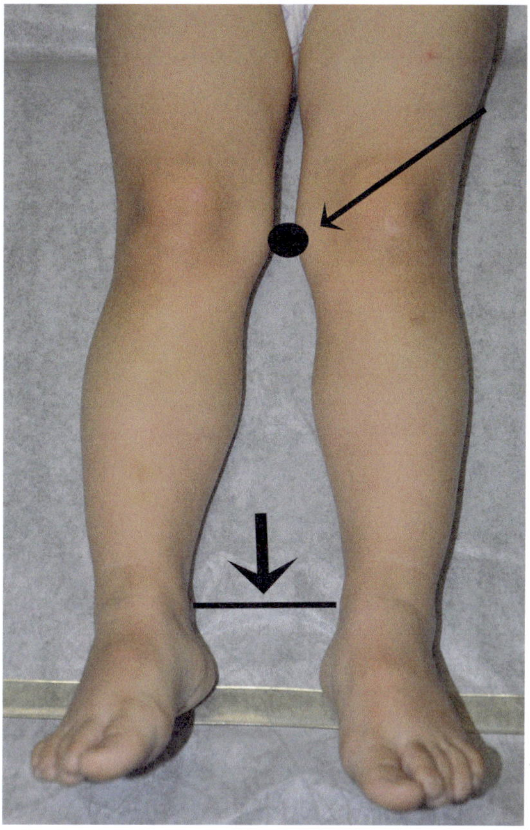

Fig. 1.17 A second method is to measure the intermalleolar distance in inches or centimeters when the knees just touch in genu valgum or the distance between the knees when the malleoli touch in tibia varum

Internal and External Rotation

Internal and external rotation should be measured first with the hip in full extension and then again with the hip flexed 90° on the trunk. When measuring the range of motion in hip extension, the posterior femoral condyles are used as reference. When the transcondylar axis (a line along the posterior surfaces of the femoral condyles) is in the frontal plane, hip rotation is in the neutral position for the purpose of measurement. Internal and external rotation of the hips should be performed on both sides at the same time in order to stabilize the pelvis and prevent inadvertent pelvic rotation that could affect amount of the true range of motion. The pelvis is first leveled, the hips are internally rotated together, and internal rotation of each of the transcondylar axes is measured with an appropriate instrument. External rotation is performed in the same manner (Fig. 1.18).

Alternatively, the child can be placed prone on the examining table and the knee flexed at right angles while the hip remains extended. The sagittal plane becomes the reference. Movement of the tibia laterally internally rotates the hip and moving medially externally rotates the hip. The angles are measured in reference to the sagittal plane (Fig. 1.19).

Hip rotation is repeated with the hips and knees each in 90° of flexion. The child is placed supine on the examining table and the pelvis is leveled. Both limbs are internally rotated at the same time. The tibia becomes one reference point and the sagittal plane of the body the second. A goniometer is placed on the tibia and the other arm is placed in the sagittal plane. The procedure is reversed for external rotation (Fig. 1.20).

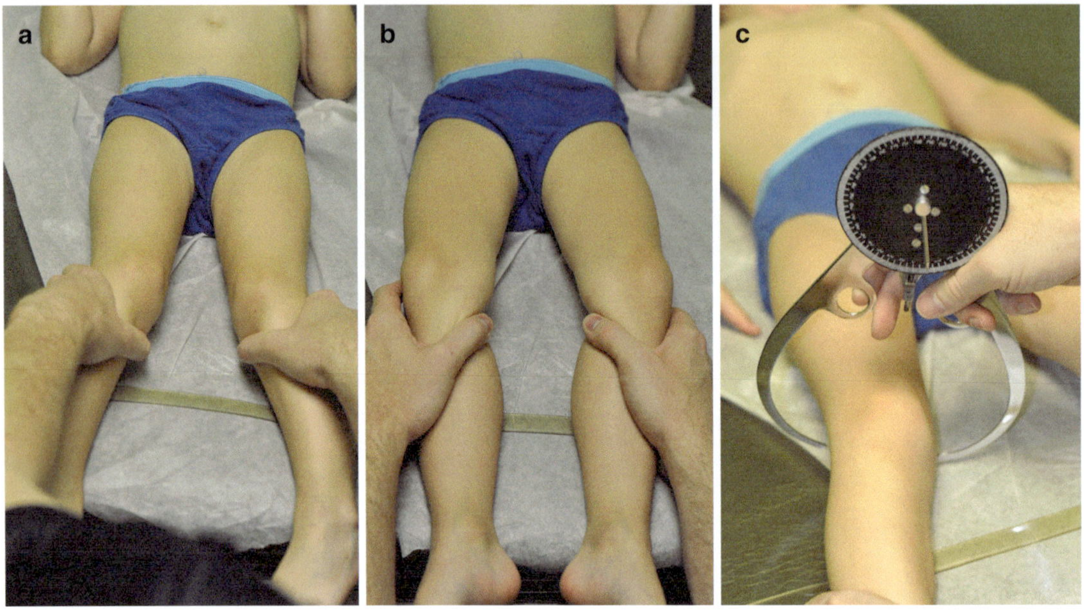

Fig. 1.18 Hip rotation in extension (**a**) and flexion (**b**) is measured and then recorded directly in degrees with an appropriate instrument (**c**)

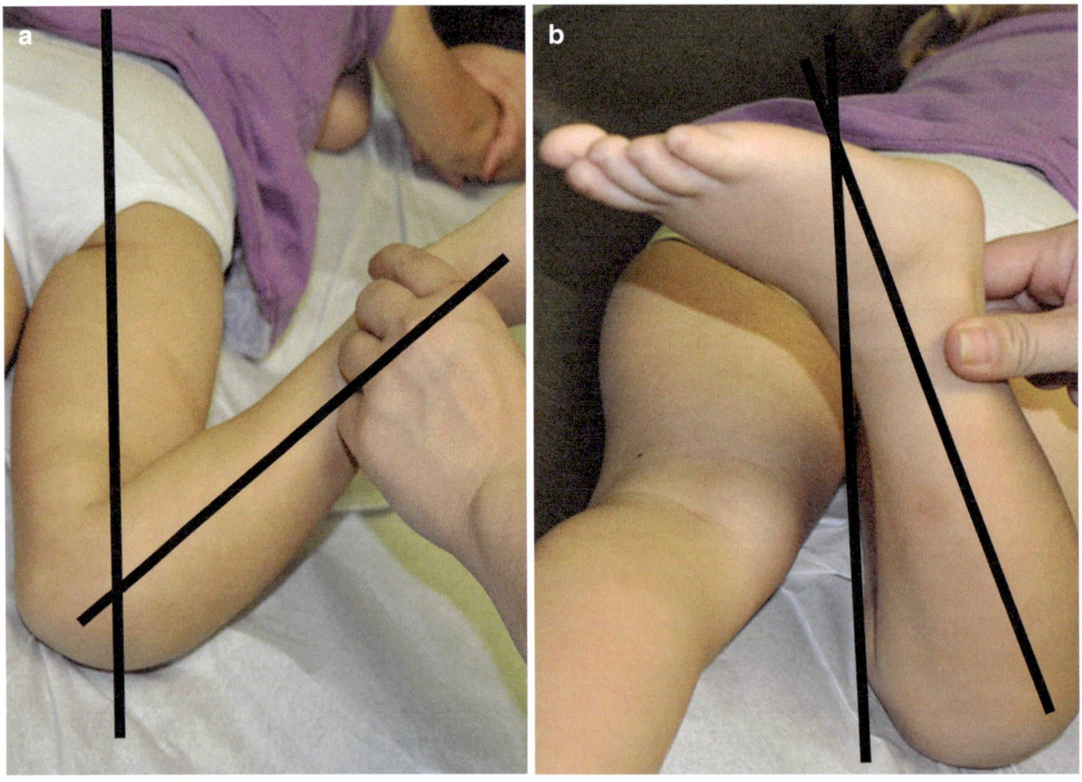

Fig. 1.19 Hip rotation in extension can be measured in the prone position using the axis of the tibia as the reference. (**a** internal rotation; **b** external rotation)

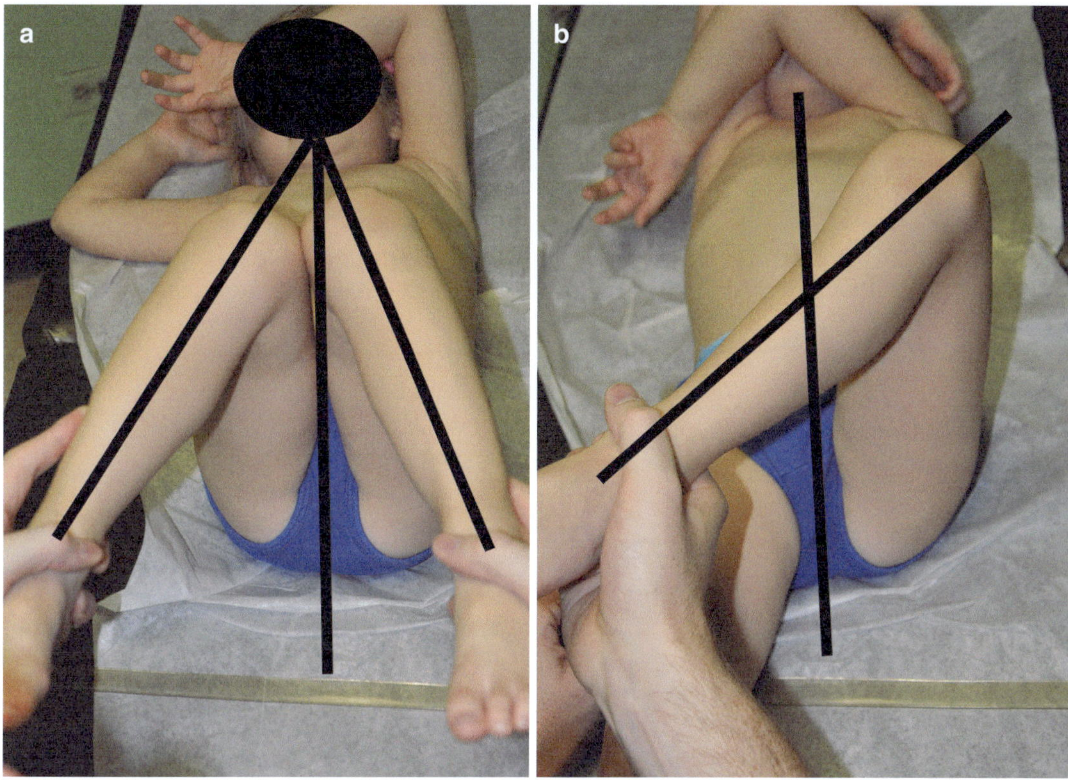

Fig. 1.20 Hip rotation in flexion is measured placing the child supine and the hips and knees flexed to 90°. (**a** internal rotation; **b** external rotation)

Adduction and Abduction

Abduction and adduction of the hip are measured first with the hip in extension and then in flexion. For abduction in hip extension, both femurs are abducted to resistance. The angle formed between the two femurs is the perineal angle in extension (Fig. 1.21). The hips are then flexed at 90° and the femurs abducted at the same time. The angle between the two femurs is the perineal angle in flexion (Fig. 1.22). In both positions, the angles between the two femurs and the sagittal plane should be symmetrical. Asymmetry in either of these two angles is usually the result of adduction contracture or subluxation/dislocation of one or both hips.

Adduction in extension and flexion performance is more problematic. In extension, it is necessary to move the side not being tested into abduction in order to allow the tested side to move past midline. The same thing is true in the flexed position (Fig. 1.23a, b).

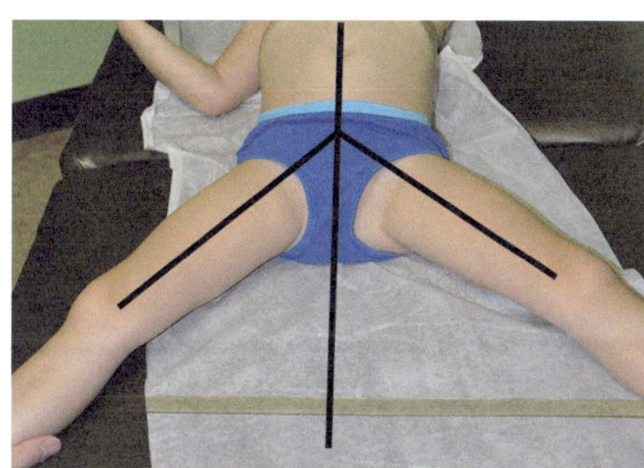

Fig. 1.21 Hip abduction in hip extension. The child is placed supine and the hips are abducted to resistance. The total angle is recorded as the perineal angle in extension. Each hip can be measured separately using the sagittal axis of the body as the reference

Hip Extension and Flexion

Hip extension is measured with the patient in the prone position. The examiner places his hand on the lumbar spine and the sacrum to stabilize the pelvis and detect any increase in lumbar lordosis from pelvic rotation during the test that could

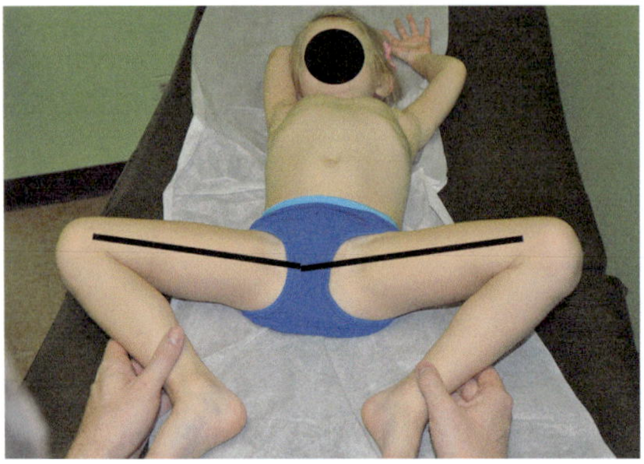

Fig. 1.22 Hip abduction in flexion. The child is placed supine with the hips and knees flexed at 90°. The hips are abducted to resistance and the angle is recorded as the perineal angle in flexion. Each hip can be measured in reference to a vertical axis

erroneously be interpreted as hip extension. The hip is extended at the hip joint. When the hip extension is complete, additional effort rotates the pelvis in the sagittal plane, and the examiner's hand on the lumbosacral spine senses rotation of the pelvis. This marks the endpoint (Fig. 1.24a).

In some cases, there may be excessive lumbar lordosis that can mask hip flexion contracture and lead to erroneous interpretation. To correct for this, Staheli modified the maneuver by allowing both lower limbs to drape over the end of the examining table [26]. This flattens out the lumbar lordosis and will unmask a hidden hip flexion contracture (Fig. 1.24b).

Hip flexion contracture is identified by the Thomas test. The patient is supine on the examining table. Both lower limbs are placed in the knee-chest position, and the limb to be tested is slowly extended and the knee allowed to extend. If the thigh can reach the examining table surface, there is no hip flexion contracture. If it does

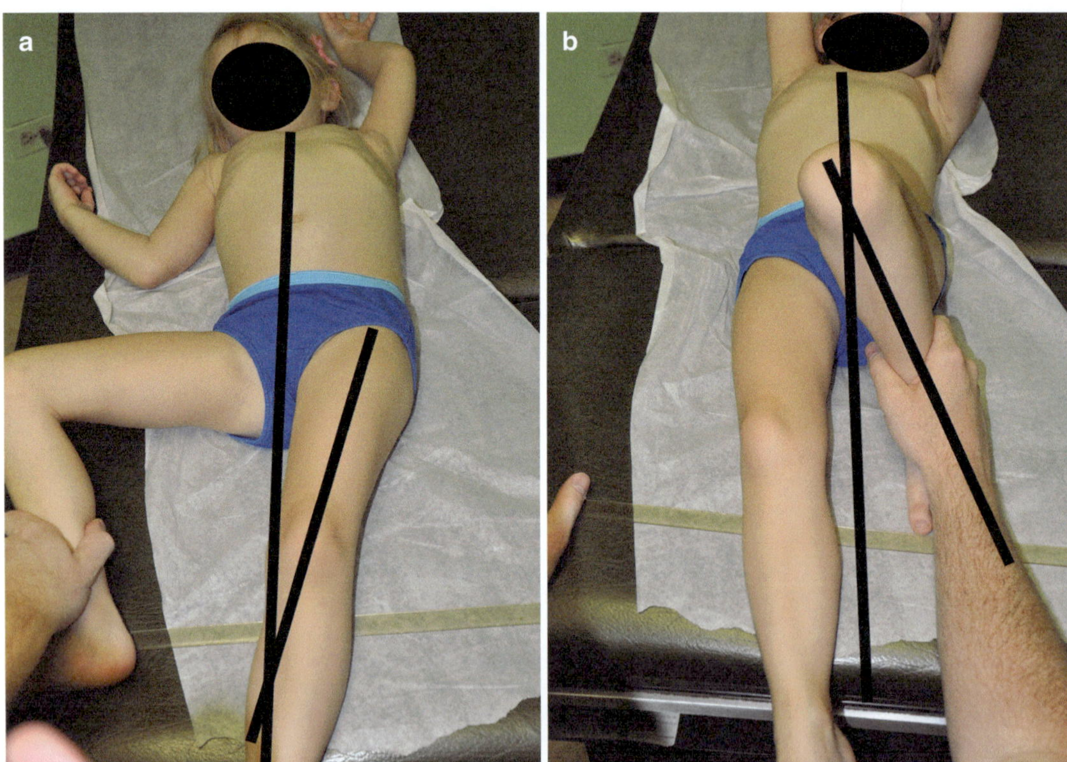

Fig. 1.23 (**a**, **b**) Hip adduction in flexion and extension. The left hip is adducted while the right thigh is moved out of the way to allow the left to clear midline (**a**). The left hip is adducted with the hip and knee flexed at 90° (**b**)

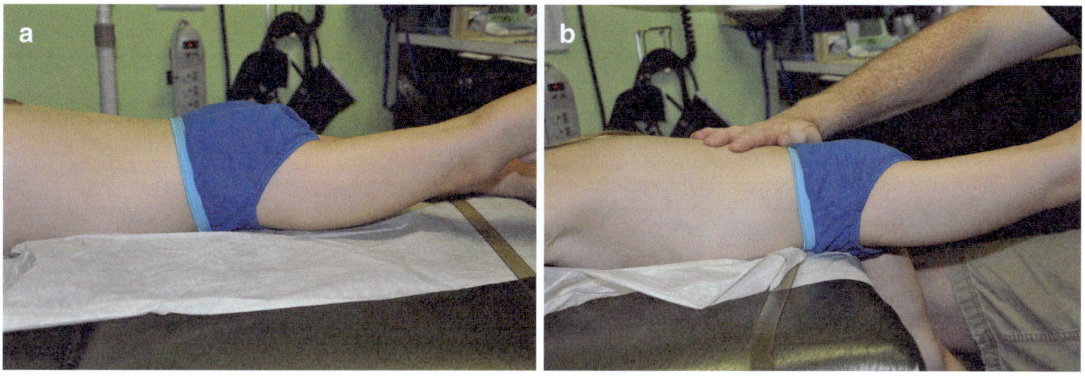

Fig. 1.24 (**a**, **b**) Hip extension is measured with the child prone and the limb to be tested extended (**a**). Staheli's modification is demonstrated in (**b**). The opposite leg is draped over the end of the examining table (arrow). Note that the lumbar lordosis under the examiner's hand has flattened out

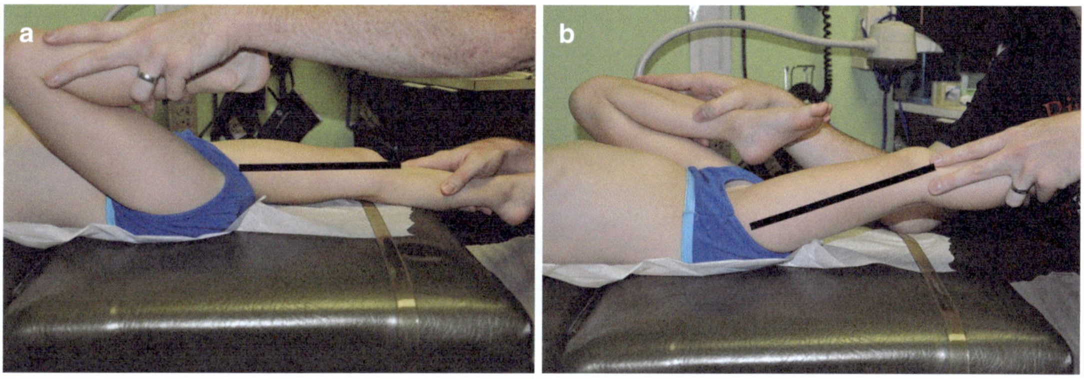

Fig. 1.25 (**a**, **b**) The Thomas test. The test begins with both lower limbs in the knee-chest position. The limb to be tested is extended at the knee and hip. In the absence of hip flexion contracture, the limb should rest on the examination table (**a**). In hip flexion contracture, the limb cannot come down to the table (**b**)

not, hip flexion contracture is present, and the angle that the thigh makes with the examining table is recorded as the angle of flexion contracture (Fig. 1.25).

Abduction contracture of the hip is rarely seen, but the Ober test identifies it. The patient is placed on the contralateral side to be tested. Both hips and knees are flexed to 90 degrees. The hip to be tested is extended both at the hip and knee, and the limb should cross midline. Abduction contracture prevents this. The procedure is repeated on the opposite side (Fig. 1.26).

Rectus femoris contraction is identified with the Ely test. The patient is placed prone and the knee is flexed. In the absence of contracture, the tibia can be brought close to the posterior thigh. If negative, the pelvis does not rotate. When positive, the pelvis rotates in the sagittal plane, the lumbar lordosis is exaggerated, and the buttock rises (Fig. 1.27).

The Ryder Maneuver

The relationship between the proximal femur and the distal femur influences the position of the remainder of the lower extremity in the transverse plane when the femoral head is in its functional position in the acetabulum. Although there are sophisticated radiographic techniques for measuring the angle between the head-neck axis and the knee axis, Ryder developed a simple

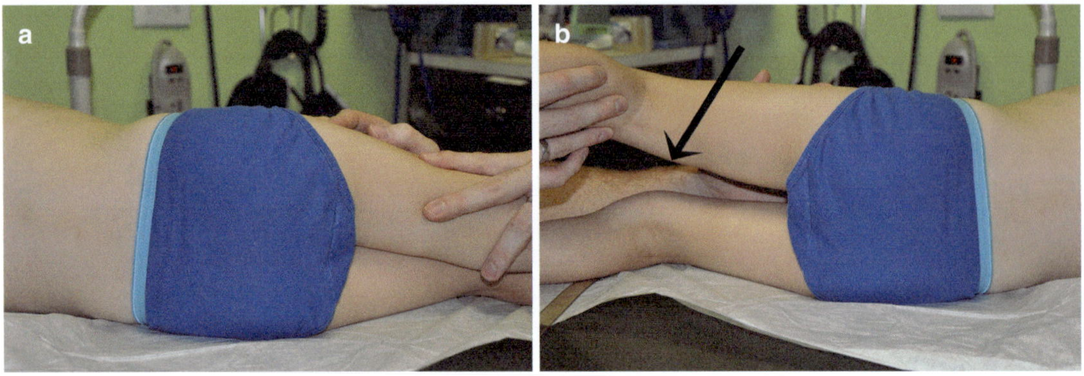

Fig. 1.26 (**a**, **b**) The Ober test. In the absence of abduction contracture, the limb to be tested should adduct past midline (**a**). In the presence of abduction contracture, the tested limb cannot cross midline (**b**)

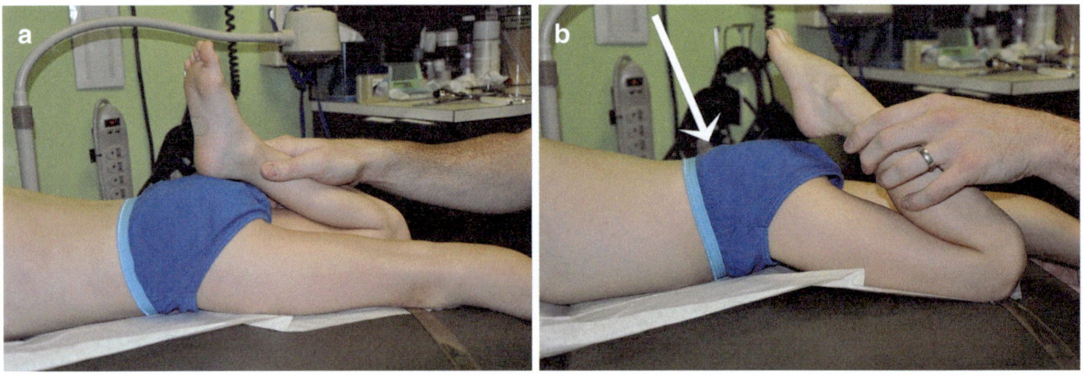

Fig. 1.27 (**a**, **b**) The Ely test. The child is placed prone. In the absence of rectus femoris contracture, the knee can be fully flexed without altering the lumbar spine position (**a**). In the presence of rectus contracture, flexing the knee increases lordosis and raises the buttock (**b**)

clinical measurement [27]. The patient is placed supine on the examining table. The examiner palpates the greater trochanter and internally and externally rotates the femur in the acetabulum several times until the contour of the greater trochanter can be identified under the examiner's hand. Once the examiner feels that he has leveled the head-neck axis in the plane of the examining table, the amount of internal (or, in rare cases, external) rotation of the knee in the transverse plane is the angle between the proximal and distal landmarks of the femur (Fig. 1.28).

The test can also be performed with the child prone and the knee flexed while the hip remains in extension. As in the supine technique, the greater trochanter is palpated while the tibia is moved medial and lateral until the proximal bony landmarks are palpated and the greater trochanter is in its most prominent lateral position (Fig. 1.29). Lateral angulation of the thigh with respect to the sagittal plane is an antetorsion value. Medial movement is a retrotorsion value.

Hip Instability and Dislocation

Examination of the hip for subluxation and dislocation should be a component of every infant and toddler physical examination. The neonatal screening program has been highly successful in

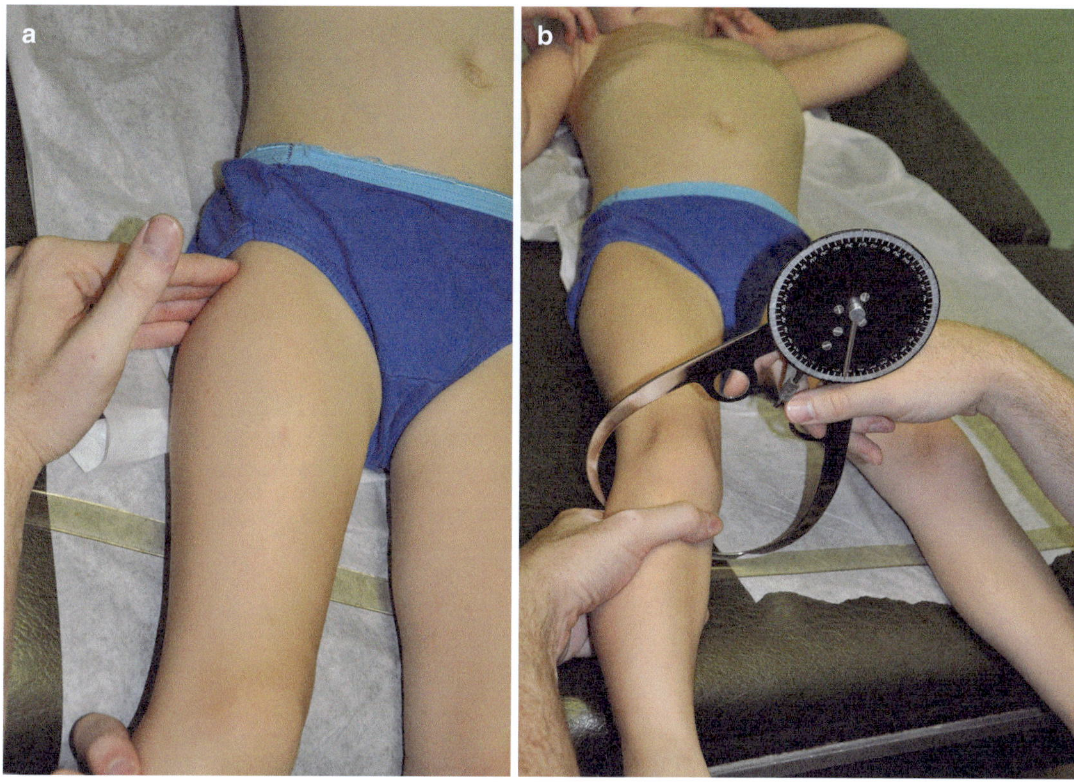

Fig. 1.28 (**a**, **b**) The Ryder maneuver to measure femoral antetorsion (anteversion). The examiner palpates the greater trochanter and rotates the thigh in and out until the greater trochanter is most prominent. The amount of knee rotation needed to level the proximal femur is the angle of antetorsion and can be measured directly in degrees with the appropriate instrument

identifying hip dysplasia and dislocation in early infancy, but it has not totally eliminated the incidence of dislocations identified in late toddlers and young children.

Barlow Test

This is a provocative test to identify a hip with a femoral head that is in the acetabulum but that can be subluxed or dislocated [28]. The infant is placed comfortably on the back. Ideally, the infant should be as relaxed as possible. Bottle-feeding the infant during this portion of the examination is recommended. The examiner flexes the thigh to be tested at right angles to the trunk and then slowly adducts the thigh past midline at the same time that he applies some downward pressure against the femur. If the hip is unstable, the examiner will feel the femoral head partly or completely slip out of the acetabulum. The feeling of subluxation is referred to as Palmen's sign (Fig. 1.30).

Ortolani Test

This test is used to identify a subluxed or dislocated hip that can still be relocated [29]. The infant is positioned as described for Barlow's test. The examiner places his fingers under the greater trochanter, the hip is abducted at the same time that longitudinal traction is placed on the femur, and an attempt is made to slip

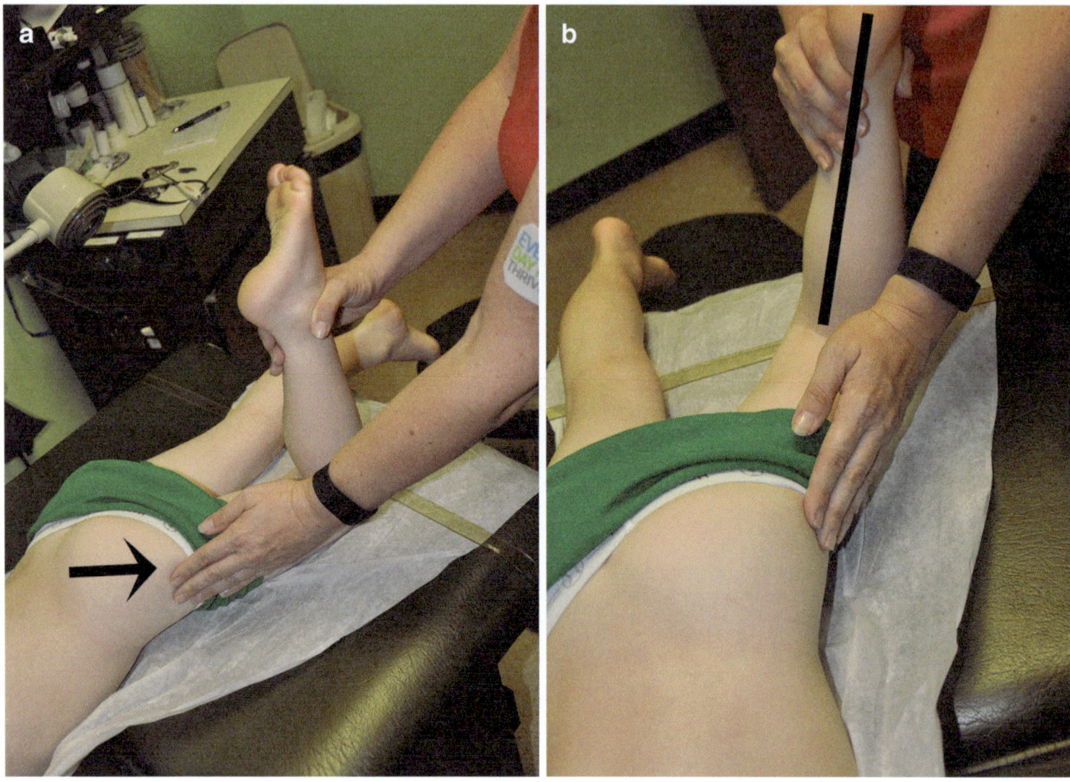

Fig. 1.29 (**a**, **b**) The Ryder test can be performed with the child prone. The examiner palpates the greater trochanter as described in the legend for Fig. 1.28, and the tibia is the reference for measurement

the femoral head back into the acetabulum if the hip is dislocated and can still be reduced (Fig. 1.31).

The Telescope Sign

The patient is placed supine on the examining table. The thigh is flexed at right angles to the trunk and is placed in the sagittal plane. In the presence of an unstable hip or a dislocated hip that can be reduced, the femoral head will be felt to slide along the lateral side of the acetabulum and ilium.

Limitation of Hip Abduction

Even after a comparatively short period of time, a dislocated hip may no longer be reducible. This decreases the reliability of the Ortolani test. However, when the contracture around the hip prevents relocation, it also limits the abduction range of motion on the involved side. The perineal angle becomes asymmetrical and smaller on the side of the dislocation (Fig. 1.32).

Galeazzi Sign

The infant is placed supine on the examining table. Hips and knees are flexed at 90°. The pelvis is leveled. The examiner sights across the distal femurs and looks for shortening of the femur. If the hip is dislocated, the proximal femur almost always moves upward and posterior. This gives the effect of a short femur on the side of the hip pathology. Placing the feet on the table at the same time will assist the examiner in determin-

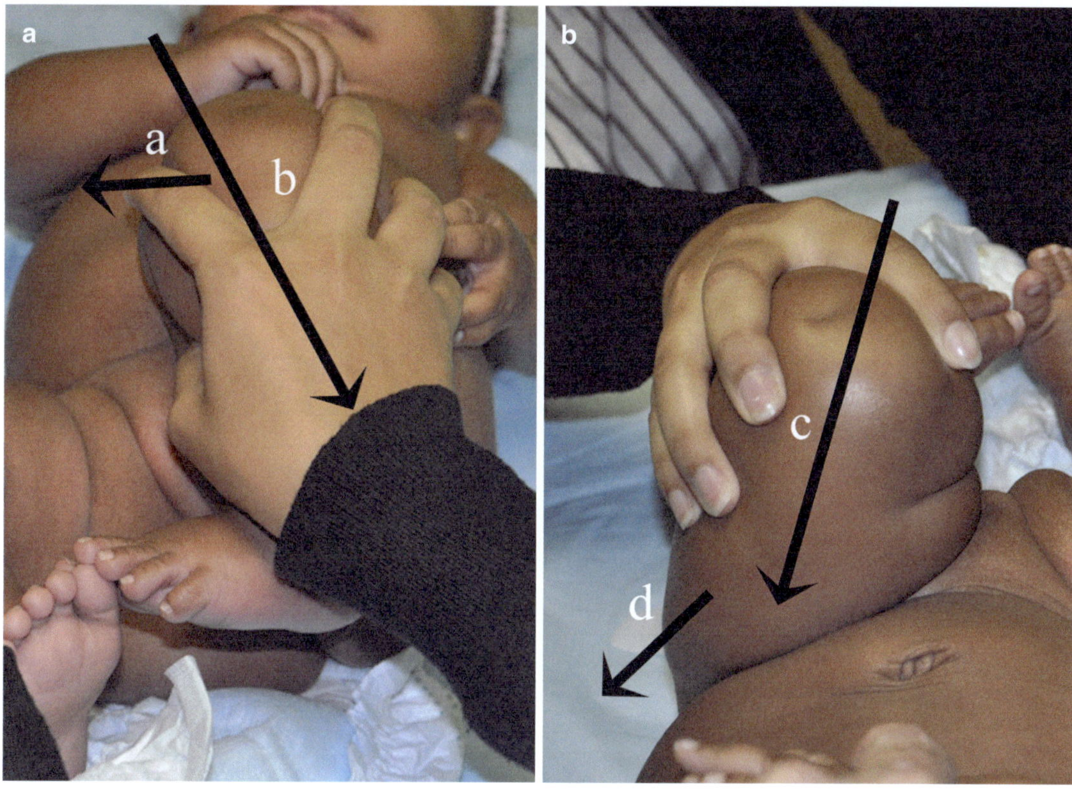

Fig. 1.30 (**a**, **b**) Barlow test. The infant is placed supine and the side to be tested is adducted (**a**). At the same time, the examiner pushes down on the femur in a lateral direction to attempt to push the femoral head out of the acetabulum (**b**)

ing whether any difference in limb length is in the tibia or the femur. Although usually associated with hip dislocation, the test will identify a short femur or tibia from any cause (Fig. 1.33).

Trendelenburg Sign

The patient stands with the back to the examiner and is requested to stand on one leg. Functioning abductors of the hip allow the child to support on one leg and raise the pelvis of the opposite side or at least keep the pelvis level. In the presence of hip abduction weakness from any cause, the pelvis drops on the non-weight-bearing side. This test is not specific for any disease, but merely indicates pelvic girdle weakness that prevents abduction on the weight-bearing side (Fig. 1.34). Trendelenburg gait is the peculiar gait disturbance produced by bilateral abductor weakness.

Gower Sign

The child is asked to lie prone on the floor and then stand without using any nearby object to support him or facilitate standing. In the absence of any hip extensor weakness, the child should be able to rise from the floor without using his hands to help extend his hips. A healthy child can perform this maneuver three times in succession without weakness. When positive, the child cannot rise from the floor without assisting himself. The classic manner is to use the hands and arms to “climb” up the limbs in order to extend the knees and hips (Fig. 1.35). Like

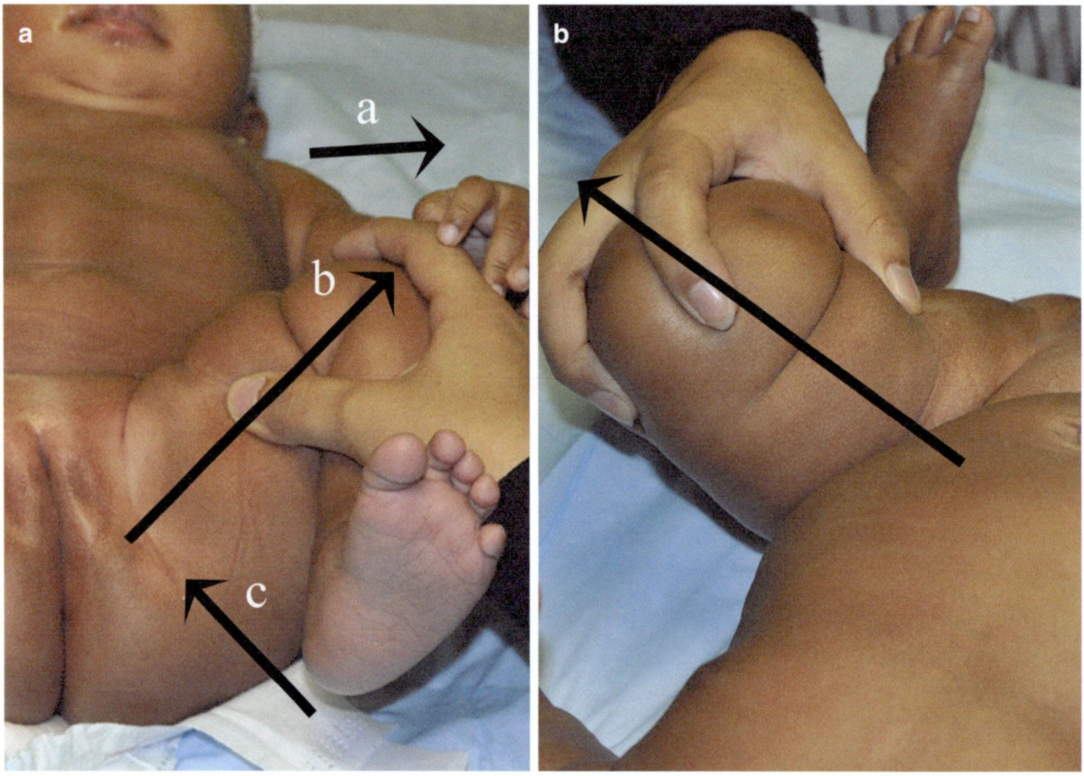

Fig. 1.31 (**a**, **b**) Ortolani test. The infant is placed supine and the side to be tested is abducted (**a**). At the same time, upward traction is placed on the femur with the fingers under the greater trochanter while the examiner attempts to "scoop" the femoral head back into the acetabulum (**b**)

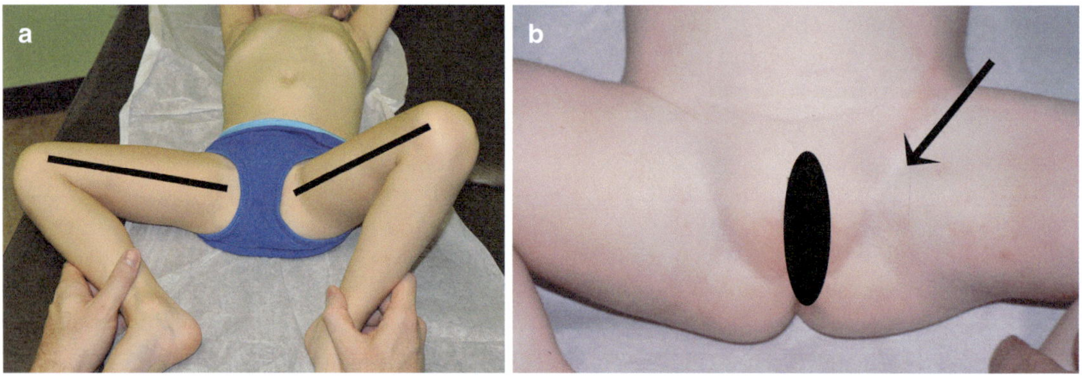

Fig. 1.32 (**a**, **b**) In hip dysplasia (**a**) there is limited hip abduction on the involved left side. On occasion, in dislocation (**b**), the adductor muscle group (arrow) is contracted

Trendelenburg sign, a positive Gower sign is not specific for any single disease. Any pathology weakening the hip extensors will result in a positive Gower sign. Gower sign may be partial, indicating some degree of weakness but not enough to totally prevent the child from rising from the ground. This may be the result of weakness on one side only or may be the initial finding of very early bilateral weakness of the hip extensors (Fig. 1.36).

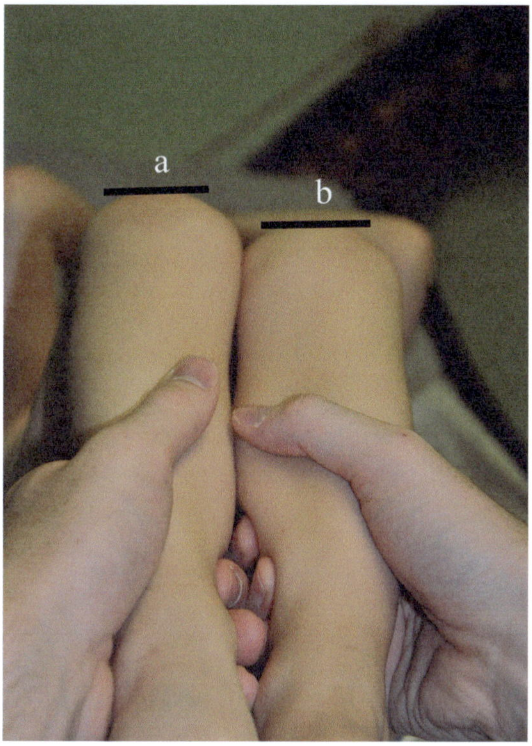

Fig. 1.33 Galeazzi sign. The child is placed supine and the knees and hips are flexed 90°. The examiner sights over the patellae. Note that line b is lower than line a indicating a short left femur

Hamstring Contracture

Contracture of the hamstrings causes inability to fully flex the hips. This may be part of a larger neurological picture or can be the result of accommodation of a painful more proximal lesion either in the hip joint itself or in the lumbar or sacral spine. This commonly occurs in patients who have spondylolisthesis. It is identified by an abnormal popliteal angle. In infancy, popliteal angles are usually zero. Normals in older children are between 35° and 45°. Hamstring contracture additionally causes decreased ability to forward bend and loss of physiologic lumbar lordosis (Fig. 1.37).

Adams Forward Bending Test

Scoliosis may be identified on routine examination in children and adolescents. Examination technique is simple and takes very little time. The child stands with the back to the examiner. The height of the shoulders is examined, followed by the iliac crest height, position of the fingertips, and the space between the torso and the arms. The back is examined for obvious scoliotic curves (Fig. 1.38). The child then bends forward from the hips facing the examiner. The back is evaluated for elevation of the ribs. The procedure is repeated with the child facing away from the examiner (Fig. 1.39). The child is examined from the side and then in forward bend to evaluate kyphosis (Fig. 1.40).

Asymmetry in shoulder height is a common finding in scoliosis but is not pathognomonic. Clinically significant scoliosis is further identified by having the child slowly bend forward. A prominent rib hump indicates vertebral body rotation (Fig. 1.41).

The convention for naming the curve is based on its anatomical location in the spine as well as the direction in which the convexity is facing. For example, a thoracic curve resulting in a lowered left shoulder means that the convexity of the curve is facing to the right side. This would then be named a right thoracic curve. Most thoracic curves are to the right. Elevation of the right ribs on forward bending indicates axial rotation of the vertebrae. In the absence of vertebral body rotation, the heights of the iliac crests, the levels of the inferior gluteal clefts, and the natal cleft may point more toward a difference in limb length.

The Neurological Examination

In most pediatric physical examinations, the purpose of the neurological component is screening for unsuspected sensory or motor conditions. Unless the chief complaint or complaints demands more detail, the neurology portion of the examination can be brief.

The examination can be divided into sensory and motor components. Sensory components include sharp dull, vibratory, and positional senses.

The motor portion can be evaluated in several different ways. The gait gives a great deal

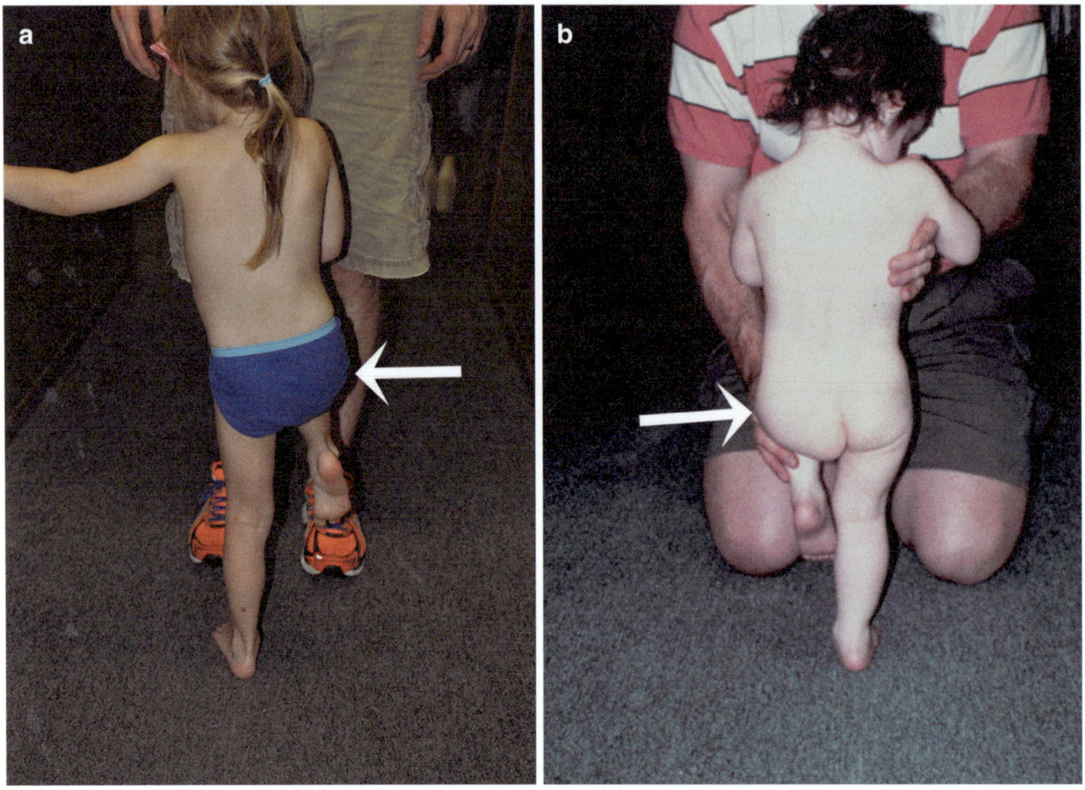

Fig. 1.34 (**a**, **b**) Trendelenburg sign. A negative finding (**a**) is shown by elevation of the right buttock when the left limb bears weight (white arrow). A positive finding (**b**) is shown when the left buttock falls when the right limb bears weight (white arrow)

of information about the integration of motor activity, the firing of the various muscles in sequence, and the relative strengths.

Strength is usually measured using the Medical Research Council grading strength [30, 31]. If there is no muscle activity at all, the grade is assigned as zero. If there is a flicker of activity, grade is assigned as grade 1. If movement can occur when gravity is neutralized by position, the grade is assigned as grade 2. If movement occurs against gravity but not resistance, the grade is assigned as grade 3. If there is movement against resistance but not full anticipated strength, the grade is assigned as grade 4. If muscle strength is age and physical size appropriate, the grade is assigned as grade 5. Upper and lower extremities should be tested (Table 1.8). Root innervations for the

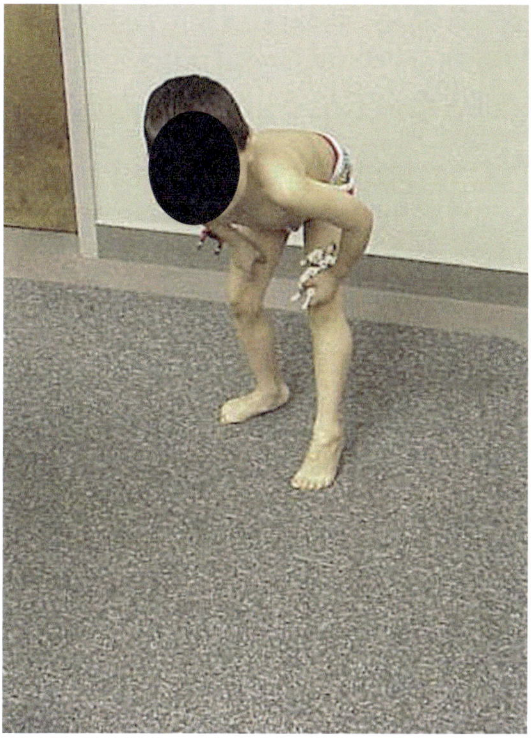

Fig. 1.35 Positive Gower sign. This male with Duchenne muscular dystrophy must use his hands and arms to help extend his hips and knees by "climbing up" the lower extremities

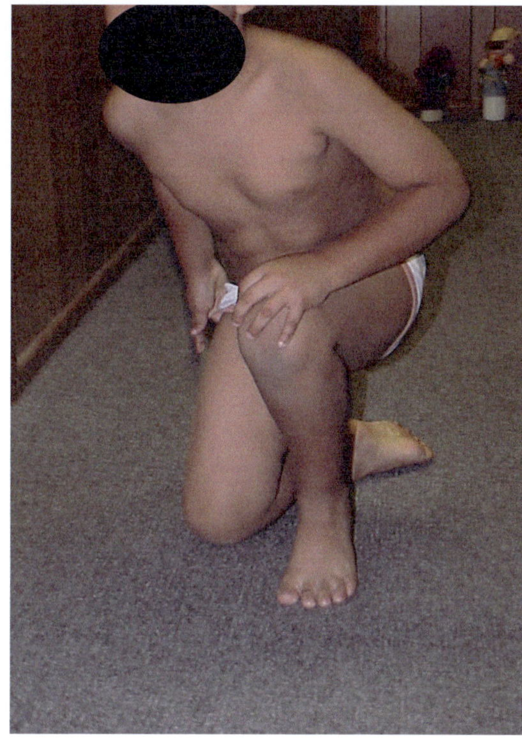

Fig. 1.36 Partial Gower sign. The child must use the left hand in the presence of left weakness to help extend the left hip and knee

major muscles below the knee are summarized in Table 1.9.

Upper and lower deep tendon reflexes should be elicited. In the upper extremity, these include biceps, triceps, and brachioradialis. In the lower extremities, patellar and tendo Achilles are elicited (Table 1.9). An attempt is made to elicit clonus and the plantar reflex is usually tested at the same time.

Sensation follows a predictable cutaneous dermatome pattern and these are summarized in Table 1.10.

Superficial reflexes include the abdominal skin reflex and the plantar reflex (Fig. 1.42).

In some complicated complaints, a more complete neurological examination is indicated as outlined above in the general physical examination.

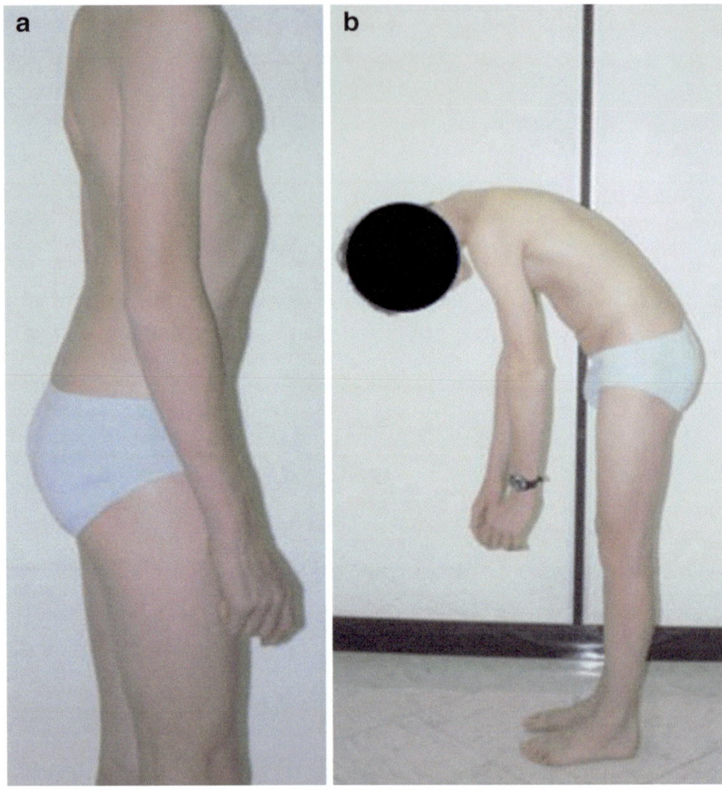

Fig. 1.37 (**a**, **b**) Spondylolisthesis. Stance is relatively normal (**a**). On forward bend, the lumbar spine flattens and limited hip flexion limits hand position to the level of the knees

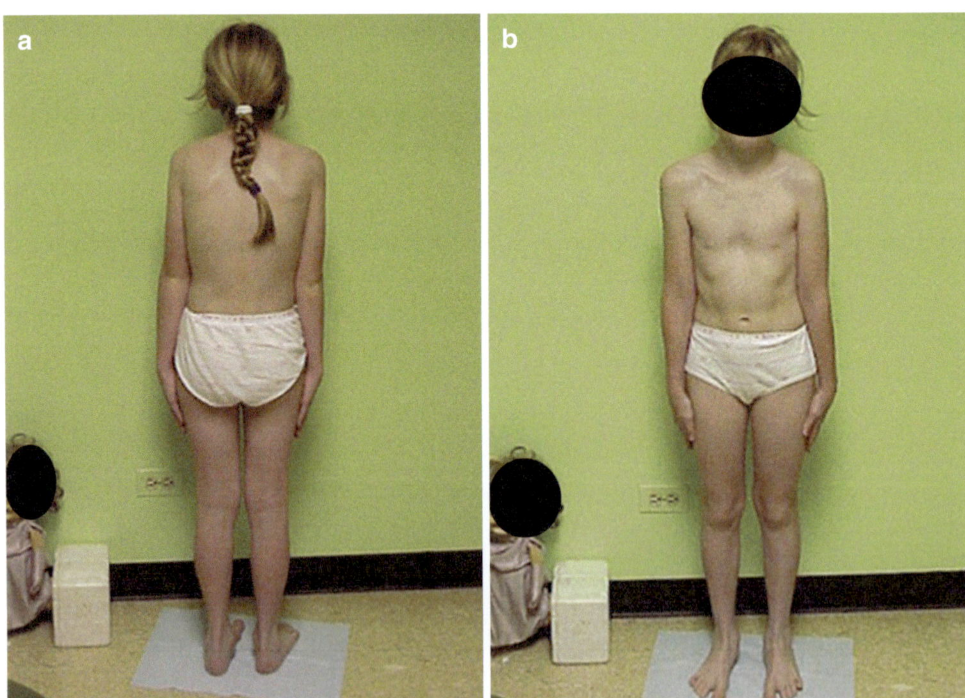

Fig. 1.38 (**a**, **b**) The Adams bending test. Evaluation for scoliosis. The child faces away from the examiner (**a**) and then toward the examiner (**b**). The examiner observes shoulder height, scapular position, arm to trunk distance, and fingertip level for symmetry. The spine is evaluated for obvious curvature

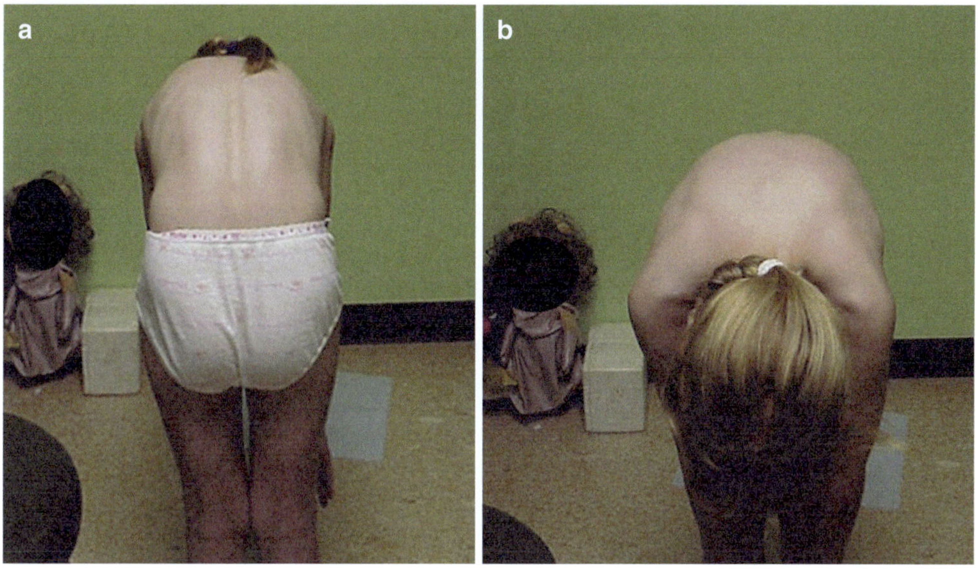

Fig. 1.39 (**a**, **b**) The Adams bending test. Evaluation for scoliosis – cont. The child bends away from the examiner (**a**) and then toward the examiner (**b**). The examiner evaluates for rib rotation. In this case it is negative

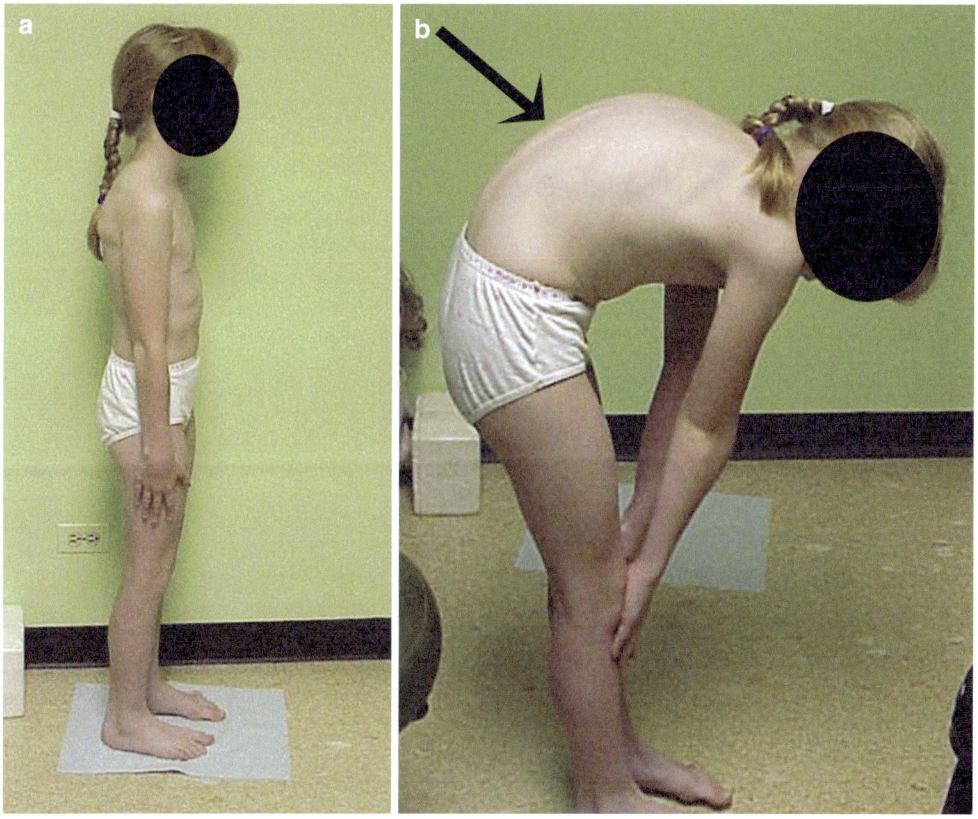

Fig. 1.40 (**a**, **b**) The Adams bending test. Evaluation for scoliosis – cont. The child's posture is evaluated from the side (**a**). The child bends forward from the waist (**b**). There is mild kyphosis (arrow)

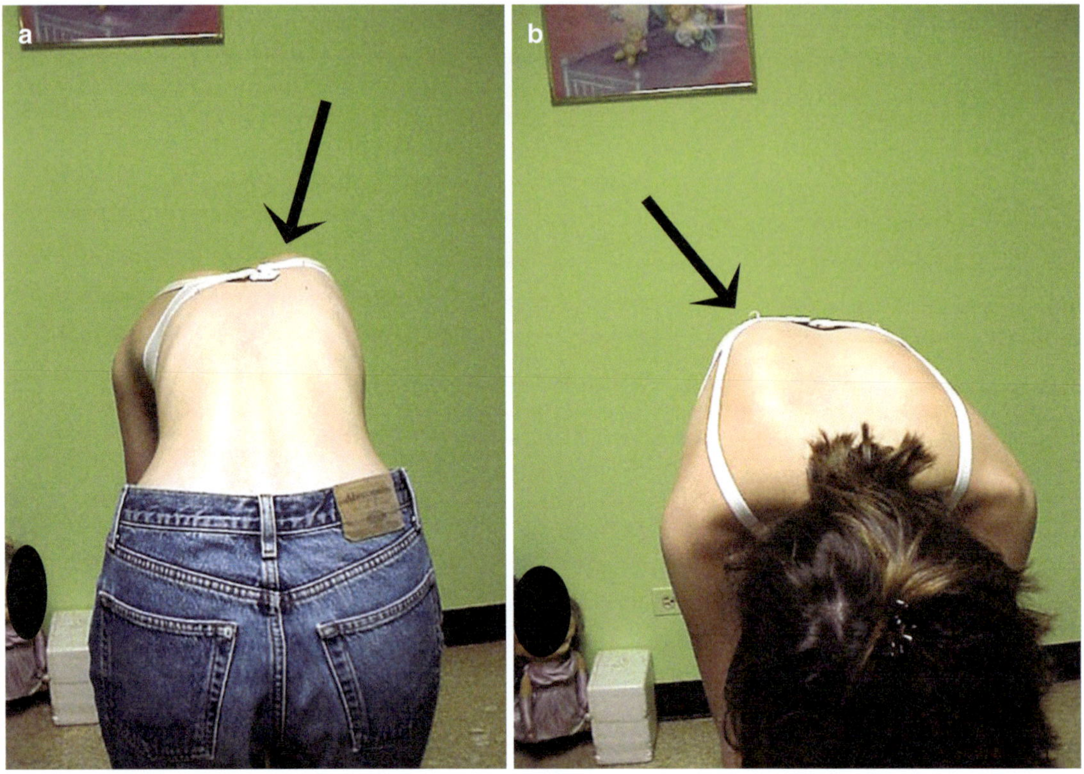

Fig. 1.41 (**a**, **b**) The Adams bending test. Evaluation for scoliosis – cont. The child bends toward (**a**) and then away (**b**) from the examiner. There is right thoracic rib prominence (arrows)

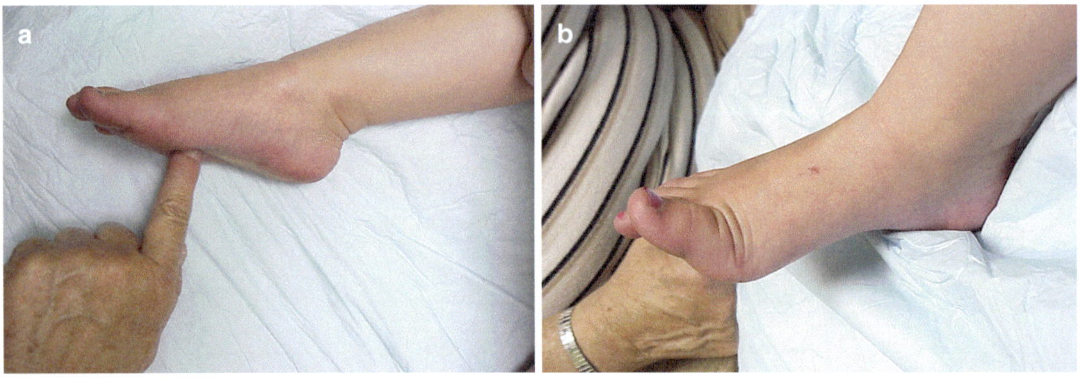

Fig. 1.42 (**a**, **b**) Plantar reflex. Positive Babinski sign. The plantar of the foot is stroked beginning on the proximal and lateral heel forward and then medially under the metatarsal heads (**a**). The hallux slowly dorsiflexes and the lesser toes fan (**b**)

Table 1.8 Grading muscle strength

0	Zero	No palpable muscle contraction
1	Trace	Palpable contraction of muscle No joint movement when gravity is eliminated
2	Poor	Muscle able to move part through full ROM, but not against gravity
3	Fair	Muscle able to move part through full ROM against gravity but not against resistance
4	Good	Muscle able to move part through full ROM against gravity with some resistance
5	Normal	Muscle able to move part through full ROM with full resistance

From Lovett and Martin [31]

Table 1.9 Deep tendon reflexes

Reflex	Muscle	Root level
Biceps	Biceps brachii	Predominantly C5, some C6
Brachioradialis	Brachioradialis	C6
Triceps	Triceps brachii	C7
Patellar	Rectus femoris, Vastus lateralis, Vastus medialis, Vastus intermedius	L4
Tendo-Achilles	Triceps surae	S1

Table 1.10 Lower extremity dermatomes

L1	Upper 1/3 of the anterior thigh below the inguinal ligament
L2	Middle 1/3 of the anterior thigh
L3	Lower 1/3 of the anterior thigh above the patella
L4	Medial 1/2 of the anterior leg and heel, medial 1/2 of posterior leg along with L3, medial plantar foot along with L5
L5	Lateral 1/2 of the leg, most of the dorsum of the foot, medial plantar foot along with L4
S1	Lateral foot, lateral 1/2 of the leg along with S2

References

1. Apgar V. A proposal for a new method of evaluation of the newborn infant. Curr Res Anesthesiol. 1953;32:260.
2. Ben-Menachem Y, Butlet JE. Arteriography of the foot in congenital deformities. J Bone Joint Surg. 1974;56A:1625–30.
3. Greider TD, Gerson P, Donovan MM. Arteriography in clubfoot. J Bone Joint Surg. 1982;64A:837–40.
4. Dobbs MB, Gordon JE, Schoenecker PL. Absent posterior tibial artery associated with idiopathic clubfoot. A report of two cases. J Bone Joint Surg. 2004;86A:599–602.
5. Hootnick DR, Levinsohn EM, Crider RJ, Packard DS. Congenital arterial malformations associated with clubfoot. A report of two cases. Clin Orthop Relat Res. 1982;167:160–3.
6. Katz DA, Albanese EL, Levinsohn EM, Hootnick DR, Packard DS, Grant WD, et al. Pulse color-flow Doppler analysis of arterial deficiency in idiopathic clubfoot. J Pediatr Orthop. 2003;23:84–7.
7. Levinsohn EM, Hootnick DR, Packard DS. Consistent arterial abnormalities associated with a variety of congenital malformations of the lower limb. Invest Radiol. 1991;26:364–73.
8. Southerland DH. Gait disorders in childhood and adolescence. Baltimore: Williams and Wilkins; 1984.
9. Silfverskiold N. Reduction of the uncrossed two-joints muscles of the leg to one-joint muscles in spastic conditions. Acta Chir Scand. 1923;56:315–30.
10. Bouchard R, Meeder PJ, Krug F, Libicher M. Evaluation of tibial torsion: comparison of clinical methods and computed tomography. Rofo. 2004;176:127–1284.
11. Clementz BG. Assessment of tibial torsion and rotational deformity with a new fluoroscopic technique. Clin Orthop Relat Res. 1989;254:199–209.
12. Eckhoff DG, Johnson KK. Three-dimensional computed tomography reconstruction of tibial torsion. Clin Orthop Relat Res. 1994;302:42–6.
13. Güven M, Akman B, Ünay K, Özturan E, Çakıcı H, Eren A. A new radiographic measurement method for evaluation of tibial torsion: a pilot study in adults. Clin Orthop Relat Res. 2009;46(7):1807–12.
14. Hudson D, Roger T, Richards J. Ultrasound measurements of torsion in the tibia and femur. J Bone Joint Surg Am. 2006;88:138–43.
15. Jakob RP, Haertel M, Stussi E. Tibial torsion calculated by computerized tomography and compared to other methods of measurements. J Bone Joint Surg Br. 1980;62:238–42.
16. Kim HD, Lee DS, Eom MJ, Hwang JS, Han NM, Jo GY. Relationship between physical examinations and two-dimensional computed tomographic findings in children with intoeing gait. Ann Rehabil Med. 2011;35(4):491–8.
17. Muhamad AR, Freitas JM, Bomar JD, Dwek J, Hosalkar HS. CT and MRI lower extremity torsional profile studies: measurement reproducibility. J Child Orthop. 2012;6(5):391–6.
18. Muhamad AR, Freitas JM, Bomar JD, Dwek J, Hosalkar HS. CT and MRI lower extremity torsional profile study: measurement reproducibility. J Child Orthop. 2012;8(6):391–6.
19. Schneider B, Laubenberger J, Jemlich S, Groenek K, Weber HM, Larger M. Measurement of femoral antetorsion and tibial torsion by magnetic resonance imaging. Br J Radiol. 1997;70:575–9.

20. Shin S, Yoon C, Lee E, Oh M, Kim A, Park M, et al. The availability of radiological measurement of tibial torsion: three-dimensional computed tomography reconstruction. Ann Rehabil Med. 2011;35(5):673–9.
21. Stuberg LT, Temme J, Kaplan P, Clark A, Fuchs R. Measurements of tibial torsion and thigh-foot angle using goniometry and computed tomography. Clin Orthop Relat Res. 1991;272:208–12.
22. Tomczak RJ, Guenther KP, Rieber A, Mergo P, Ros PR, Brambs HJ. MR imaging measurements of the femoral antetorsional angle as a new technique: comparison with CT in children and adults. Am J Roentgenol. 1997;168(3):791–4.
23. Upadhyay SS, O'Neil T, Burwell RG, Moulton A. A new method using medical ultrasound for measuring femoral anteversion (torsion): technique and reliability. An intra-observer and inter-observer study on dried bones from human adults. J Anat. 1987;155:119–32.
24. Brenner D, Elliston C, Hall E, Berdon W. Estimated risks of radiation-induced fatal cancer from pediatric CT. Am J Roentgenol. 2001;176(2):289–96.
25. Brenner DJ, Hall EJ. Computed tomography – an increasing source of radiation exposure. N Engl J Med. 2007;357(22):2277–84.
26. Staheli LT. The prone hip extension test: a method of measuring hip flexion deformity. Clin Orthop Relat Res. 1977;123:12.
27. Ryder CT, Crane L. Measuring femoral anteversion: the problem and a method. J Bone Joint Surg. 1953;35-A(2):321–8.
28. Barlow T. Early diagnosis and treatment of congenital dislocation of the hip. J Bone Joint Surg. 1962; 44:292.
29. Ortolani M. Un segno poco noto e sue importanza per la diagnosi precoce di preussssasione congenita dell'anca. Pediatria. 1937;45:129.
30. Lovett RW, Martin EG. Certain aspects of infantile paralysis with a description of a method of muscle testing. JAMA. 1916;66:729.
31. Lovett RW. Fatigue and exercise in treatment of infantile paralysis: study of one thousand eight hundred and twenty-six cases. JAMA. 1917;69:168.

Recommended Reading

Herring JA. Tachdjian's pediatric orthopaedics. 4th ed. Philadelphia: Saunders Elsevier; 2008.

Hoppenfeld S. Orthopaedic neurology a diagnostic guide to neurologic levels. J. B. Lippincott Company: Philadelphia; 1977.

Mosca VS. Principles and management of pediatric foot and ankle deformities and malformations. Philadelphia: Wolters Kluwer; 2014.

Southerland DH. Gait disorders in childhood and adolescence. Baltimore: Williams and Wilkins; 1984.

Zitelli BJ, Davis HW. Atlas of pediatric physical diagnosis. 3rd ed. St. Louis: Mosby-Wolfe; 1997.

Radiology of the Pediatric Foot and Ankle

2

Robert A. Christman

Radiographic interpretation of the pediatric foot and ankle is challenging. Not only do radiographic presentations vary at different ages, but variation occurs from patient to patient even at the same age, especially between male and female. Furthermore, several bones are not yet visible radiographically in the infant, which can confound observation and determination of osseous relationships and alignment. This chapter will provide guidance to address these challenges by discussing normal developmental anatomy, developmental variants, positioning techniques (including radiation protection and safety), and alignment relationships.

Normal Anatomy and Development

Because bone initially develops from cartilage, large "spaces" are seen between the bones, especially in the younger child. This is because cartilage is not visible radiographically and cannot be distinguished from adjacent soft tissues [1]. As bones mature, these spaces become smaller until only the joint spaces are visible. Bones will change in size and shape as they develop, especially when secondary growth centers appear. However, primary ossification centers, especially in the tarsus, are not small representations of a cartilaginous anlage's shape and position, nor does ossification proceed symmetrically throughout childhood [2].

Epiphyses and apophyses are secondary ossification centers. The epiphysis is found at the end of a long bone and articulates with an adjacent bone (Fig. 2.1a) [3]. It typically does not have muscle or tendon attachment. The epiphysis distributes pressure from an adjacent bone and has, therefore, also been referred to as the "pressure epiphysis." The adjacent physis (or growth plate) is perpendicular to the long axis of the primary ossification center and contributes to longitudinal bone growth.

The apophysis is found at the future site of a tubercle, tuberosity, or process [3]. It has also been referred to as a "traction epiphysis," since it serves as the site for tendon insertion (Fig. 2.1b). In contrast to the epiphysis, the physis adjacent to an apophysis may be parallel or oblique to the primary ossification center's axis. Apophyses in the foot are located at the fifth metatarsal proximally and the calcaneus posteriorly. They do not participate in longitudinal growth of long bones nor do they articulate with an adjacent long bone.

The radiolucent zone located between the epiphysis and metaphysis of a long bone is known as the physis (Fig. 2.2). At the metaphyseal edge of the physis is an area of increased density referred to as the zone of provisional calcification. Their appearances vary with each bone

R. A. Christman (✉)
College of Podiatric Medicine, Western University of Health Sciences, Pomona, CA, USA
e-mail: rchristman@westernu.edu

M. L. Butterworth, J. T. Marcoux (eds.), *The Pediatric Foot and Ankle*,
https://doi.org/10.1007/978-3-030-29788-6_2

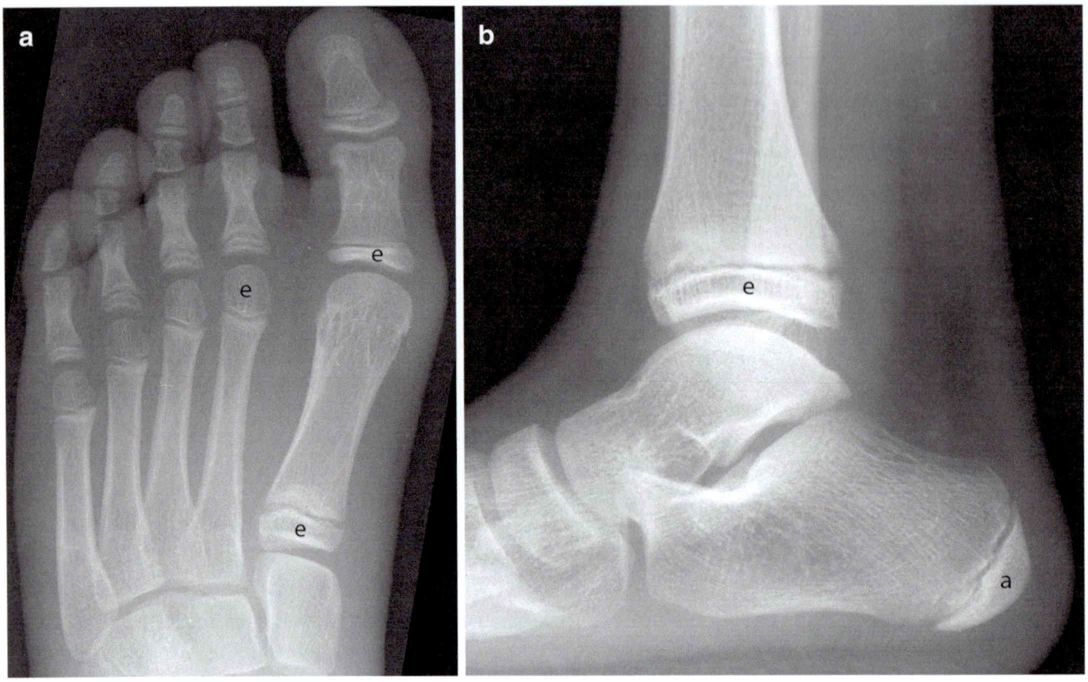

Fig. 2.1 Epiphyses. (**a**) Pressure epiphysis (e). (**b**) Traction epiphysis (aka apophysis) (a)

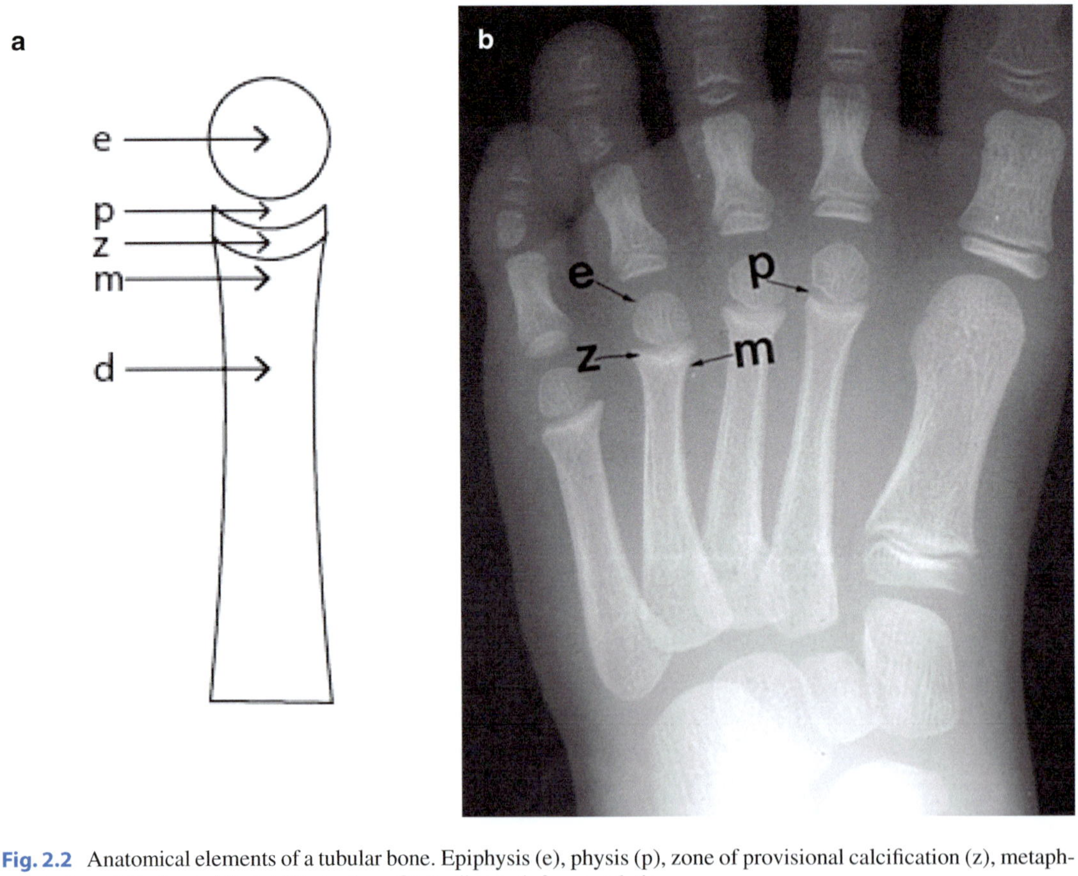

Fig. 2.2 Anatomical elements of a tubular bone. Epiphysis (e), physis (p), zone of provisional calcification (z), metaphysis (m), and diaphysis (d). (**a**) Illustration. (**b**) Radiograph for correlation

as well as with age and sex [4]. However, excessive narrowing or widening of a physis should be considered abnormal, as should irregularity of the zone of provisional calcification [4].

Ranges for ossification dates (i.e., when an ossification center is first visible radiographically) are available in a number of publications [5–7]. However, when viewed side to side, variability between sources is noted [8]. Tables 2.1, 2.2, 2.3, and 2.4 provide a general guideline as to times of appearance; however, be aware that the range of appearance (before and after the average date of appearance) may span months or even years. Therefore, don't focus on the exact ossification center time periods as much as on the relative nature of them and their sequence of appearance.

Most, if not all, ossification centers appear earlier in females than in males, even before birth. However, the difference is less the earlier an ossification center appears. The cuboid, for example, appears in the male about the same time as it does in the female. But, the sex difference increases as age advances; the calcaneal apophysis appears, on average, 2 years earlier in the female than in the male [5]. Also, skeletal maturity is achieved earlier in females than in males [9]. Ossification stops at approximately 12 years of age in the female and 14 years of age in the male [10].

Two methods have been used to determine the skeletal age of infants and utilize a lateral radiograph of the foot and leg [11]. The Erasmie method [12] (for up to 1 year of age) first determines the sum of the length and height of the talus and calcaneus ossification centers and assesses the appearance (maturity) of the cuboid, third cuneiform, and distal tibial and fibular epiphyses; these values are then plotted on a nomogram relative to the child's weight. The Hernandez method [13] (for up to 2 years of age) assigns maturity

Table 2.1 Ossification dates: primary centers

Bone	Avg. date of appearance
Talus, calcaneus, metatarsals	Present at birth
Cuboid	Present at birth to 1 mo
Lateral cuneiform	4 mo
Medial cuneiform	1.5 y
Intermediate cuneiform	2 y
Navicular	2.5 y
Sesamoid	10 y

The dates in this table are AVERAGES of the COMBINED male and female times of appearance and closure; generally speaking, the average female time of appearance will be earlier than this date, the male later

Table 2.2 Ossification dates: major epiphyses

Epiphysis	Avg. date of appearance	Avg. date of closure
Distal tibia	4 mo	15 y
Distal fibula	11 mo	15 y
Calcaneus (apophysis)	6.5 y	15 y
Posterior talus	9.5 y	11.5 y
Fifth metatarsal (apophysis)	11 y	14.5 y

The dates in this table are AVERAGES of the COMBINED male and female times of appearance and closure; generally speaking, the average female time of appearance will be earlier than this date, the male later

Table 2.3 Ossification dates: metatarsal epiphyses

Epiphysis	Avg. date of appearance	Avg. date of closure
1st metatarsal (base)	2 y	15 y
1st metatarsal (head)	2.5 y	10.5 y
2nd metatarsal	2.5 y	15 y
3rd metatarsal	3 y	15 y
4th metatarsal	3.5 y	15 y
5th metatarsal	4 y	15 y

The dates in this table are AVERAGES of the COMBINED male and female times of appearance and closure; generally speaking, the average female time of appearance will be earlier than this date, the male later

Table 2.4 Ossification dates: phalangeal epiphyses

Epiphysis	Avg. date of appearance	Avg. date of closure
Hallux (distal phalanx)	1 y	15 y
Hallux (proximal phalanx)	2 y	15 y
Lesser toe 2–4 (proximal)	1.5 y	14.5 y
Lesser toe 5 (proximal)	2 y	15 y
Lesser toe 2–3 (distal)	4 y	13 y
Lesser toe 4 (distal)	3.5 y	13 y

The dates in this table are AVERAGES of the COMBINED male and female times of appearance and closure; generally speaking, the average female time of appearance will be earlier than this date, the male later scores to the calcaneus, cuboid, third cuneiform, and distal tibial and fibular epiphyses; this score is then plotted on a nomogram relative to the child's age.

Ossification of the foot is fast during the first 5 years and slows thereafter. The foot reaches one half of the adult size by 5 years of age [10]. Hoerr et al. [14] have provided a standard of reference for skeletal development of the foot and will not be duplicated here. Figures 2.3, 2.4, 2.5, 2.6, 2.7, and 2.8 focus on what the author considers the major ossification centers, primary and secondary, that are useful for determining the approximate age of a patient based upon radiographs alone.

The tarsal bones present (or visible radiographically) at birth include the talus and calcaneus and usually the cuboid (Fig. 2.3); occasionally, the cuboid may not appear until up to 6 months after birth. Though the talus and calcaneus ossification centers are consistently visible at birth, a large portion remains cartilaginous [15]. No secondary ossification centers are present at birth [16].

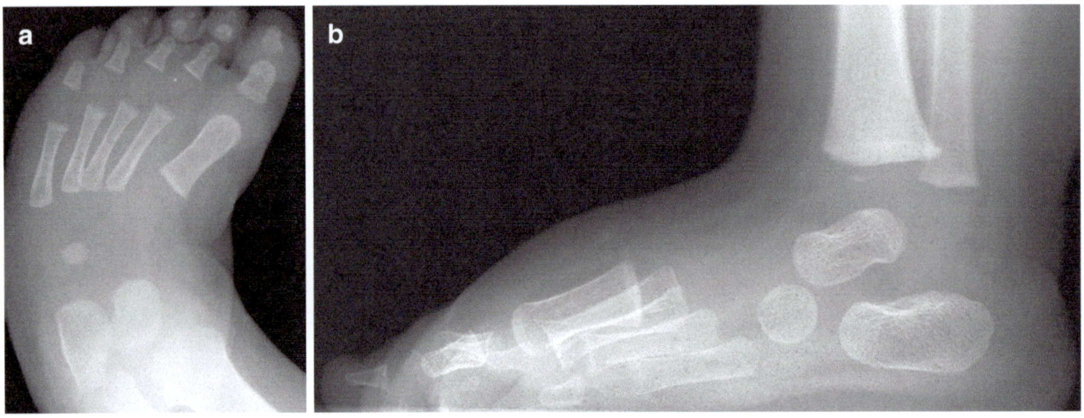

Fig. 2.3 Major ossification centers, primary and secondary: Birth–3 months. (**a**) Dorsoplantar view. (**b**) Lateral view. Talus, calcaneus, and cuboid

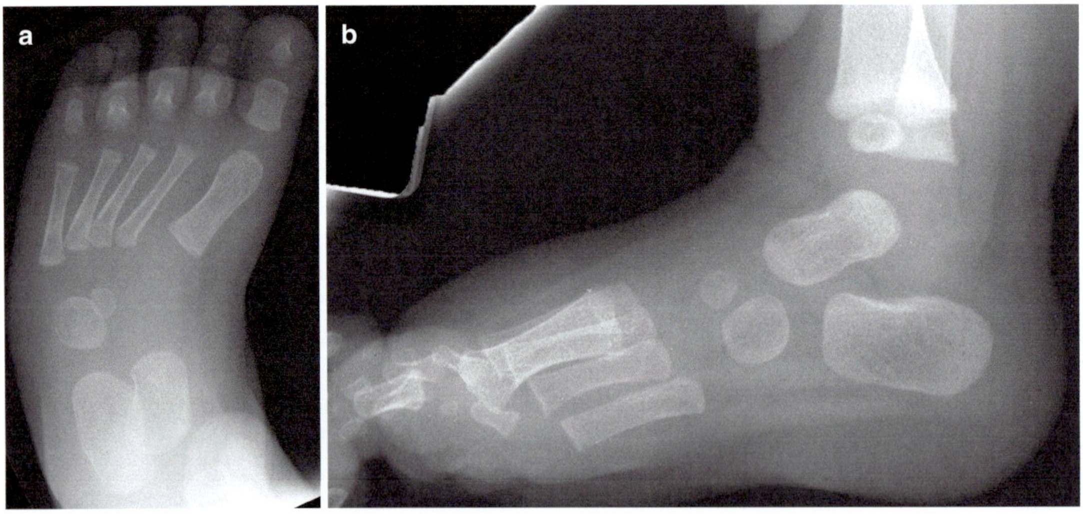

Fig. 2.4 Major ossification centers, primary and secondary: 3–9 months. Lateral cuneiform and distal tibial epiphysis. (**a**) Dorsoplantar view. (**b**) Lateral view

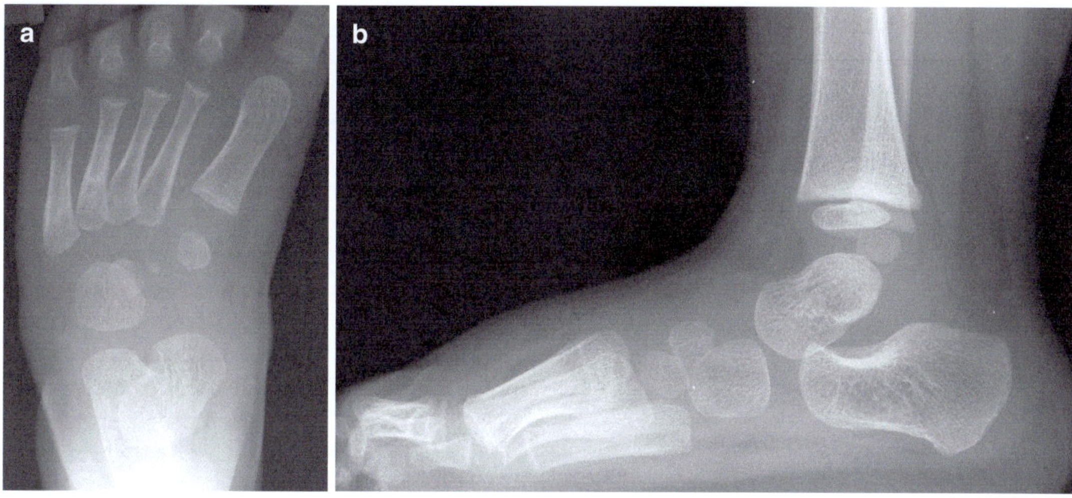

Fig. 2.5 Major ossification centers, primary and secondary: 9 months–2 years. The distal fibular epiphysis and medial cuneiform appear prior to the intermediate cuneiform and 1st metatarsal and proximal phalangeal basal epiphyses, which are just beginning to ossify. (**a**) Dorsoplantar view. (**b**) Lateral view

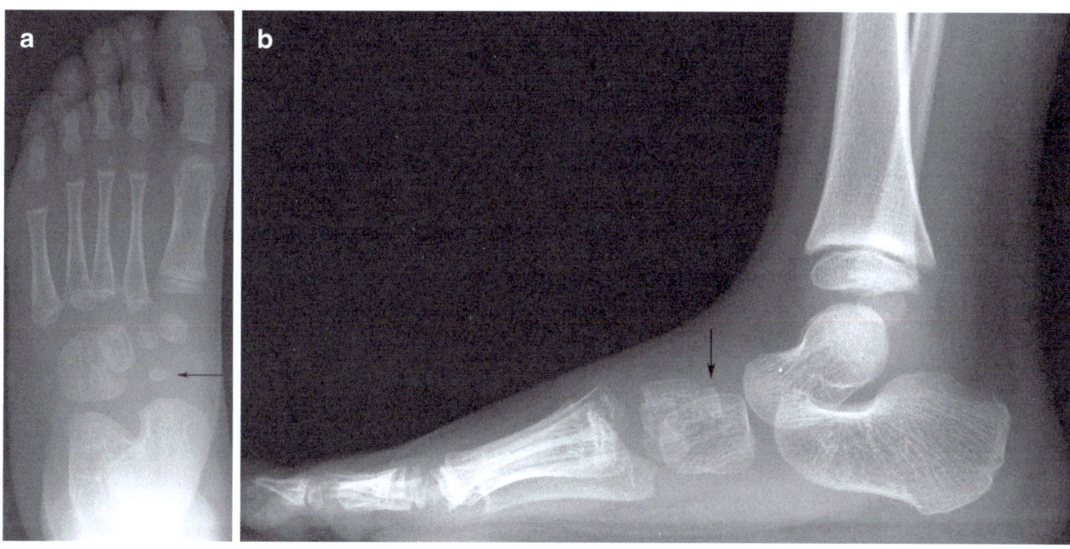

Fig. 2.6 Major ossification centers, primary and secondary: 2–5 years. Navicular (arrows) and lesser metatarsal head. Also note variant pseudoepiphyses at all lesser metatarsal bases. (**a**) Dorsoplantar view. (**b**) Lateral view

The next group of ossification centers appears between 3 and 9 months, including the lateral cuneiform and the distal tibial epiphysis (Fig. 2.4). The distal tibial and fibular growth plates provide most lower leg bone growth during infancy, but after 30% of the bone growth is achieved, it slows down and bone length comes from the proximal growth plates [10].

The distal fibular epiphysis and medial cuneiform ossification centers ossify around 9 months to 2 years, followed by the intermediate cuneiform and the 1st metatarsal and proximal phalangeal basal epiphyses (Fig. 2.5). Though the most common ossification sequence order after ossification of the cuboid and lateral cuneiform bones is medial cuneiform-middle cuneiform-navicular, at least six tarsal sequences may be encountered (Table 2.5). This is probably due to genetic differences but also could be attributed to disease or malnutrition [17]. Distal fibular epiphyseal ossification always appears after ossification of the distal tibial epiphysis [18].

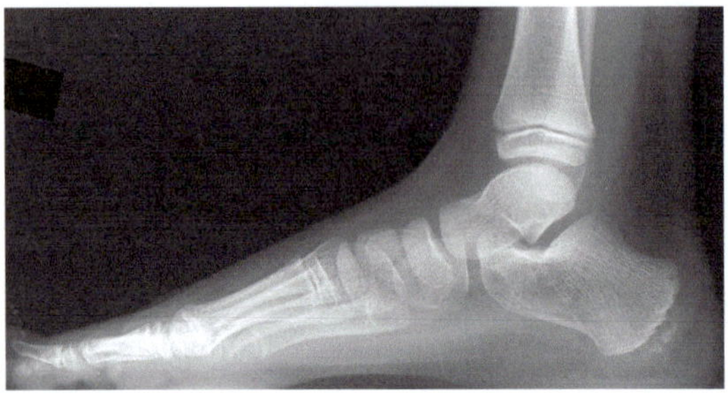

Fig. 2.7 Major ossification centers, primary and secondary: 5–9 years. Calcaneal apophysis. Lateral view: small calcifications/ossifications are present posteroinferior to the calcaneus

Table 2.5 Sequence of ossification: tarsal bones (after cuboid – lateral cuneiform)

Medial cuneiform	Middle cuneiform	Navicular	Average % of cases (Boys and girls)
1	2	3	70.5
1	3	2	13.5
2	1	3	6
2	3	1	5.5
3	1	2	4
3	2	1	0.5

Modification of Table 3 from: Garn et al. [17]

The navicular and the lesser metatarsal head epiphyseal ossification centers appear in the 2- to 5-year range (Fig. 2.6). The fibular physis is located more proximally, at the midlevel of the tibial epiphysis, in infancy [19, 20]; it is at or below the ankle joint after 4 years of age [10], which is probably related to weight bearing [20].

The calcaneal apophysis begins to ossify somewhere between 5 and 9 years of age (Fig. 2.7). The fifth metatarsal apophyseal ossification center and the sesamoids ossify between 9 and 12 years of age (Fig. 2.8).

In 1966, Kump [21] described a hump along the medial and anterior aspects of the distal tibial physis (Fig. 2.9). This is a normal developmental feature and has been referred to as the "Kump hump" since then by other authors [18, 22, 23].

Developmental Variants

Developmental variants may be misinterpreted as abnormal findings (e.g., fracture). Some are common; others are rare. Multipartite ossification centers are probably the best example and may involve primary or secondary ossification centers

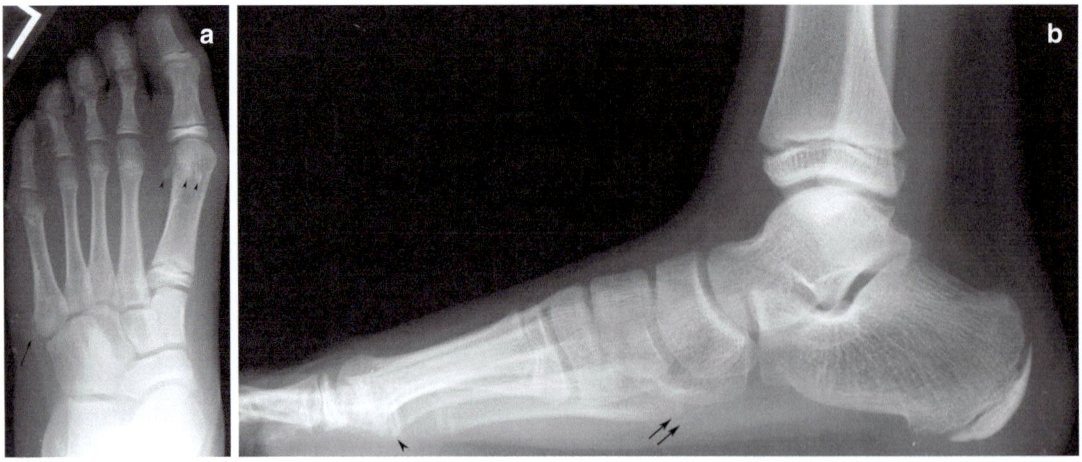

Fig. 2.8 Major ossification centers, primary and secondary: 9–12 years. Fifth metatarsal apophyseal ossification center (arrows) and sesamoids (arrowheads). (**a**) Dorsoplantar view. The tibial sesamoid ossification center is multipartite. (**b**) Lateral view. The fifth metatarsal apophyseal ossification center is multipartite

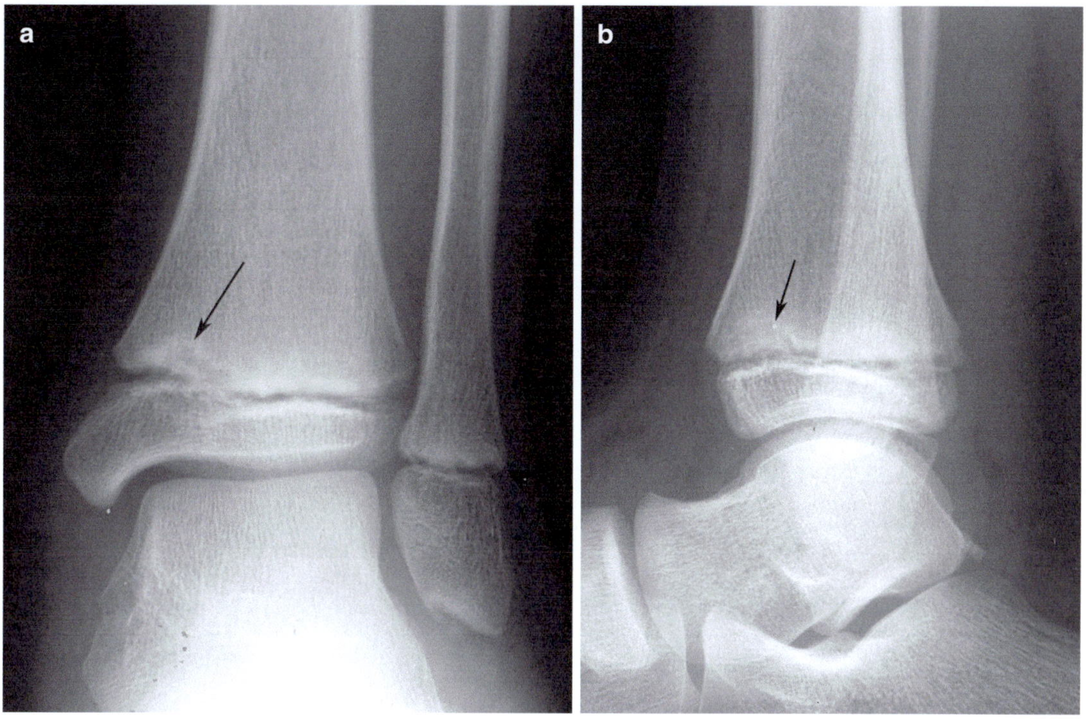

Fig. 2.9 Kump hump (arrows). (**a**) Mortise ankle view. (**b**) Lateral ankle view

(Fig. 2.10). Sometimes the partition dividing an ossification center is referred to as a "fissure" [24].

Clefts and the cone-shaped epiphysis are commonly encountered in the phalanges (Fig. 2.11). They frequently are bilateral, though not necessarily symmetrical. The term "bracket epiphysis" (aka longitudinal epiphyseal bracket and delta phalanx) describes the presence of an epiphysis along the side of a phalanx (Fig. 2.12), not at its base [10]. It is usually an isolated finding associated with skeletal dysplasias and syndromes [25–27].

The term "pseudoepiphysis" is applied to an apparent secondary ossification center located at the non-epiphyseal end of a long bone. It also has been referred to as an accessory bone and supernumerary epiphysis. The pseudoepiphysis, when present, is more mature and precedes formation and enlargement of the true epiphysis at the other end of the bone [28, 29]. In contrast to the true epiphysis and physis, the pseudoepiphysis is characterized by a direct extension of metaphyseal bone through a physeal variant [30]. A pseudoepiphysis frequently is seen at the distal end of the first metatarsal (Fig. 2.13). It appears between 2 and 4 years of life; it later appears as a cleft before it fully unites with the adjacent metaphysis by 11 years of age. A pseudoepiphysis may also be seen at a lesser metatarsal base (Fig. 2.6a). Also, the posterior margins of the lesser metatarsals (their bases) may appear very irregular and undulating, with or without a pseudoepiphysis (Fig. 2.10a).

Because the calcaneal apophyseal ossification center is so large, its appearance at varying stages of development can look considerably different (Fig. 2.14). When it is just beginning to ossify, multiple small calcific densities will be seen. And, the inferior half of the apophysis usually ossifies prior to the superior half. The normally developing calcaneal apophysis will appear sclerotic relative to the calcaneal body [31]. As development continues, the calcaneal apophysis is often multipartite. The inferior tubercles (medial and lateral) are also formed within this apophysis and may be seen as separate ossification centers.

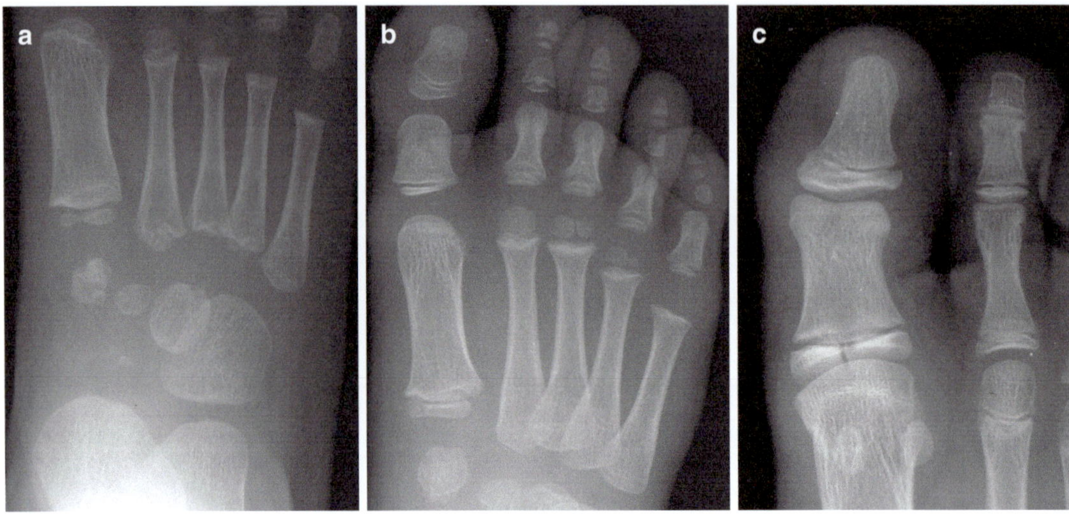

Fig. 2.10 Multipartite ossification centers. (**a**) Multipartite secondary ossification centers involving the first metatarsal base and multipartite primary ossification centers for the navicular and medial cuneiform bones. The bases of the second through fourth metatarsals are irregular, and pseudoepiphyses are also seen. (**b**) Bipartite epiphyses of the third and fourth metatarsal heads. The second toe middle phalangeal epiphysis is cone-shaped. (**c**) Bipartite basal epiphysis of the hallux proximal phalanx, which could easily be misinterpreted as fracture (this particular patient had no history of trauma nor were there any symptoms)

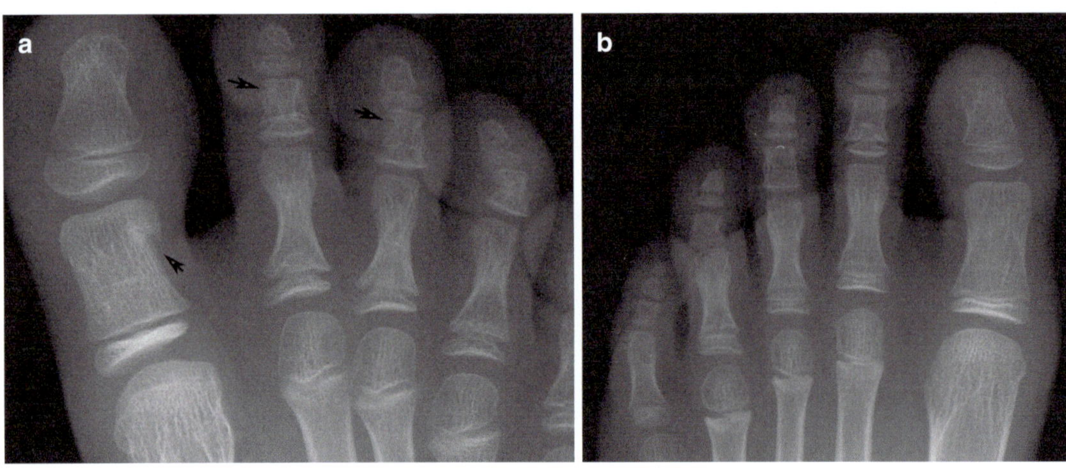

Fig. 2.11 Phalangeal variants of development. (**a**) Clefts (arrows) are seen along the lateral aspect of the hallux proximal phalanx head and the medial aspects of the second and third toe middle phalangeal heads. The basal epiphyses of the second and third toe proximal phalanges are cone-shaped. (**b**) Cone-shaped epiphysis of the second toe middle phalanx

(Persistence of a separate tubercle ossification center is rare but has been reported as the os subcalcis.) Generally speaking, the margins of each partite ossification center are well-defined; ill-defined decreased densities separating a "partite" ossification center would suggest pathology (e.g., fracture). Another variation includes a jagged metaphysis, sometimes having a "saw tooth" appearance [10].

Sever disease is defined as inflammation of the calcaneal apophysis. The typical presentation is of an adolescent male involved in sports

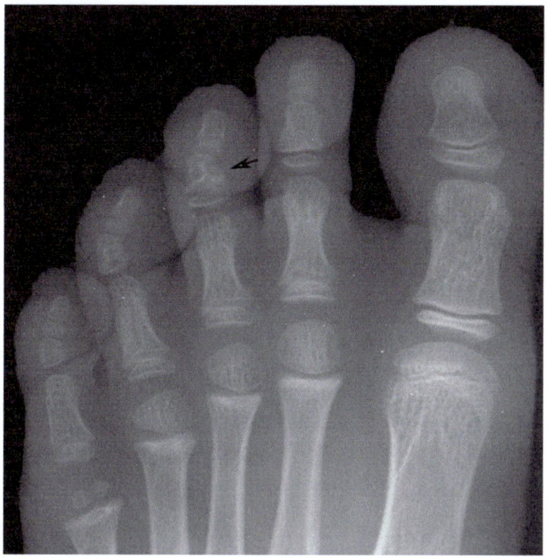

Fig. 2.12 Longitudinal epiphyseal bracket. Though this is not a classic example (a basal epiphysis is present), the epiphysis (arrow) does appear to encompass nearly the entire medial aspect of the third toe middle phalanx

who has a very painful heel. The disorder has been associated with the radiographic presentation of a sclerotic apophysis with fragmentation (the radiographic appearance of osteochondrosis). However, as noted above, the calcaneal apophysis is normally sclerotic, and "fragmentation" or partitioning is a normal variant that is often reported in children who have no symptoms. Because of this, Sever disease is considered a clinical diagnosis, and the radiographic features are considered a variation of ossification. The debate lingers on as to whether or not these findings are significant; in the author's experience, these particular findings have been seen in many patients who had no associated heel pain. However, according to Scharfbillig et al. [32], this has not been investigated in a scientific manner, and therefore, the jury is still out, so to speak.

The fifth metatarsal proximal apophysis (Fig. 2.15) is only visible radiographically for a short period of time before it unites with the base. And, its appearance is not necessarily bilateral or symmetrical during ossification. This apophysis appears as a small fleck of bone and may be shell-shaped; it is longitudinally oriented or slightly oblique to the long axis of the metatarsal shaft along the plantar-lateral aspect of the base [33, 34]. An irregular-shaped apophysis may be normal. Although the apophysis can appear fragmented (partitioned), this is a variant finding, not pathologic. In bilateral studies, the apophysis may appear slightly enlarged in symptomatic patients, with slight separation of the chondro-osseous junction [33]. Radiographically, the secondary center of ossification is best seen in the medial oblique view.

Iselin disease is an apophysitis of the fifth metatarsal tuberosity [35]. It is a clinical diagnosis based on pain at the region of the fifth metatarsal apophysis and is related to overuse. Radiographs are unremarkable but are obtained to rule out metatarsal fracture. Osteochondrosis of the fifth metatarsal apophysis has the typical radiographic appearance of sclerosis and fragmentation (partitioning) and is considered a normal variant, similar to Sever disease. Positive findings for apophyseal pathology (not Iselin disease) include ill-defined decreased density and/or distraction from the tuberosity. In this case, images of the opposite extremity might be useful for comparison.

On occasion, the apophysis may not unite to the base and persist into adulthood; this is known as the persistent fifth metatarsal apophysis. It may be bilateral or unilateral (Fig. 2.16). This has erroneously (in the author's opinion) been referred to as the os vesalianum.

Numerous accessory ossicles can be seen in the adult and have been described elsewhere [36]. Therefore, corresponding ossification centers may be seen at the same locations in the child. More common examples include the accessory navicular (which ossifies between 7 and 11 years of age), the os trigonum (appearing about 5 years of age), and the os subtibiale (ossifying from 7 to 8 years of age) [10].

Small accessory ossicles may develop along the distal fibular zone of provisional calcification, medially and/or laterally [20]. A larger ossification center is often seen adjacent to and lateral to the distal fibular metaphysis, referred to as the "fibular ossicle" [37]. It appears around 6 years of age and eventually unites with the fibula.

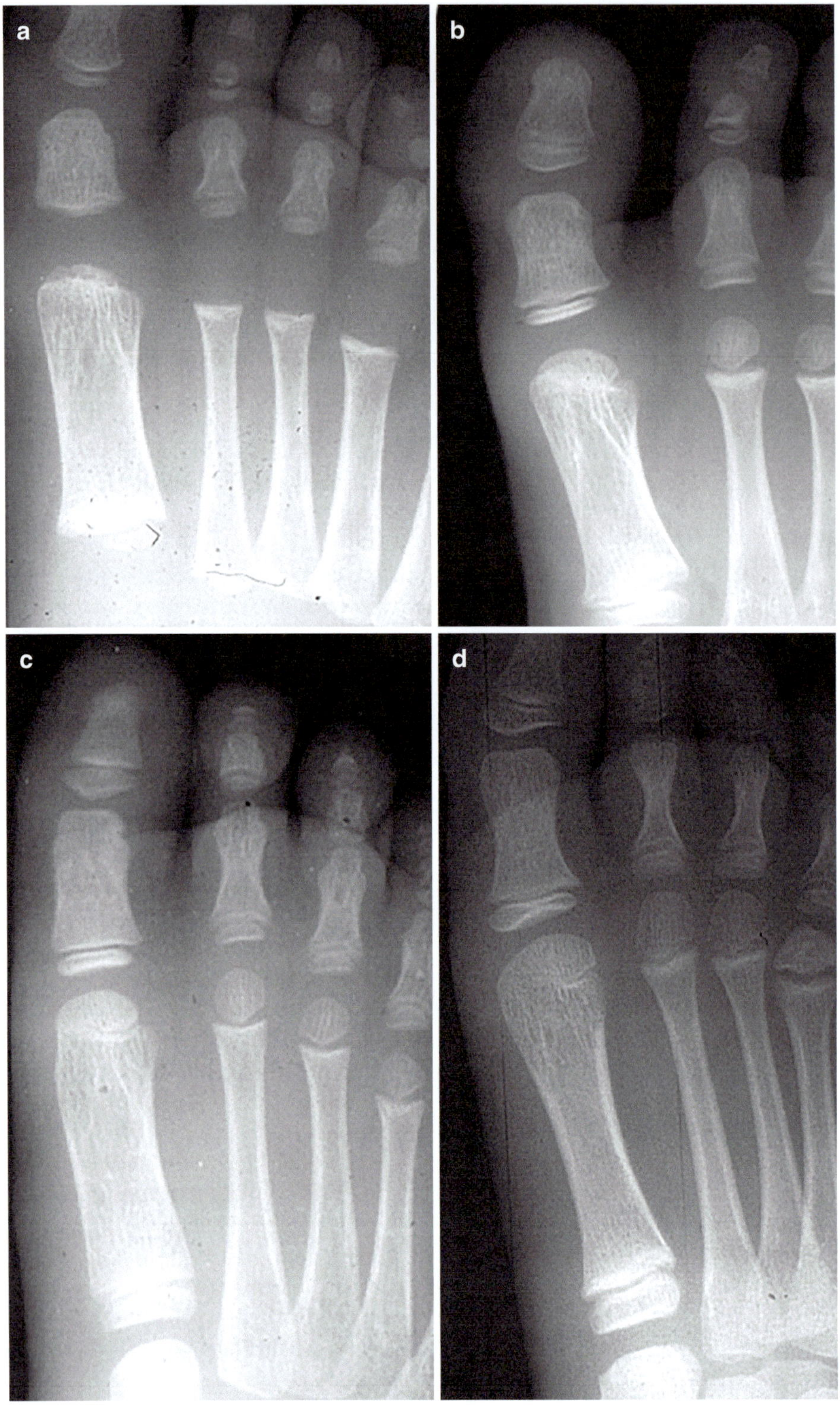

Fig. 2.13 First metatarsal distal pseudoepiphysis. (**a**) Early development of the pseudoepiphysis from small ossifications. (**b**) Appearance as a full "epiphysis", though it is most likely attached to the metaphysis centrally. (**c**) Asymmetrical union with the adjacent metaphysis. (**d**) Appearing as a cleft as it continues to unite

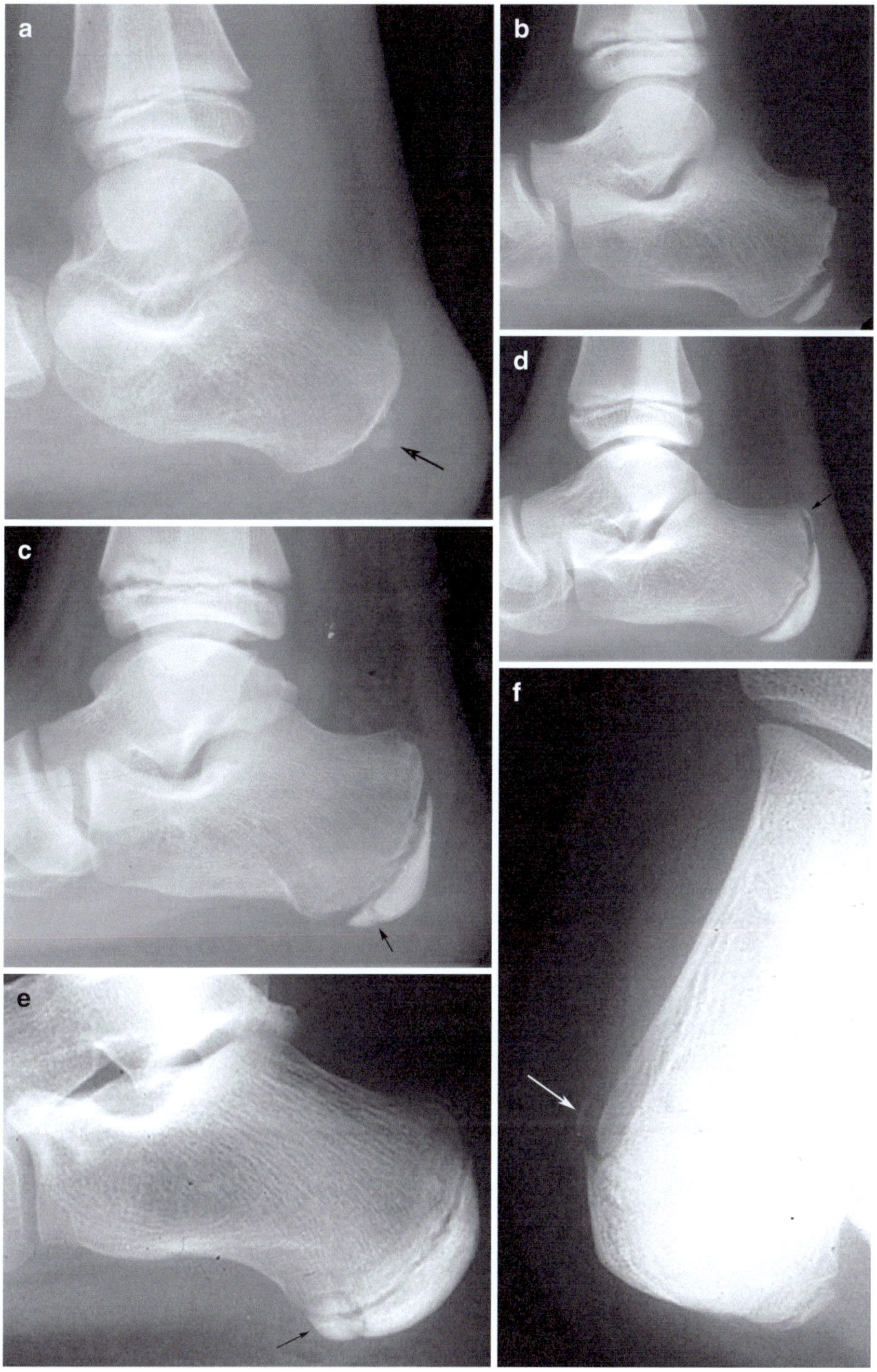

Fig. 2.14 Calcaneal apophyseal ossification center. (**a**) Ossification center is just beginning to ossify, and multiple small calcific densities can be seen. (**b**) Inferior half of the apophysis usually ossifies prior to the superior half. The adjacent metaphysis is often jagged, as seen here; this should not be considered pathologic. (**c**) The apophysis is normally sclerotic relative to the calcaneal body. It often is partite (arrow) and develops from multiples centers of ossification, as seen here. (**d**) Ossification of the bursal projection (arrow) and inferior tubercles are also formed within the apophysis and occur last. (**e**) Ossification center for the medial tubercle (arrow). (**f**) Medial oblique foot view; separate ossification center for the lateral tubercle is identified (arrow)

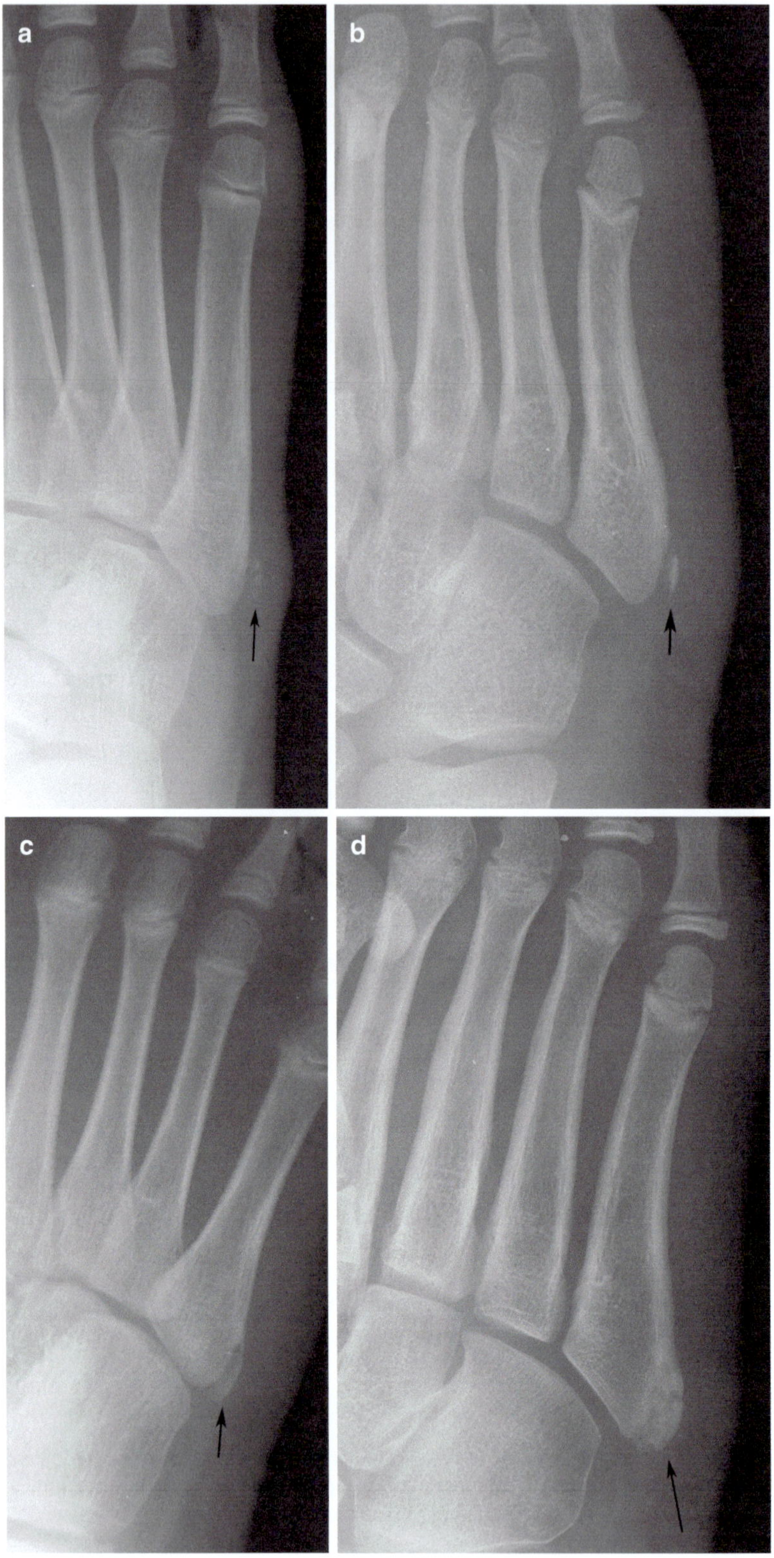

Fig. 2.15 Fifth metatarsal apophysis. (**a**) DP view of very early ossification from multiple centers. (**b**) Medial oblique view demonstrating sclerosis. (**c**) DP view; this apophysis is smooth and homogeneous in density. (**d**) Medial oblique view; though it is irregular, multipartite, and sclerotic, this apophysis was asymptomatic and symmetrical in appearance bilaterally

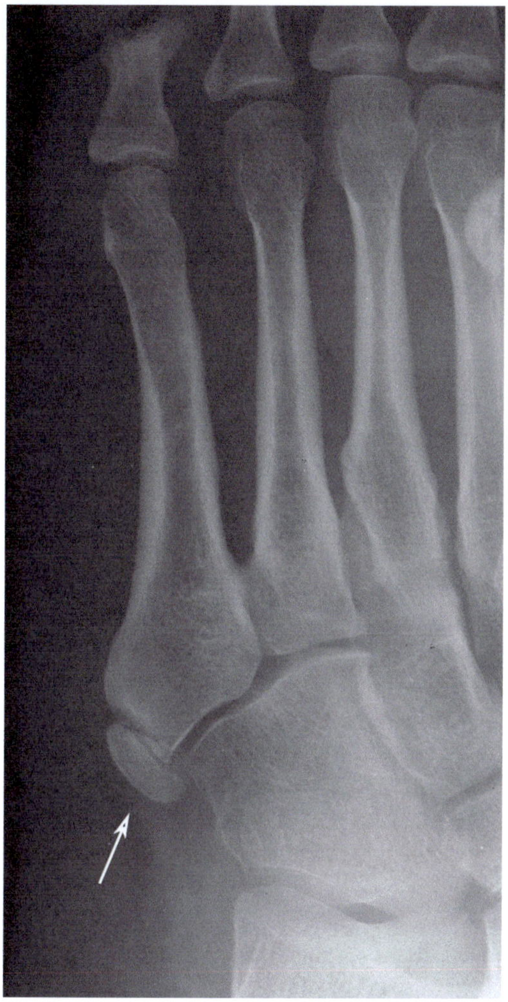

Fig. 2.16 Persistent 5th metatarsal apophysis

Some rare examples of developmental variation include the reverse calcaneal spur and the bifid calcaneus (Fig. 2.17).

Positioning Techniques

A pediatric radiographic study should be justified and documented. Because children have higher radiation sensitivity than adults, apply appropriate shielding to the gonads, collimate the primary x-ray beam, and lower the kVp, mA, and time settings accordingly for a child versus an adult. Immobilization devices (sandbags) may be necessary and should be considered in advance of the procedure. If the child is to be restrained and/or comforted during the study, a non-pregnant parent, family member, or guardian should be used, not a staff member. One could also arrange to perform the study after feeding time, while the child is asleep or under sedation, if warranted. A parent may question the risk of the radiographic study; consider having a handout (or video) available that explains the procedure and risks. One can also refer the parent to a medical physicist for estimation of the radiation dose [38].

Radiography is valuable for both the diagnosis and treatment of pediatric foot deformities [39]. Standard foot radiographic images include the dorsoplantar (DP) and lateral views. Other views, such as oblique, axial, and lateral ankle flexion,

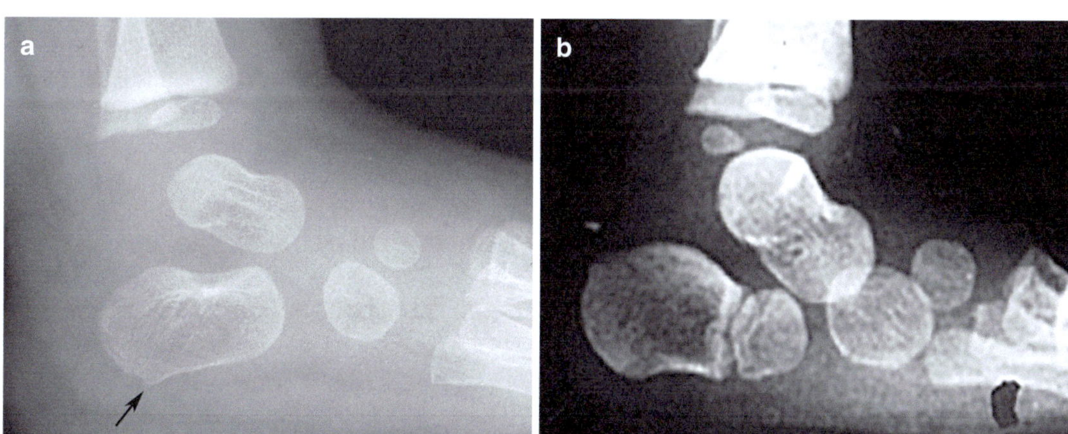

Fig. 2.17 Calcaneal variants of development. (**a**) Reverse calcaneal spur. (**b**) The bifid calcaneus. The two calcaneal ossification centers in **b** eventually united as one ossification center, which appeared entirely normal

are ordered depending upon the specific indications [40], which may include any of the following: fracture, tarsal coalition, infection, and post-operative, to name a few [10, 31]. Routine bilateral studies are not justified for comparison, nor for unilateral trauma, but may be useful in select cases (e.g., occult fracture) and may eliminate the need for other studies such as nuclear medicine, MRI, and CT [41].

Whenever possible, radiographs of the feet (except oblique positions) should be taken with the child standing [42]. In particular, DP and lateral positioning techniques should be performed weight bearing for assessment of osseous alignment relationships [31]; non-weight-bearing views are not adequate for assessing alignment [43]. Effort should be made to apply plantar stress to infants and those unable to stand [15]; this may require the assistance of a positioning device or a guardian wearing lead shielding. A non-infant patient could be seated and bearing partial weight (simulating weight bearing) while the foot is placed against the image detector. However, for infants and toddlers (3–12 months of age), simulated weight-bearing radiographs may result in a wide variation in angular measurements unless the lower extremity and foot are positioned at 90° [44]. Non-weight-bearing DP and lateral views should be reserved for evaluating trauma; oblique views may also be indicated in this case.

Generally speaking, positioning techniques for the child are performed the same way they are for the adult and are described in detail elsewhere [45]. However, it is important to note special considerations when positioning the child, especially the infant; these are described below. Also, suggestions are made on how to correct for alignment abnormalities during positioning, which is preferred by some practitioners.

Dorsoplantar Foot Techniques

The foot is positioned such that it is perpendicular to the leg; it also should not be forcibly pronated or supinated [40]. As noted above, this may necessitate a sitting or supine position for the infant or young child. If seated, the hips and knees should also be flexed at 90° (Fig. 2.18a) [46]. The lateral aspect of the hindfoot (or rearfoot) should be placed parallel to the edge of the image receptor. If bilateral images are required for an infant, one image can be obtained of both feet to limit exposure. In this case, the knees should be held together so that the lower extremities are not rotated; the legs should be perpendicular to the image receptor and parallel to one another [47]. (If forefoot adduction is present, the knees may need to be slightly separated to accommodate the forefoot deformity.)

For clubfoot deformity, Simons [46] also recommends forcing the foot into a 15° dorsiflexed position (which may require that the tube head be angulated 30° from vertical). He believes that, by holding the pre-operative foot as close as possible to the maximally corrected position, the talocalcaneal angle will be more accurate. Kite [48] performed the standard technique with no correction; in fact, *Merrill's Atlas of Radiographic Positioning & Procedures* [49] recommends that no attempt be made to correct the deformity.

Clues have been identified to determine if the foot was not positioned properly for the DP positioning technique [46, 50]. If the tibial and fibular shafts are identified, and/or the anterior ends of the talus and calcaneus are greater than 2–3 mm apart from one another longitudinally, then the foot was probably positioned in plantarflexion. The foot may have been inverted or supinated if the metatarsals are overlapping significantly. In all cases, one must correlate the radiographic image to the foot itself to verify if the technique was performed properly.

Lateral Foot Techniques

The lateral foot projection can be performed such that the medial side of the foot is placed against the image receptor. However, if the forefoot is adducted, such as in a clubfoot, the ankle and hindfoot will become externally rotated relative to the image receptor; the result is the appearance of a flattened talar dome (this can be confirmed as a positional "deformity" if the fibular malleolus is identified posteriorly relative to the tibial malleolus). In this case, the lateral projection can be performed as one would position the extremity for the lateral ankle projection, such that the ankle joint axis is perpendicular to the image receptor or the hindfoot is parallel to the edge of it [10, 15, 31]. For clubfoot deformity, since hindfoot measurement is most important, Simons [46] additionally recommends full dorsiflexion of the ankle joint (while the heel stays on the cassette). This technique holds the foot as close as possible to the maximally corrected position (pre-operatively). If the technique is performed as simulated weight bearing, the lateral side of the foot can be positioned against the image receptor, which negates any forefoot effect on the position of the hindfoot. If seated, the hips and knees are flexed at 90°.

For the infant or young child that is seated or supine, the leg and foot should be positioned perpendicular to one another (i.e., the ankle joint is at 90°). To achieve this, a plastic board can be used to push against the sole of the foot with one hand while stabilizing the leg with the other hand (Fig. 2.18b) [43, 47]. Radiographs of each foot should be obtained separately, not simultaneously as in the "frog leg" position.

Clues have been identified to determine if the foot was not positioned properly for the lateral positioning technique [46, 50]. As mentioned above, if the fibular malleolus is located posterior to the tibial malleolus in the radiograph, then the hindfoot was externally rotated relative to the image receptor. If the metatarsals appear stacked upon one another (i.e., they are not overlapped), then the foot may have been inverted or supinated. If the tibia is not perpendicular to the foot, then the foot was either dorsiflexed or plantarflexed. As with the DP view, one must correlate the radiographic image to the foot itself to verify if the technique was performed properly.

There are times when one will want to obtain lateral views with the foot maximally flexed. The lateral forced dorsiflexion technique is used to assess vertical talus and clubfoot; the lateral forced plantarflexion technique is used for vertical talus evaluation [42].

Calcaneal Axial Techniques

Several tube head angulations have been recommended for the calcaneal axial projection. The standard technique positions the tube head at 25° from vertical. However, this technique may not produce visibility of the posterior and middle talocalcaneal joints. In order to view these joints, Harris and Beath [51] positioned the tube head at 45° while the patient dorsiflexed the ankle and flexed the knee. Grissom [40] recommends a 25° tube head angulation with the foot dorsiflexed and 40° if not.

Melamed [52] recommended a modification of the Harris-Beath technique for viewing an avulsion fracture of the navicular tuberosity or the accessory navicular. The extremity is internally rotated approximately 20–25° such that the forefoot is pointed inward. The tube head is angulated at 45°

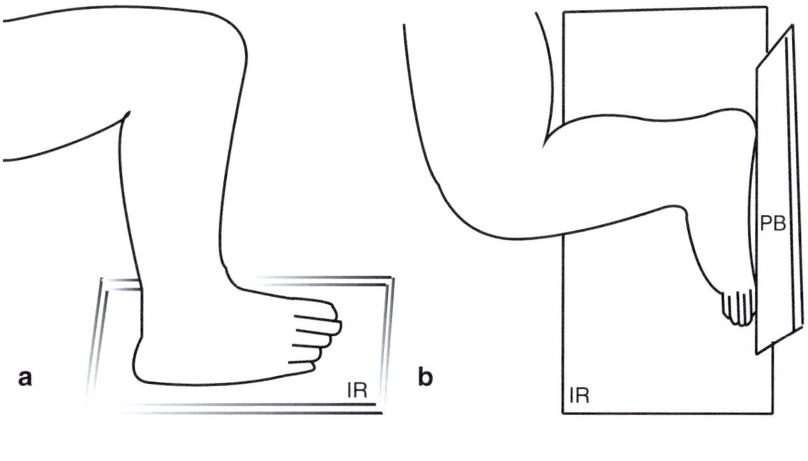

Fig. 2.18 Simulated weight-bearing views in an infant (IR = image receptor). (**a**) DP view. (**b**) Lateral view. A plastic board (PB) is pushed against the sole as the other hand stabilizes the leg. The lateral side of the foot is positioned against the image receptor

from vertical, and the central beam is directed toward the navicular. However, a similar image of the accessory navicular can be obtained with the non-weight-bearing lateral oblique foot view [36].

Hindfoot varus or valgus has been measured by using one of two specialty views, the hindfoot alignment view or the long leg calcaneal axial view [53].

Hindfoot Alignment Techniques

Cobey [54] described a posterior view of the foot, modifying the Harris-Beath calcaneal axial view such that distortion was minimized (by directing the x-ray beam perpendicular to the image receptor). The patient stood on a radiolucent platform, and a 14 × 17-inch image receptor was positioned anterior to the patient and extending partially below the platform such that it was tilted 15–20° from vertical (Fig. 2.19a). The x-ray tube head angulation was 15–20° from horizontal and directed caudally, which positioned the x-ray beam parallel to the forefoot axis (i.e., the foot was positioned pointing straight ahead). The central beam is directed toward the ankle. Mendicino et al. [55] modified the Cobey technique such that the feet are placed in angle and base of gait.

Buck et al. [56] modified Cobey's technique by placing the image receptor perpendicular to the floor (vertically) such that the x-ray beam is angled at 20° from horizontal (not perpendicular to the image receptor). The foot was still positioned pointing straight ahead (Fig. 2.19b). They preferred this technique because they felt that the resultant tibial and calcaneal axes would be more accurate and that it eliminated the forefoot and midfoot from the image. Johnson et al. [57] further modified the Buck et al. technique such that the foot was placed in a natural position of stance (angle and base of gait), which they believed "more closely measures 'true' coronal hindfoot alignment" compared to the techniques described by Cobey and Buck et al., where the foot was positioned pointing straight ahead.

Long Leg Axial Technique

The long leg axial study (Fig. 2.19c), derived from the Harris-Beath, posterior tangential, and suroplantar views [51, 58, 59], is performed (preferably) with a 14 × 17-inch image receptor to include the lower leg; the tube head is angled 45° caudally, and the central beam is directed toward the subtalar joint [55]. The foot may be dorsiflexed at the ankle; however, Kleiger and Mankin [58] found that the subtalar joint is seen just as well without dorsiflexion. Care must be taken by the radiographer not to supinate or pronate the foot when positioning. Reilingh et al. [53] believe that the long axial view is more reliable than the hindfoot alignment view (better interobserver reliability).

Ankle Positioning Techniques

The standard ankle views are anteroposterior (AP) and lateral. Oftentimes mortise and/or 45-degree medial oblique views are acquired. For alignment assessment, ankle techniques should be performed weight bearing or, if an infant, simulated. Osseous detail is better assessed non-weight bearing [10].

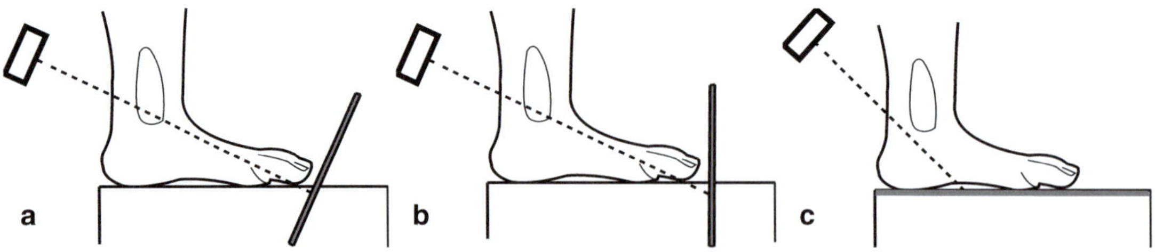

Fig. 2.19 Calcaneal axial techniques. (**a**) Hindfoot alignment view, Cobey method. The tube head is angled 15–20° from horizontal and the image receptor is angled 15–20° from vertical. (**b**) Hindfoot alignment view, Buck modification. The tube head is angled 20° from horizontal, but the image receptor is vertical. (**c**) Long axial view. The tube head is angled 45°, and the image receptor is horizontal

Alignment Relationships

Terminology

Alan Oestreich [60] published a short primer to evaluate and measure foot positional relationships in the two-dimensional radiograph. Some of the definitions differ when compared to the same terms used for the three-dimensional, clinical biomechanical analysis of the foot. The following explanations and examples are drawn from his primer, applying the terms universally.

Varus and valgus refer to angulation of a distal bony segment to the proximal segment relative to the body's midline. (The coronal plane of the leg translates to the transversal or axial plane in the foot.) Hindfoot varus and valgus refer to the position of the calcaneus relative to the talus. Forefoot varus and valgus refer to the position of the first metatarsal relative to the talus. Metatarsus primus adductus refers to the first metatarsal being in varus relative to the medial cuneiform. And, hallux valgus refers to the position of the hallux relative to the first metatarsal.

Adduction and abduction do not represent a relationship between different adjacent segments (or bones) of the body, as do varus and valgus. They refer to a deviation of a body part toward or away from the body's midline. Therefore, metatarsus adductus refers to the forefoot deviating toward the midline of the body.

The term hallux abductovalgus combines these concepts: abducto meaning that the hallux deviates away from the body's midline, and valgus refers to the position of the hallux relative to the first metatarsal (if the first metatarsal is aligned with the body's midline, then the hallux would be pointing away from it, i.e., in valgus).

Axes

For assessment of alignment, the foot is divided radiographically into three segments: hindfoot, midfoot, and forefoot [10, 61, 62]. The hindfoot is composed of the calcaneus and talus and includes the tibiotalar and talocalcaneal joints. The midfoot is made up of the navicular, cuboid, and cuneiform bones and includes the talonavicular and calcaneocuboid joints. The metatarsals and phalanges make up the forefoot, which also includes the cuneiform-metatarsal and cuboid-metatarsal joints. There also are two columns, medial and lateral. The medial column includes the talus, navicular, three cuneiforms, and first and second metatarsals. The lateral column includes the calcaneus, cuboid, and third through fifth metatarsals. Osseous axes, for the most part, are drawn in a fashion similar to that of the adult. However, there may be some special considerations, especially in the young child, which are outlined below.

DP View

The talar axis is commonly drawn as a bisection of the talus (Fig. 2.20a). However, Howard and Benson [63] warn that the ossification center in infants, which is in the anterior talus, may not reflect the true axis but that of the neck. Furthermore, Bleck [64] states that, in the newborn, the talar neck is more medially deviated relative to the body than in the adult (30° in the newborn versus 18° in the adult). As a result, some have endorsed drawing the axis along the medial aspect of the ossification center in the younger child [43, 61].

Relative to the first metatarsal base, the bisected talar axis should run through it or just medially [10, 43]. The talar axis, in an older child, also can be represented by a bisecting perpendicular line to a line that connects two points along the medial and lateral margins of the talar head articular margins [62]. This is also known as the talar head articulation axis (Fig. 2.21).

The calcaneal axis (Fig. 2.20a) could be drawn as a bisection in the younger child. However, Howard and Benson [63] again caution that, since the ossified nucleus of the calcaneus is obliquely oriented in the infant, its axis may be skewed. Drawing the axis along the lateral aspect of the calcaneus ossification center has been advocated by some [43, 61]. The calcaneal (mid-body) axis should nearly bisect the cuboid and should parallel the fourth metatarsal or pass through the fourth metatarsal base [10, 43].

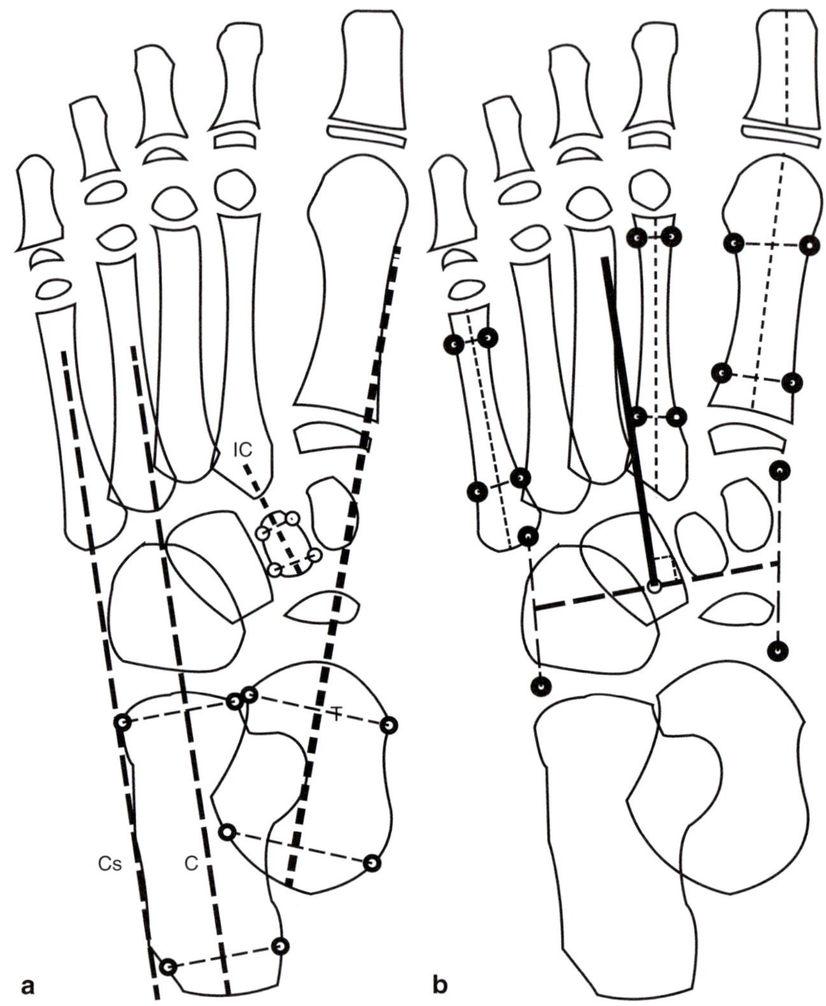

Fig. 2.20 DP view axes. (**a**) Talus (T), calcaneus (C), and intermediate cuneiform (IC) bisections; lateral calcaneal surface (Cs) axis. (**b**) Lesser tarsus (solid line), metatarsal, and phalanx axes

The navicular articulation axis (Fig. 2.21) is a bisecting perpendicular line to the line that connects two points at the medial and lateral margins of the navicular articular surface for the talar head [62]. The intermediate cuneiform axis is drawn as a bisection (Fig. 2.20a).

The lesser tarsus axis (Fig. 2.20b) is drawn as follows:

- Connect the following medial two points by a straight line: the most medial aspect of the first metatarsal-medial cuneiform articulation and the most medial aspect of the talonavicular articulation.
- Mark a point representing the bisection of this line.
- Connect the following lateral two points by a straight line: the most lateral aspect of the fourth metatarsal-cuboid articulation and the most lateral aspect of the calcaneocuboid articulation.
- Mark a point representing the bisection of this line. A line connecting the two bisections plotted above is the lesser tarsus transection.
- Draw a perpendicular to this line to obtain the lesser tarsus longitudinal axis.

Each metatarsal axis is drawn centrally and parallel to its shaft as a bisection (Fig. 2.20b). Plotting points at the proximal and distal ends of the shaft, forming lines between the distal points and proximal points, marking bisections on these lines, and connecting the bisections is the method

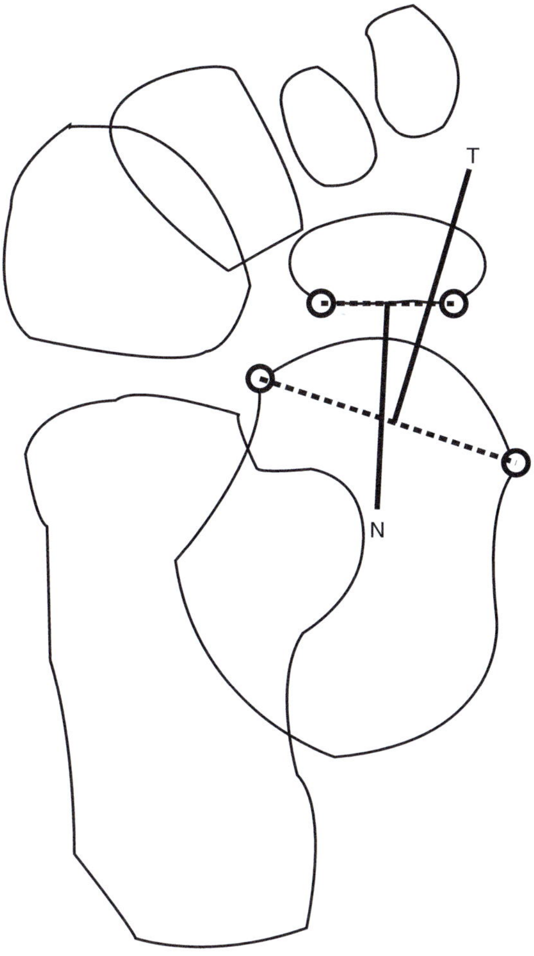

Fig. 2.21 DP view, talar axis (T) perpendicular to talar head articular surface; navicular articular surface axis (N) perpendicular to the navicular articular surface

used to draw the axis. Phalangeal axes are drawn in the same manner (Fig. 2.20b).

Lateral View (Fig. 2.22)

The talar axis is drawn through its midsection. The talus is directed more vertical at birth but is less so by 4 years of age [10]. The talus will then point toward or parallel the first metatarsal shaft [43]. The calcaneal axis can be drawn through its midsection or along its inferior surface; the two lines should run parallel to one another [43]. The first metatarsal axis is drawn through its shaft and is nearly parallel to its superior border. The tibial axis is drawn parallel to its shaft.

Calcaneal Axial Views (Including Hindfoot Alignment and Long Leg)

In the newborn, the calcaneal ossification center is oriented vertically and beneath the fibula; the talus ossification center is oriented horizontally and beneath the tibia [59].

There have been different methods for drawing the calcaneal axis. Sensiba et al. [65] and Cobey and Sella [66] chose the simplest methods, i.e., using a line parallel to either the lateral or medial aspect of the calcaneus, respectively (Fig. 2.23a). The medial side is used on a posterior coronal MRI image since it is less variable [67]. The other methods are more complicated. For example, Johnson et al. [57] used an overlaid egg-shaped elliptical to determine the coronal axis of the calcaneus. Robinson [68] accounts for both the calcaneal body and the posterior calcaneus by using a 60:40 bisection point for the posterior calcaneus, which compensates for the prominent medial expansion of the medial tuberosity, based upon their anatomical anthropometric results; Reilingh et al. [53] defined levels for the marks from the inferior calcaneal edge at 7 mm for the posterior calcaneus and 20 mm for the calcaneal body (Fig. 2.23b). And, Buck et al. [69] drew the calcaneal axis on the long calcaneal axial view in this manner: a line was formed between two points plotted at the lateral and medial aspects of the lateral and medial tubercles, respectively; a second line was formed between points plotted at the lateral aspect of the posterior talocalcaneal joint and at the spot where the sustentaculum tali joins the calcaneal body medially; a third line connecting the bisections of the first two lines represented the calcaneal axis (Fig. 2.23c).

The tibial axis runs centrally and parallel to the tibial shaft (Fig. 2.23).

Angles and Other Positional Relationships

Radiographs are a valuable adjunct for effective diagnosis and treatment of pediatric foot deformities [39]. The radiographic diagnosis is, for the most part, based upon angular (quantitative)

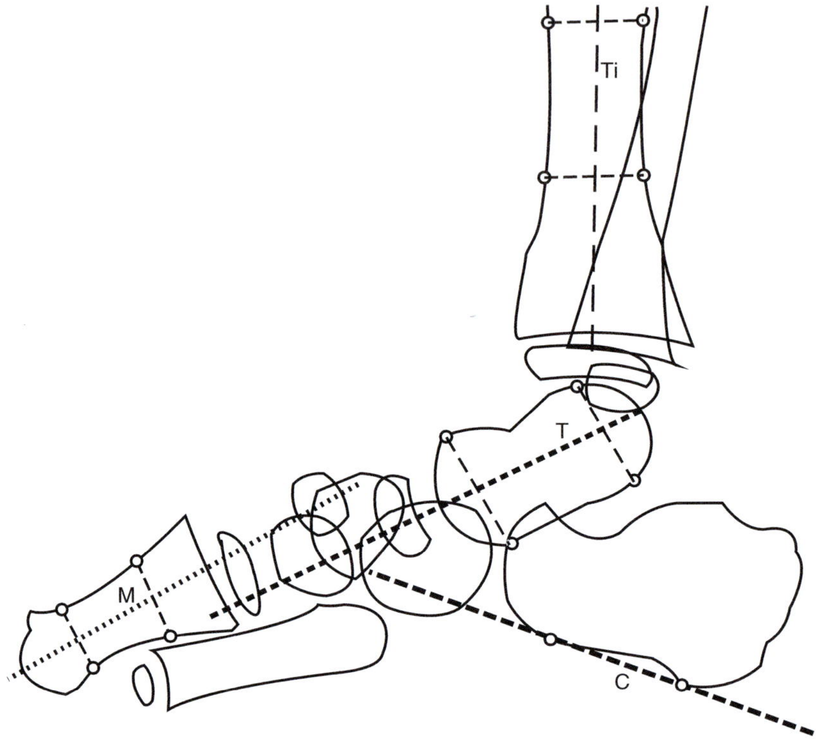

Fig. 2.22 Lateral view axes. Talar (T), calcaneal (C), first metatarsal (M), and tibial (Ti) axes

relationships. Due to developmental ossification, bones are not fully visible and the relationships (anatomic and functional) between bones, especially in the tarsus, may change [15]. Talus, calcaneus, and navicular bone ossification does not begin in the center of the bones' cartilaginous anlagen [2]; this helps explain why the talocalcaneal angles in the DP and lateral views decrease with age, as you will see below. Also, each measurement technique has varying degrees of reliability and validity. For example, Radler et al. [44] found high, sometimes as much as 30%, interobserver discrepancy in measurement of the pediatric foot, especially in the infant; therefore, quantitative values alone should not be used to make a definitive diagnose nor to indicate surgical intervention in the very young, though they are useful for comparison during treatment and follow-up. As patient age increased, however, interobserver reliability tended to improve. Despite their limitations, radiographic measurements are useful for describing malalignment in the pediatric foot and may aid in clinical decision-making and outcome assessment [62, 70, 71].

DP Foot View

Talocalcaneal Angle (Fig. 2.24a)

The talocalcaneal angle assesses hindfoot alignment. It is formed by the talar and calcaneal axes. The standard range varies between 10° and 55°: Dobbs and Beaty [72] use between 30° and 55°, Grissom [40] between 25° and 50°, and Templeton [47] between 15° and 50°, and Beatson and Pearson [73] reported a range between 10° and 50°.

Even though the range for this angle varies in the literature, there is consensus that the angle is higher at birth and decreases with age: Vanderwilde [74] reported a linear decrease with age, averaging 42° in the 6-month-old (ranging between 27° and 56° at 2 standard deviations (SD)) and decreasing to 24° in the 9+ year old (ranging between 12° and 35°); Simons [75] reported between 20° and 40° in the young child less than 5 years of age; and Templeton [47] reported between 30° and 50° in infants and young children and between 15° and 30° in children older than 5 years of age. Radler et al.

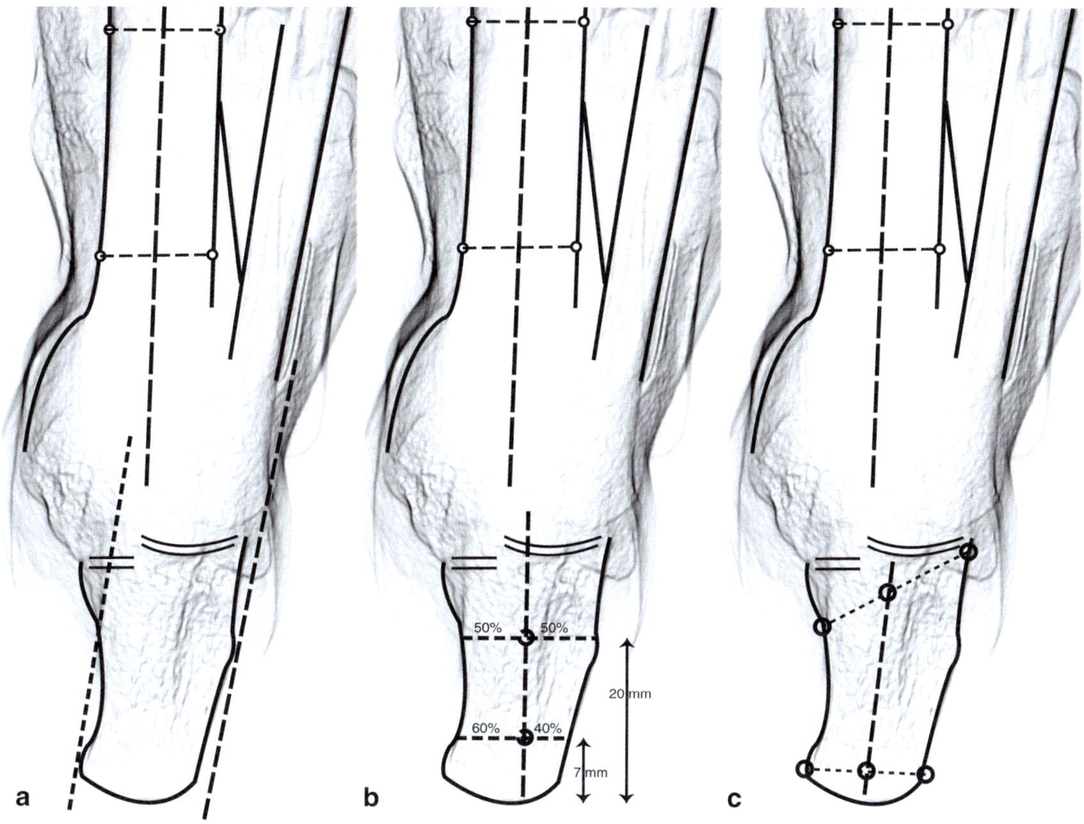

Fig. 2.23 Calcaneal axial view, calcaneal axes. (**a**) Lines parallel to either the medial or lateral surfaces. (**b**) Method according to Reilingh et al. (**c**) Method according to Buck et al.

[44] reported 35 ± 9° in the birth to 3-month age group, 36 ± 9° in the 3-month to 3-year-old group, 28 ± 7° in the 3–7-year group, and 23 ± 4 in the 7–14-year group.

Talus-First Metatarsal Angle (Fig. 2.24a)
The talus-first metatarsal angle assesses hindfoot/forefoot alignment. It has also been used to measure metatarsus adductus in infants. This angle is formed between the talar and first metatarsal axes. Lee et al. [70] determined that the talus-first metatarsal angle is a reliable and valid measure for discriminating between hindfoot varus and valgus deformity.

Generally speaking, the first metatarsal axis is either parallel to the talar axis or slightly valgus, ranging from 0 to 20 degrees valgus [75]. (The terms varus and valgus are preferable to negative and positive values due to discrepancies in the literature and to avoid confusion.) Taking into account 2 SD, Vanderwilde [74] reported the range to extend from 10° varus to 30° valgus, decreasing with age (between 6 months and 9+ years old) and averaging between 5° and 20° valgus. Others list the normal angle between 5° and 15° valgus [72, 76] and averaging 10 ± 7° (range of −3 to 28°, between ages 5–17 years) [62]. Xu et al. [77] reported an average of 16 ± 10° with a range between −5 and 49° (mean age, 10 years; range, 8–16 years). Radler et al. [44] reported a slightly valgus first metatarsal axis from birth to 7 years of age (between 5 and 9 ± 8 to 13°) and approximately 0 ± 9° from 7 to 14 years of age. Ideally, the angle approaches 0° in the adolescent, and the talar axis will be collinear with the first metatarsal axis.

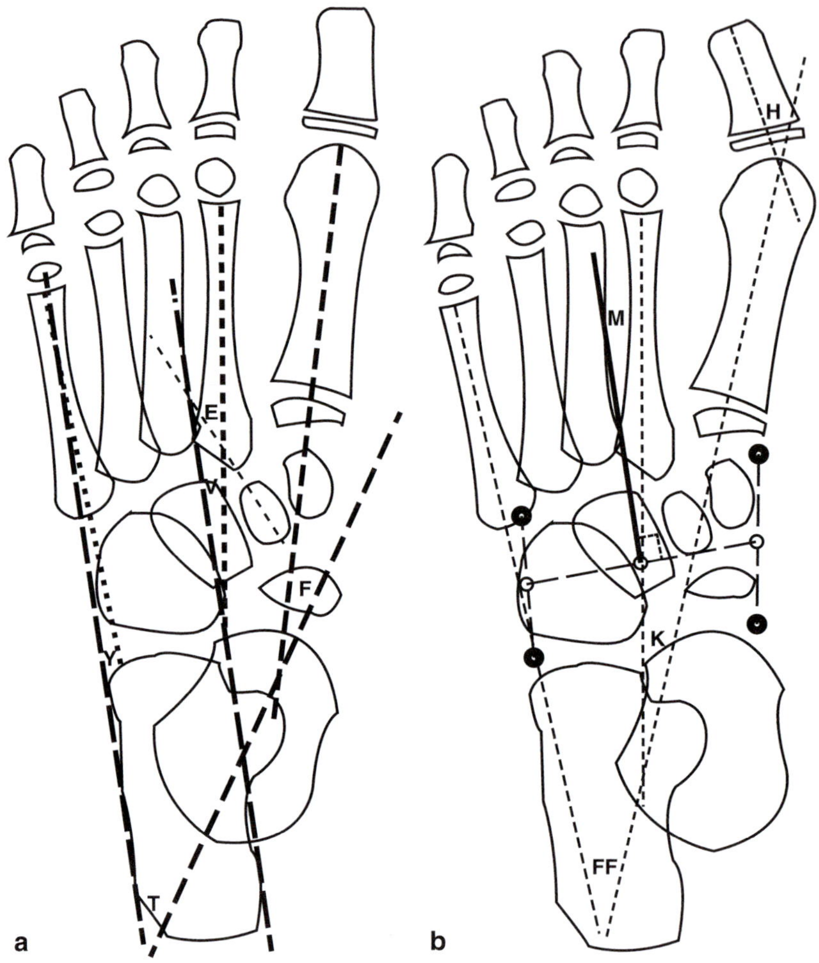

Fig. 2.24 DP view angles. (**a**) Talocalcaneal (T), talus-first metatarsal (F), second metatarsal-intermediate cuneiform (E), calcaneus-fifth metatarsal (Y), and calcaneus-second metatarsal (V) angles. (**b**) Hallux abductus (H), intermetatarsal 1–2 (K), metatarsus adductus (M), and first-fifth metatarsal angles (FF)

Metatarsus Adductus Angle (Fig. 2.24b)

The traditional metatarsus adductus angle utilizes the lesser tarsus bisection relative to the second metatarsal. This method is better applied in the older child when the tarsal bones are all ossified. Normally this measurement is 22–25° at birth but decreases to 10–21° in the adult [78].

Second Metatarsal-Intermediate Cuneiform Angle (Fig. 2.24a)

A simplified method for measuring the metatarsus angle uses the second metatarsal relative to the intermediate cuneiform. This angle is 3° greater than the traditional method (abnormal would be greater than 24°) [79]. Crawford and Green [80] caution against using the intermediate cuneiform due to poor correlation compared to traditional techniques of metatarsus adductus measurement.

Calcaneus-Fifth Metatarsal Angle (Fig. 2.24a)

The calcaneus-fifth metatarsal angle, like the talus-first metatarsal angle, has been used to measure hindfoot/forefoot alignment as well as to assess metatarsus adductus in infants. Vanderwilde [74] found this measurement to average between 0° and 4° in children between 6 months and 10 years of age. La Reaux [78] states that the calcaneus-fifth metatarsal angle is normally 5° and considered abnormal if greater than 10°. Radler et al. [44] reported a negative average in younger children that later became positive: −4 ± 11° (in the birth to 3-month-old group), −3 ± 10° (in the 3- to 12-month-old group), −4 ± 8° (in the 1- to 3-year-old group), 2 ± 7° (in the 3- to 7-year-old group), and 1 ± 5° (in the 7- to 14-year-old group).

First-Fifth Metatarsal Angle (Fig. 2.24b)

Another method used to measure the metatarsus adductus angle in infants is the first-fifth metatarsal angle. Normally this angle is around 22°; a measurement greater than 27° is considered abnormal [81].

Calcaneus-Second Metatarsal Angle (Fig. 2.24a)

Ganley [82] preferred using the calcaneus-second metatarsal angle to assess the forefoot adductus relationship in the infant (normally 12–18°). Simons [83] uses a slightly higher normal range for this angle: 15–20°.

Talonavicular Coverage Angle (Fig. 2.25)

The talonavicular coverage angle is formed between the talar and navicular articulation axes. The angle has been used to assess both hindfoot and midfoot alignment [70, 84]. In patients ranging between 5 and 17 years of age (mean age 10 years), the average is 20 ± 10° (range 5–39°) [62]. The talonavicular coverage angle was determined to be a reliable and valid measure for discriminating between hindfoot varus and valgus deformity [70]. Xu et al. [77] reported an average of 25 ± 11° with a range between 2 and 51° (mean age, 10 years; range, 8–16 years).

Talocalcaneal Divergence/Overlap (Fig. 2.26)

Talocalcaneal divergence was described by Simons [83] and refers to the position of the anterior ends of the talus and calcaneus relative to one another. Normally, a small cleft will be seen between the two bones [50]; there should be no overlap or separation, which is measured in 1/4 increments.

Cuboid Position (Fig. 2.27)

LeNoir [85] described abnormal alignment of the cuboid relative to the calcaneal axis as the "cuboid sign." Simons [86] took this a step further and described a radiographic grading system for calcaneocuboid malalignment. The calcaneal axis (bisection) normally runs through the midsection of the cuboid ossification center; this is considered grade 0. A second line along the

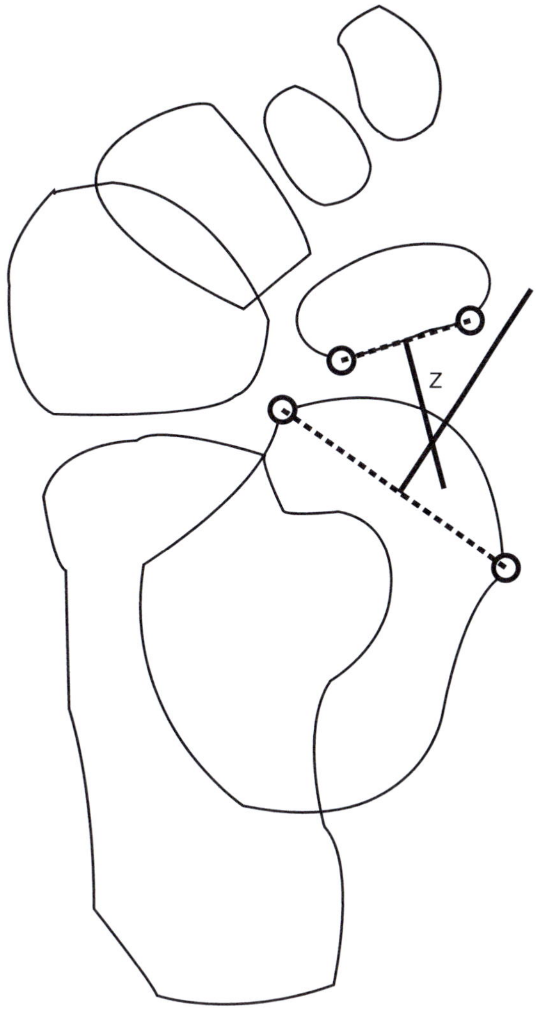

Fig. 2.25 Talonavicular coverage angle (Z)

medial border of the calcaneus and parallel to the calcaneal axis, referred to as the medial tangent, lays along the medial aspect of the cuboid. Malalignment occurs when the cuboid midsection is positioned medial to the calcaneal longitudinal axis. The position of the cuboid midpoint relative to the calcaneal longitudinal axis and medial tangent are used to grade the malalignment (Table 2.6).

Navicular Position (Fig. 2.28)

The navicular (if visible) and talar head should be directly opposite to one another [43]. As with the cuboid position, Simons [83] expands upon the relationship between the navicular bone and talar head.

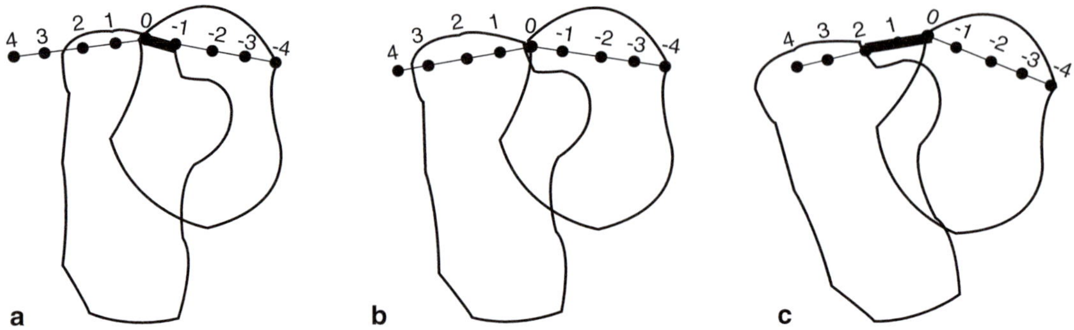

Fig. 2.26 Talocalcaneal divergence/overlap. (**a**) Varus (−1 overlap). (**b**) Normal (0, no overlap or divergence). (**c**) Valgus (+2 divergence). (Adapted from Figure 2 in: Simons [83])

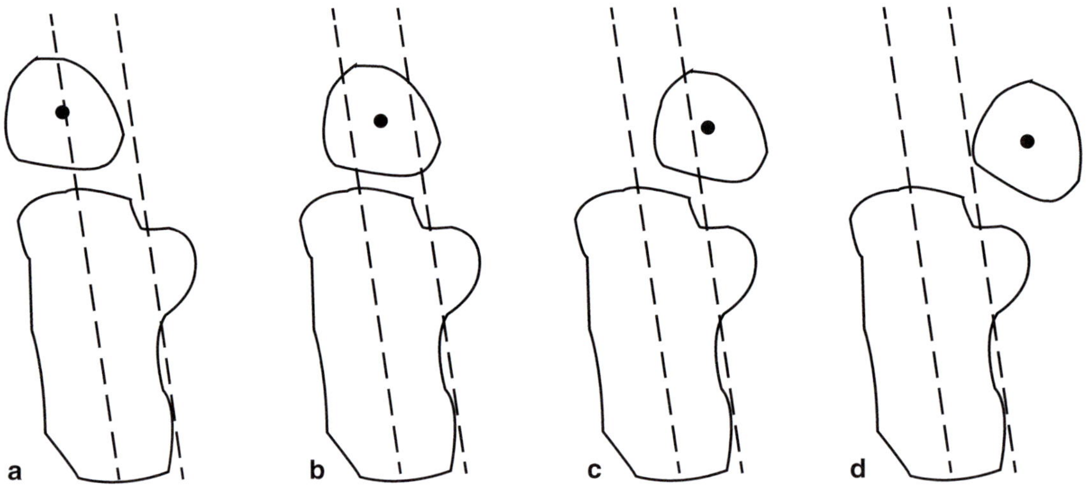

Fig. 2.27 Cuboid position. (**a**) Normal alignment. (**b**, +1 grade. (**c**) +2 grade. (**d**) +3 grade

Table 2.6 Cuboid position (grading system according to Simons, 1995)

Grade	Cuboid midpoint relative to calcaneal longitudinal axis	Cuboid midpoint relative to medial tangent
0	Centered	Lateral
1	Medial (axis runs thru lateral half)	Lateral (tangent runs thru medial half)
2	Medial (entire cuboid medial to axis)	Medial (tangent runs thru lateral half)
3	Medial (entire cuboid medial to axis)	Medial (entire cuboid medial to tangent)

Grading is based upon the position of the navicular relative to the diameter of the talar head which is divided into quarters. A grade of 0 is assigned when the center of the navicular aligns with the center of the talar head (Fig. 2.28b). A grade of −1 is used if the navicular is displaced medially by 1/4 of the talar head diameter, −2 if 1/2, etc. (Fig. 2.28a); a laterally displaced navicular is either a grade of +1, +2, etc. if displaced laterally (Fig. 2.28c). A grade of −2 to +2 is considered satisfactory.

If the navicular bone is not yet ossified, the position of the talar axis relative to the first metatarsal is used. A grade of 0 is when the talar axis passes through the first metatarsal base and is considered normal (Fig. 2.28b). If it passes lateral to the base by 1/2 the latter's width, a grade of −1 is given, a grade of −2 if lateral by the full width of the metatarsal base (Fig. 2.28a). The same parameters are applied if the talar axis passes medial to the base, but a positive (+) number is applied (Fig. 2.28c).

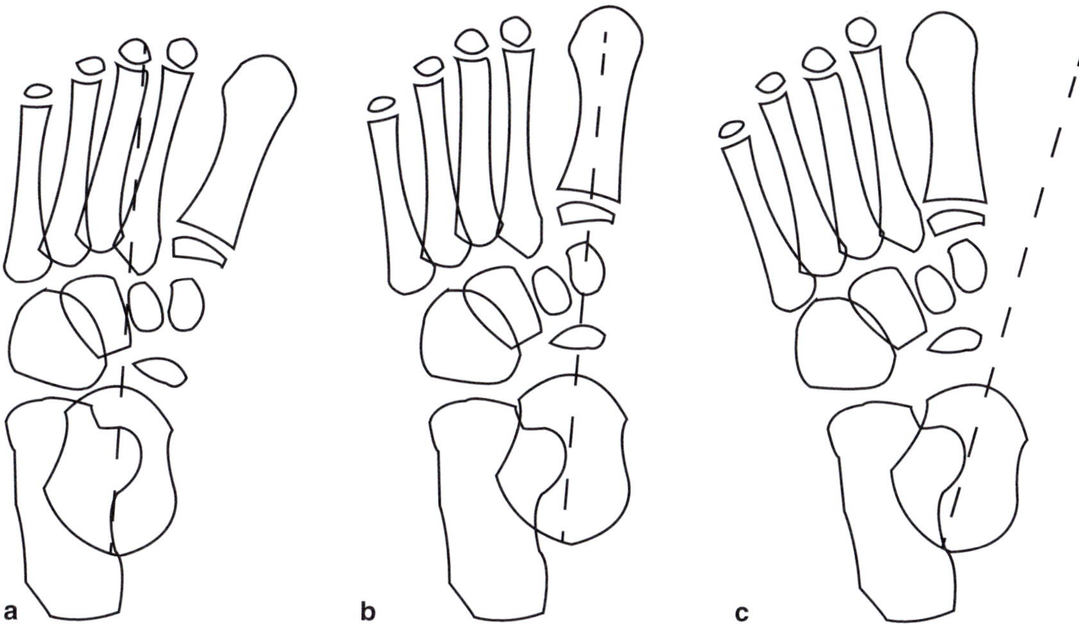

Fig. 2.28 Navicular position, dorsoplantar view. (**a**) −2 grade. (**b**) grade 0 (normal). (**c**) +2 grade

Hallux Abductus Angle (Fig. 2.24b)

The hallux abductus angle is formed between the first metatarsal and hallux proximal phalanx axes. Hardy and Clapham [87, 88] reported normal values for children between the ages of 4 and 15 years: 10 ± 4° (4–5 years old), 10 ± 5° (6–7 years old), 12 ± 5° (8–9 years old), 13 ± 5° (10–11 years old), and 14 ± 5° (12–15 years old). The average between 4 and 15 years of age was 12 ± 5°, with an expected range (at 2 SD) of 2–22°; in the adult the average was 15 ± 6°.

Piggott [89] used 15° as an "artificial" division between normal and abnormal in the adolescent; he felt that the normal foot was better differentiated from pathologic hallux valgus based on congruity of the first metatarsophalangeal joint surfaces (versus deviated or subluxated).

Intermetatarsal Angle (Fig. 2.24b)

The intermetatarsal angle is formed between the first and second metatarsal axes. Hardy and Clapham [87, 88] reported the following normal values: 7 ± 2° (4–11 years old) and 8 ± 2° (12–15 years old). The average between 4 and 15 years of age was 7 ± 2°, with an expected range (at 2 SD) of 3–12°; in the adult the average was 9 ± 3°.

Hallux Interphalangeal Angle

The interphalangeal angle is formed between the hallux proximal and distal phalanx axes. Hardy and Clapham [87, 88] used an arbitrary displacement measurement; no angular measurement was used.

Other Positional Relationships

The metatarsal bases converge and overlap slightly near the midfoot; there also is mild splaying of the metatarsals [40]. The calcaneal axis normally intersects the fourth metatarsal base, and the talar axis parallels the first metatarsal [10].

Aside from Hardy and Clapham, very little attention has focused on the radiographic angles used to assess hallux valgus in the child. In fact, most literature addresses the adolescent (10 years of age and older), whose foot has nearly fully achieved the adult form [71, 90, 91].

Lateral Foot View

Talocalcaneal Angle (Fig. 2.29)

The lateral view talocalcaneal angle assesses hindfoot alignment, as does that same angle in

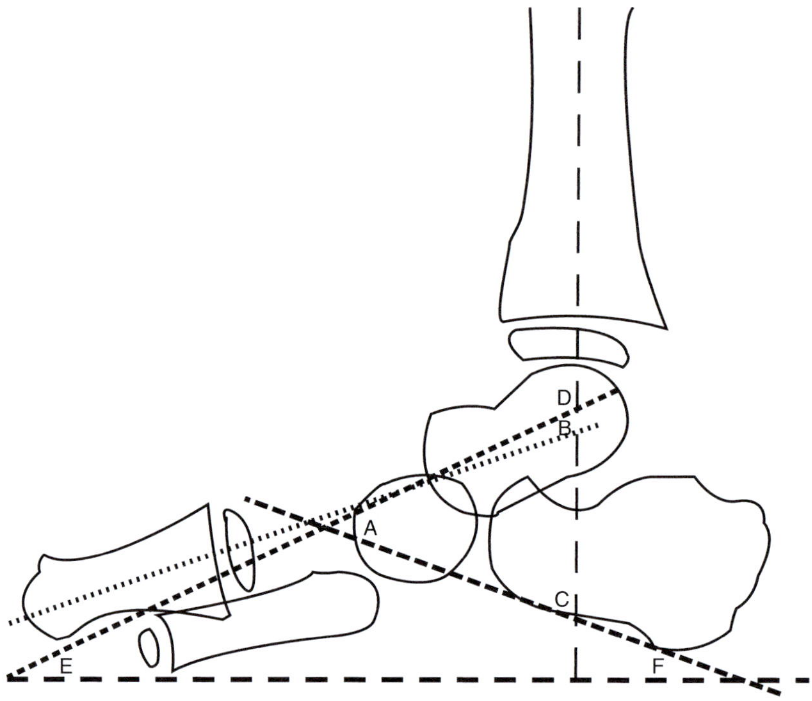

Fig. 2.29 Lateral view angles. Talocalcaneal (**A**), talus-first metatarsal (**B**), tibiocalcaneal (**C**), tibiotalar (**D**), talar declination (**E**), and calcaneal declination (**F**)

the DP view. The angle averages between 38° and 45°, according to Vanderwilde [74]; the range is between 25° and 55° at 6 months of age and 30–50° at 9+ years of age. Simons [75, 83] lists the normal range as 35 to either 50° or 55°; Heywood [92] reported between 35° and 50° also but states that 20–40° is normal. Templeton [47] uses 25–50°; Beatson and Pearson [73] reported a range between 15° and 55°. Radler et al. [44] reported the following values: 46 ± 11° (3–12 months), 43 ± 6° (1–3 years), 47 ± 7° (3–7 years), and 43 ± 7° (7–14 years). Davids et al. [62] reported an average of 49 ± 7°, ranging between 36° and 61° in children between the ages of 5 and 17 years. Xu et al. reported an average of 39 ± 8° with a range between 13 and 62° (mean age, 10 years; range, 8–16 years).

The maximum dorsiflexion talocalcaneal angle is used to measure the cumulative effects of equinus and varus in the clubfoot [74]. Dobbs [72] lists the range as 25–50°. According to Hammer [10], this angle is largest from birth to 2 years of age, averaging 45°, and decreases to approximately 33°. Vanderwilde [74] demonstrated an average between 45° at 6 months of age (23–55° range) and 41° at 9+ years of age (31–51° range), a slight decrease over time. However, Radler et al. [44] did not see an age-related decrease and found that dorsiflexion did not influence the talocalcaneal angle significantly: 47 ± 9° (birth to 3 months), 48 ± 7° (3–12 months), 48 ± 8° (1–3 years), 45 ± 8° (3–7 years), and 44 ± 8° (7–14 years).

Talocalcaneal Index

The talocalcaneal index is the sum of the DP and lateral view talocalcaneal angles. Beatson and Pearson [73] first reported its use for evaluation of clubfoot deformity; they found considerable overlap between normal and clubfoot talocalcaneal angles (DP and lateral), but not with the summation of the two. Their reported normal range was between 40° and 85° for the talocalcaneal index; less than 40° was considered abnormal. Vanderwilde [74] reported a range between 45° and 103°, averaging between 65° and 85°.

Talus-First Metatarsal Angle (Fig. 2.29)

As in the DP view, the lateral talus-first metatarsal angle is used to assess hindfoot/forefoot alignment [62]. The normal range is higher in the infant and decreases thereafter. The angle, according to Vanderwilde [74], averages from 18° at 6 months of age (range − 2 to 39°) to 5° at 9+ years of age (range 18 to −7°). (A negative value results when the first metatarsal axis is plantarflexed relative to the talar axis.) Simons [83] and Katz [39] use the range of 0–20°. In children 5–17 years of age, Davids et al. [62] found an average of 13 ± 8° (range 1–35°). Radler et al. [44] reported averages of 16 ± 15° (3 to 12 months old), 8 ± 6° (1–3 years old), 10 ± 7° (3–7 years old), and 5 ± 6° (7–14 years old). Xu et al. [77] reported an average of 3 ± 11° with a range between −33 and 29 (mean age, 10 years; range, 8–16 years).

Tibiocalcaneal Angle (Fig. 2.29)
The tibiocalcaneal angle is used to assess equinus and hindfoot alignment [62]. It is normally less than 80° [42]. According to Vanderwilde [74], the angle averages 77° at 6 months of age (range of 60–95°) and 67° at 10 years of age (range 64–75°). In children ranging between 5 and 17 years of age, Davids et al. [62] reported an average of 69 ± 8° (ranging from 44 to 86°). Radler et al. [44], mentioning that the measurement is very dependent on foot position, reported the following: 73 ± 15° (ages 3–12 months), 77 ± 9° (ages 1–3 years), 68 ± 11° (ages 3–7 years), and 67 ± 7° (7–14 years). Xu et al. [77] reported an average of 71 ± 10° with a range between 50 and 101° (mean age, 10 years; range, 8–16 years).

At maximum dorsiflexion, the tibiocalcaneal angle averages 41° at 6 months of age (range of 25–60) and 50° at 9+ years of age (range of 40–60°) [74].

Tibiotalar Angle (Fig. 2.29)
The tibiotalar angle measures the position of the talus relative to the tibia and can also be used to determine ankle joint range of motion. It averages 116° (range of 86–145°) at 6 months of age and slightly decreases to 108° (range of 95–123°) at 10 years of age [74]. Radler et al. [44] reported an overall average of 115° that is very dependent on ankle joint position with the following breakdown: 121 ± 10° (ages 3–12 months), 119 ± 8° (ages 1–3 years), 114 ± 11° (ages 3–7 years), and 110 ± 8° (7–14 years).

Ankle range of motion should normally be greater than 30°; this can be determined by measuring the tibiotalar angle with the foot in both dorsiflexion and plantarflexion (and subtracting the former from the latter). In dorsiflexion, the normal range is 70 to 100° and 120 to 180° in plantarflexion [50].

Talar Declination (Talohorizontal) Angle (Fig. 2.29)
The talar declination angle is formed between the talar axis and the plane of support; it decreases slightly over time. Vanderwilde et al. [74] reported an average of 35° (range of 14–55°) at 6 months of age and 25° (range of 15–36°) in the 10-year-old. Radler et al. [44] reported 37 ± 13° (3–12 months old), 33 ± 6° (1–3 years old), 30 ± 7° (3–7 years old), and 26 ± 6° (7–14 years old).

Calcaneal Declination (Pitch) Angle (Fig. 2.29)
The calcaneal declination angle is formed between the calcaneal axis and the plane of support. Though the measurement is widely used and reliable, it is not as valid as other measurements for assessing hindfoot alignment [70]. In children between the ages of 5 and 17 years, Davids et al. [62] reported an average angle of 17 ± 6° (range of 5–32°). Radler et al. [44] reported the following averages: 9 ± 14° (ages 3–12 months), 10 ± 4° (ages 1–3 years), 16 ± 5° (ages 3–7 years), and 18 ± 4 (7–14 years). Xu et al. [77] reported an average of 12 ± 5° with a range between 1 and 23° (mean age, 10 years; range, 8–16 years).

Naviculocuboid Overlap (Fig. 2.30)
Naviculocuboid overlap is used to assess hindfoot/midfoot alignment [70]. It is measured in the following manner: a line is made between two points (*a*, *b*) plotted at the superior and inferior margins of the cuboid, respectively; a third point (*c*) is plotted at the inferior margin of the navicular; naviculocuboid overlap = *ac*/*ab* × 100% [62]. Lee et al. [70] determined that naviculocuboid overlap is both a reliable and valid method for distinguishing between hindfoot varus and valgus; however, they caution that the measurement does not distinguish

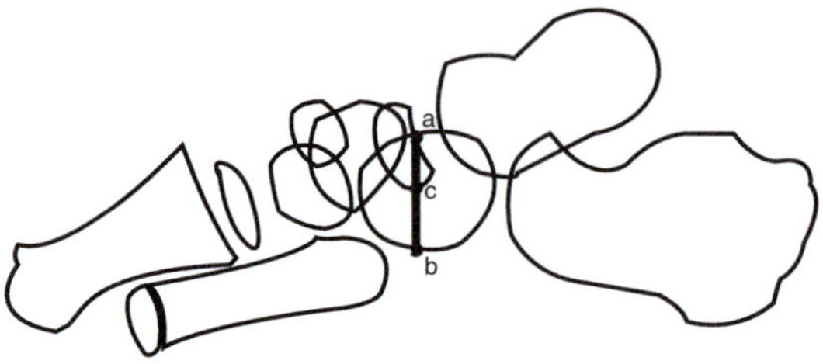

Fig. 2.30 Naviculocuboid overlap. (See text for further description)

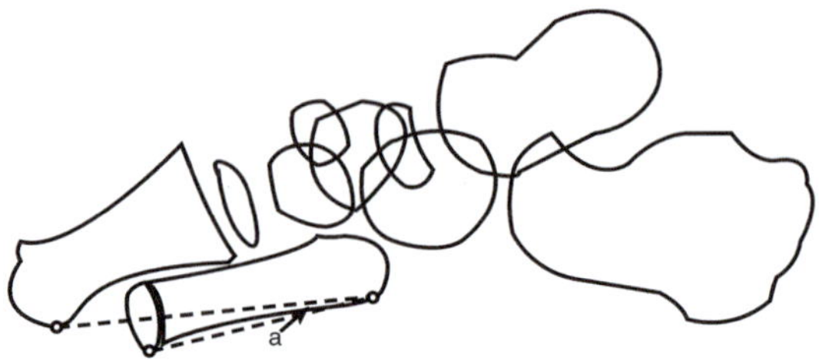

Fig. 2.32 Metatarsal stacking angle (a)

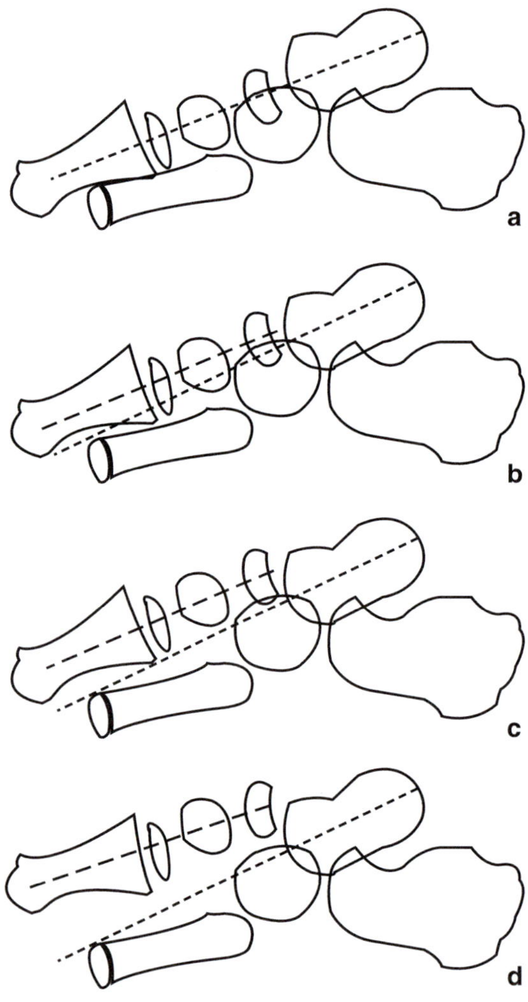

Fig. 2.31 Navicular position, lateral view. (**a**) Grade 0 (normal). (**b**) +1 grade. (**c**) +2 grade. (**d**) +3 grade. The grading can be based on the navicular bone, if visible, or the first metatarsal axis, if not visible

between the severity of a severe varus or valgus deformity. Davids et al. [62] reported an average 47 ± 14% (ranging between 22 and 85%). Xu et al. [77] reported an average of 40 ± 20% with a range between −8 and 103% (mean age, 10 years; range, 8–16 years).

Navicular Position (Fig. 2.31)

The center of the talar head should normally align with the center of the navicular. Simons [83] also described a grading scale for the position of the navicular bone relative to the talar axis in the lateral view. Normal is grade 0. If the navicular is displaced superiorly 1/3 of its height, grade + 1 is applied, +2 for 2/3, and + 3 for 100% displacement (dislocation) superiorly. If the navicular is not yet ossified, then the first metatarsal axis is compared to the position of the talar axis in a similar fashion.

Metatarsal Stacking Angle (Fig. 2.32)

The axes used to determine the metatarsal stacking angle are made as follows: points are plotted at the inferior aspects of the first and the fifth metatarsal heads and at the inferior aspect of the fifth metatarsal base; the metatarsal head points are each connected to the fifth metatarsal base point to form two lines. The angle is used to describe forefoot alignment. Davids [62] reported an average of 8 ± 3° with a range between 1° and 13° (mean age 10 years, range 5–17 years). Xu et al. [77] reported an average of 1 ± 8° with a range between −30° and 25° (mean age, 10 years; range, 8–16 years).

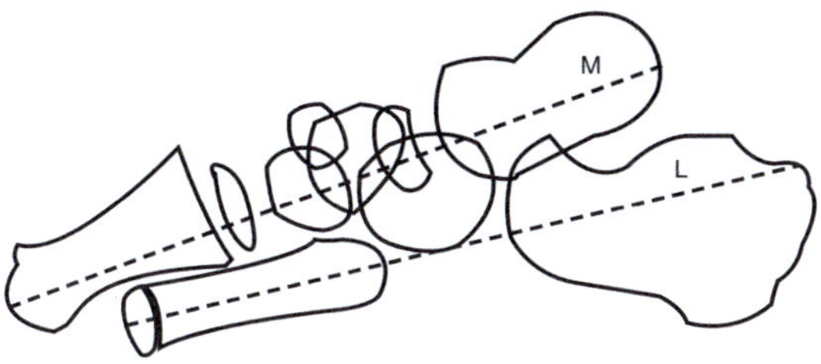

Fig. 2.33 Medial-lateral column ratio. The medial column (M) length in this example is 4.45 inches, and the lateral column (L) length is 4.42 inches. The ratio is, therefore, 4.45/4.42 = 1.01

Medial-Lateral Column Ratio (Fig. 2.33)

The medial–lateral column ratio describes the relative lengths of the medial and lateral columns. The medial column line is formed between two points marked at the anterior end of the first metatarsal and the posterior-inferior edge of the talar dome. The lateral column line is formed between two points marked at the anterior end of the fifth metatarsal head and the posterior-superior corner of the calcaneal bursal projection [62]. The ratio is the length of the medial column line divided by the lateral column line. Davids [62] reported an average ratio of 0.9 ± 0.1, with a range between 0.8 and 1.1 (mean age 10 years, range 5–17 years). Xu reported an average ratio of 1.0 ± 0.1, with a range between 0.9 and 1.2 (mean age, 10 years; range, 8–16 years).

Other

The metatarsals normally overlap distally; it should be difficult to trace out metatarsals two through four. The metatarsals should not appear ladder-like [10, 40].

Hindfoot Alignment Views

Hindfoot Alignment Angle (Fig. 2.34)

The tibial shaft axis and the calcaneal axis are used to form the hindfoot alignment angle. The normal angle is between 0° and 5° valgus; any amount of hindfoot varus is considered abnormal [93].

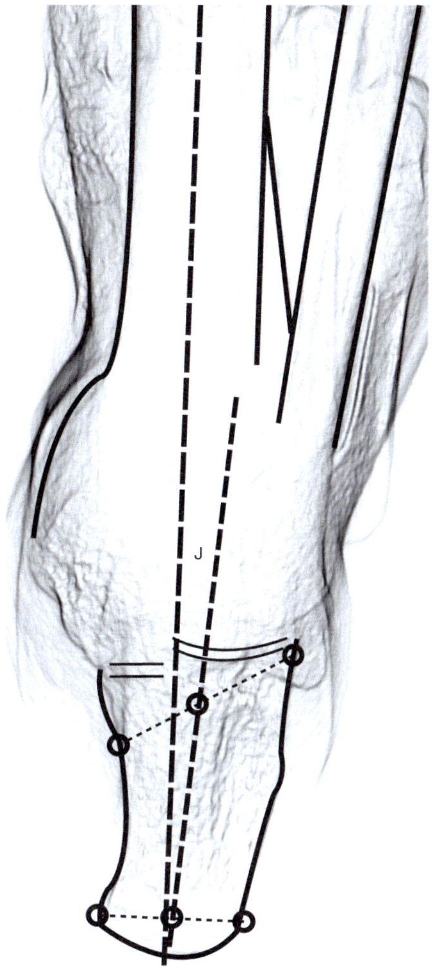

Fig. 2.34 Hindfoot alignment angle. This angle (J) is formed between the tibial and calcaneal axes

Coronal Plane Tibiocalcaneal Displacement (Fig. 2.35)

Saltzman and El-Khoury [94] modified a measurement technique used by Cobey and Sella [66] to quantify heel valgus. They measured the perpendicular distance between the tibial axis and the most inferior point of the calcaneus (i.e., the “apparent moment arm” or tibial/calcaneal displacement). If the tibial axis was medial to the inferior calcaneal point, a positive value was

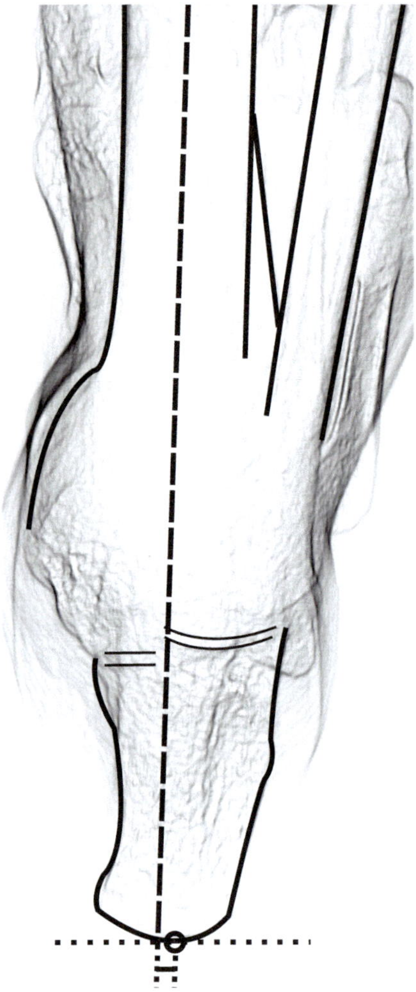

Fig. 2.35 Coronal plane tibiocalcaneal displacement. It is the distance (horizontally) between the tibial axis (dashed line) and the most inferior aspect of the calcaneal tuberosity (o)

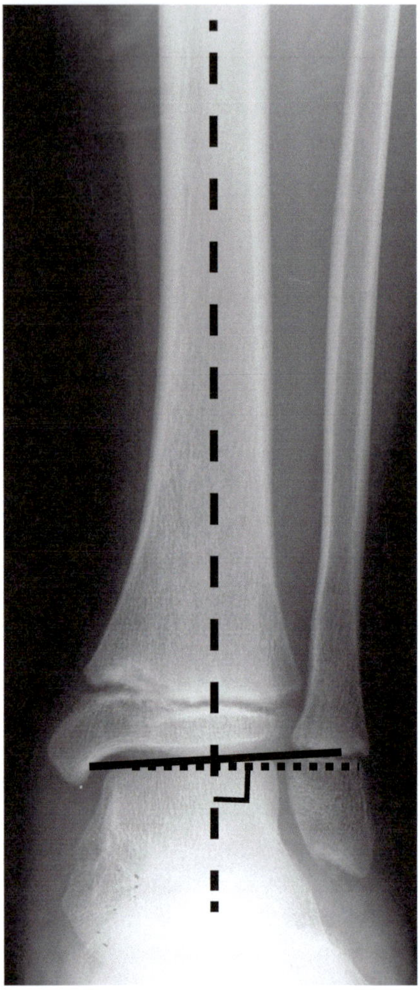

Fig. 2.36 Tibiotalar angle. The angle is formed between the talar dome superior surface (solid line) and a perpendicular to the tibial axis (dotted line; dashed line is the tibial axis). In this instance, since the talus is in valgus relative to the tibia, the resultant measurement will be a positive value

assigned; if the tibial axis was lateral, a negative value was used. With the foot pointing straight ahead, the mean apparent moment arm length was −3.2 mm. With the foot in its natural position (angle and base of gait), the mean apparent moment arm length was −1.6 mm.

Ankle AP View

There may be slight valgus angulation of the distal tibial articular surface relative to the tibial shaft axis at birth and in young children [95]. It should approach a 90-degree angulation by 10 years of age [10], though a slight varus position may be seen at maturity [95].

Tibiotalar Angle (Fig. 2.36)

The tibiotalar angle is formed between a line along the superior aspect of the talar dome and a perpendicular to the tibial axis [62]. Davids et al. [62] used this angle to assess hindfoot alignment and, in children between 5 and 17 years of age, reported an average of 1 ± 4° in children between the ages of 5 and 17 years. The range was between −9° and 12°; a negative value is assigned to a varus attitude of the talus relative to the tibia; a positive value is valgus. Beals and Skyhar [96] reported an average of 90 (or, 0) degrees at 1 year of age, which increased to about 8° (valgus) at 12 years of age, ranging between −6 and 14°. Xu et al. [77] reported an average of $-6 \pm 6°$, with a range between −20° and 8° (mean age, 10 years; range, 8–16 years).

References

1. Oestreich AE, Crawford AH. Atlas of pediatric orthopedic radiology. Stuttgart/New York: Thieme; 1985.
2. Hubbard AM, Meyer JS, Davidson RS, Mahboubi S, Harty MP. Relationship between the ossification center and cartilaginous anlage in the normal hindfoot in children: study with MR imaging. AJR Am J Roentgenol. 1993;161(4):849–53.
3. Dorland's illustrated medical dictionary. 31st ed. Philadelphia: Saunders; 2007.
4. Kumar R, Madewell JE, Swischuk LE. The normal and abnormal growth plate. Radiol Clin North Am. 1987;25(6):1133–53.
5. Garn SM, Rohmann CG, Silverman FN. Radiographic standards for postnatal ossification and tooth calcification. Med Radiogr Photogr. 1967;43(2):45–66.
6. Acheson R. Maturation of the skeleton. In: Falkner F, editor. Human development. Philadelphia: Saunders; 1966.
7. Sarrafian S, Kelikian A. Development of the foot and ankle. In: Kelikian A, editor. Sarrafian's anatomy of the foot and ankle. 3rd ed. Philadelphia: Lippincott Williams & Wilkins; 2011.
8. Christman RA, Truong J. Normal development. In: Christman RA, editor. Foot and ankle radiology. 2nd ed. Philadelphia: Wolters Kluwer Health; 2015.
9. Whitaker JM, Rousseau L, Williams T, Rowan RA, Hartwig WC. Scoring system for estimating age in the foot skeleton. Am J Phys Anthropol. 2002;118(4):385–92.
10. Hammer M, Pai D. The foot and ankle: congenital and developmental conditions. In: Stein-Wexler R, editor. Pediatric orthopedic imaging. Berlin: Springer; 2015.
11. Waldt S, Woertler K. Skeletal age. Measurements and classifications in musculoskeletal radiology. New York: Thieme; 2014.
12. Erasmie U, Ringertz H. A method for assessment of skeletal maturity in children below one year of age. Pediatr Radiol. 1980;9(4):225–8.
13. Hernandez M, Sanchez E, Sobradillo B, Rincon JM, Narvaiza JL. A new method for assessment of skeletal maturity in the first 2 years of life. Pediatr Radiol. 1988;18(6):484–9.
14. Hoerr NL, Pyle SI, Francis CC. Radiographic atlas of skeletal development of the foot and ankle. CC Thomas: Springfield; 1962.
15. Ozonoff M. The foot. Pediatric orthopedic radiology. 2nd ed. Philadelphia: WB Saunders; 1992. p. 397–460.
16. Gray's anatomy. The anatomical basis of clinical practice. 39th ed. London: Elsevier; 2005.
17. Garn SM, Rohmann CG, Blumenthal T. Ossification sequence polymorphism and sexual dimorphism in skeletal development. Am J Phys Anthropol. 1966;24(1):101–15.
18. Chung T, Jaramillo D. Normal maturing distal tibia and fibula: changes with age at MR imaging. Radiology. 1995;194(1):227–32.
19. Love SM, Ganey T, Ogden JA. Postnatal epiphyseal development: the distal tibia and fibula. J Pediatr Orthop. 1990;10(3):298–305.
20. Ogden JA, McCarthy SM. Radiology of postnatal skeletal development. VIII. Distal tibia and fibula. Skeletal Radiol. 1983;10(4):209–20.
21. Kump WL. Vertical fractures of the distal tibial epiphysis. Am J Roentgenol Radium Ther Nucl Med. 1966;97(3):676–81.
22. Ecklund K, Jaramillo D. Imaging of growth disturbance in children. Radiol Clin North Am. 2001;39(4):823–41.
23. Keats TE, Anderson MW. Atlas of normal roentgen variants that may simulate disease. 9th ed. Philadelphia: Saunders; 2013.
24. Lyritis G. Developmental disorders of the proximal epiphysis of the hallux. Skeletal Radiol. 1983;10(4):250–4.
25. Johnson JM, Higgins TJ, Lemos D. Appearance of the delta phalanx (longitudinally bracketed epiphysis) with MR imaging. Pediatr Radiol. 2011;41(3):394–6.
26. Yucel A, Kuru I, Bozan ME, Acar M, Solak M. Radiographic evaluation and unusual bone formations in different genetic patterns in synpolydactyly. Skeletal Radiol. 2005;34(8):468–76.
27. Calif E, Stahl S. Complex bilateral polysyndactyly featuring a triplet of delta phalanges in a syndactylised digit. Eur Radiol. 2002;12 Suppl 3:S140–2.
28. Ogden JA, Ganey TM, Light TR, Belsole RJ, Greene TL. Ossification and pseudoepiphysis formation in the "nonepiphyseal" end of bones of the hands and feet. Skeletal Radiol. 1994;23(1):3–13.
29. Ogden JA, Ganey TM, Light TR, Greene TL, Belsole RJ. Nonepiphyseal ossification and pseudoepiphysis formation. J Pediatr Orthop. 1994;14(1):78–82.
30. Laor T, Clarke JP, Yin H. Development of the long bones in the hands and feet of children: radiographic and MR imaging correlation. Pediatr Radiol. 2016;46(4):551–61.
31. Oestreich AE. Radiology. In: Drennan JC, editor. The child's foot and ankle. New York: Raven Press; 1992.
32. Scharfbillig RW, Jones S, Scutter SD. Sever's disease: what does the literature really tell us? J Am Podiatr Med Assoc. 2008;98(3):212–23.
33. Canale ST, Williams KD. Iselin's disease. J Pediatr Orthop. 1992;12(1):90–3.

34. Gillespie H. Osteochondroses and apophyseal injuries of the foot in the young athlete. Curr Sports Med Rep. 2010;9(5):265–8.
35. Schwartz B, Jay RM, Schoenhaus HD. Apophysitis of the fifth metatarsal base. Iselin's disease. J Am Podiatr Med Assoc. 1991;81(3):128–30.
36. Christman RA. Normal variants and anomalies. In: Christman RA, editor. Foot and ankle radiology. 2nd ed. Philadelphia: Wolters Kluwer Health; 2015.
37. Freyschmidt J, Wiens J, Brossman J, Sternberg A. Freyschmidt's "Koehler/Zimmer" borderlands of the normal and early pathological findings in skeletal radiography. 5th revised ed. New York: Thieme; 2003.
38. Radiation protection in paediatric radiology. Vienna: IAEA International Atomic Energy Agency; 2012.
39. Katz MA, Davidson RS, Chan PSH, Sullivan RJ. Plain radiographic evaluation of the pediatric foot and its deformities. Uni Pa Orthop J. 1997;10(Spring):30–9.
40. Grissom L. Imaging of the normal foot. In: McCarthy JJ, Drennan JC, editors. Drennan's the child's foot & ankle. 2nd ed. Philadelphia: Lippincott Williams & Wilkins; 2010.
41. Don S, Slovis TL. Musculoskeletal imaging strategies and controlling radiation esposure. In: Stein-Wexler R, Wooten-Gorges SL, Ozonoff MB, editors. Pediatric orthopedic imaging. New York: Springer; 2015.
42. Staheli LT. Foot. Fundamentals of pediatric orthopedics. 5th ed. Philadelphia: Lippincott Williams & Wilkins; 2016.
43. Thapa MM, Pruthi S, Chew FS. Radiographic assessment of pediatric foot alignment: review. AJR Am J Roentgenol. 2010;194(6 Suppl):S51–8.
44. Radler C, Egermann M, Riedl K, Ganger R, Grill F. Interobserver reliability of radiographic measurements of contralateral feet of pediatric patients with unilateral clubfoot. J Bone Joint Surg Am. 2010;92(14):2427–35.
45. Baron RL, Strugielski CF, Christman RA. Positioning techniques and terminology. In: Christman RA, editor. Foot and ankle radiology. 2nd ed. Philadelphia: Wolters Kluwer Health; 2015.
46. Simons GW. A standardized method for the radiographic evaluation of clubfeet. Clin Orthop Relat Res. 1978;135:107–18.
47. Templeton AW, McAlister WH, Zim ID. Standardization of terminology and evaluation of osseous relationships in congenitally abnormal feet. Am J Roentgenol Radium Ther Nucl Med. 1965;93:374–81.
48. Kite JH. Principles involved in the treatment of congenital clubfoot. JBJS. 1939;21:595–606.
49. Long WL, Rollins JH, Smith BJ. Merrill's atlas of radiographic positioning & procedures. 13th ed. St. Louis: Mosby; 2016.
50. Thompson GH, Simons GW. Congenital talipes equinovarus (clubfeet) and metatarsus adductus. In: Drennan JC, editor. The child's foot and ankle. New York: Raven Press; 1992.
51. Harris RI, Beath T. Etiology of peroneal spastic flat foot. J Bone Joint Surg Br. 1948;30B(4):624–34.
52. Melamed EA. Intoeing Harris view for accessory navicular visualization and hindfoot alignment: technique tip. Foot Ankle Int. 2010;31(12):1122–4.
53. Reilingh ML, Beimers L, Tuijthof GJ, Stufkens SA, Maas M, van Dijk CN. Measuring hindfoot alignment radiographically: the long axial view is more reliable than the hindfoot alignment view. Skeletal Radiol. 2010;39(11):1103–8.
54. Cobey JC. Posterior roentgenogram of the foot. Clin Orthop Relat Res. 1976;118:202–7.
55. Mendicino RW, Catanzariti AR, John S, Child B, Lamm BM. Long leg calcaneal axial and hindfoot alignment radiographic views for frontal plane assessment. J Am Podiatr Med Assoc. 2008;98(1):75–8.
56. Buck P, Morrey BF, Chao EY. The optimum position of arthrodesis of the ankle. A gait study of the knee and ankle. J Bone Joint Surg Am. 1987;69(7):1052–62.
57. Johnson JE, Lamdan R, Granberry WF, Harris GF, Carrera GF. Hindfoot coronal alignment: a modified radiographic method. Foot Ankle Int. 1999;20(12):818–25.
58. Kleiger B, Mankin HJ. A roentgenographic study of the development of the calcaneus by means of the posterior tangential view. JBJS. 1961;43-A(7):961–9.
59. Kandel B. The suroplantar projection in the congenital club foot of the infant; its clinical and radiological significance. Acta Orthop Scand. 1952;22(2):161–73.
60. Oestreich AE. How to measure angles from foot radiographs: a primer. New York: Springer; 1990.
61. Ozonoff M. The foot. Pediatric orthopedic radiology. 1st ed. Philadelphia: WB Saunders Company; 1979.
62. Davids JR, Gibson TW, Pugh LI. Quantitative segmental analysis of weight-bearing radiographs of the foot and ankle for children: normal alignment. J Pediatr Orthop. 2005;25(6):769–76.
63. Howard CB, Benson MK. The ossific nuclei and the cartilage anlage of the talus and calcaneum. J Bone Joint Surg Br. 1992;74(4):620–3.
64. Bleck EE, Minaire P. Persistent medial deviation of the neck of the talus: a common cause of in-toeing in children. J Pediatr Orthop. 1983;3(2):149–59.
65. Sensiba PR, Coffey MJ, Williams NE, Mariscalco M, Laughlin RT. Inter- and intraobserver reliability in the radiographic evaluation of adult flatfoot deformity. Foot Ankle Int. 2010;31(2):141–5.
66. Cobey JC, Sella E. Standardizing methods of measurement of foot shape by including the effects of subtalar rotation. Foot Ankle. 1981;2(1):30–6.
67. Donovan A, Rosenberg ZS. Extraarticular lateral hindfoot impingement with posterior tibial tendon tear: MRI correlation. AJR Am J Roentgenol. 2009;193(3):672–8.
68. Robinson I, Dyson R, Halson-Brown S. Reliability of clinical and radiographic measurement of rearfoot alignment in a patient population. Foot. 2001;11:2–9.
69. Buck FM, Hoffmann A, Mamisch-Saupe N, Espinosa N, Resnick D, Hodler J. Hindfoot alignment measurements: rotation-stability of measurement techniques on hindfoot alignment view and long axial view radiographs. AJR Am J Roentgenol. 2011;197(3):578–82.

70. Lee KM, Chung CY, Park MS, Lee SH, Cho JH, Choi IH. Reliability and validity of radiographic measurements in hindfoot varus and valgus. J Bone Joint Surg Am. 2010;92(13):2319–27.
71. Benedetti MG, Berti L, Straudi S, Ceccarelli F, Giannini S. Clinicoradiographic assessment of flexible flatfoot in children. J Am Podiatr Med Assoc. 2010;100(6):463–71.
72. Dobbs MB, Beaty JH. Congenital foot deformities. In: Coughlin MJ, Saltzman CL, Anderson RB, editors. Mann's surgery of the foot and ankle. 2. 9th ed. Philadelphia: Saunders; 2014.
73. Beatson TR, Pearson JR. A method of assessing correction in club feet. J Bone Joint Surg Br. 1966;48(1):40–50.
74. Vanderwilde R, Staheli LT, Chew DE, Malagon V. Measurements on radiographs of the foot in normal infants and children. J Bone Joint Surg Am. 1988;70(3):407–15.
75. Simons GW. Analytical radiography of club feet. J Bone Joint Surg Br. 1977;59-B(4):485–9.
76. Somppi E. Clubfoot. Review of the literature and an analysis of a series of 135 treated clubfeet. Acta Orthop Scand Suppl. 1984;209:1–109.
77. Xu J, Park KW, Kang QL, Jung YJ, Song HR. How reliable are standard radiographic measures of the foot and ankle in children with achondroplasia? Clin Orthop Relat Res. 2013;471(9):3021–8.
78. La Reaux RL, Lee BR. Metatarsus adductus and hallux abducto valgus: their correlation. J Foot Surg. 1987;26(4):304–8.
79. Engel E, Erlick N, Krems I. A simplified metatarsus adductus angle. J Am Podiatry Assoc. 1983;73(12):620–8.
80. Crawford M, Green D. Metatarsus adductus: radiographic and pathomechanical analysis. Update 2014 – the proceedings of the annual meeting of the Podiatry Institute. Tucker: The Podiatry Institute, Inc.; 2014.
81. French S, Niespodziany J, Wysong D, Zahari D. A radiographic study of infant metatarsus adductus treatment by serial casting. J Foot Surg. 1985;24(3):222–9.
82. Ganley JV, Ganley TJ. Metatarsus adductus deformity. In: McGlamry ED, editor. Comprehensive textbook of foot surgery. 2nd ed. Baltimore: Lippincott Williams & Wilkins; 1992.
83. Simons GW. Complete subtalar release in club feet. Part II--comparison with less extensive procedures. J Bone Joint Surg Am. 1985;67(7):1056–65.
84. Westberry DE, Davids JR, Roush TF, Pugh LI. Qualitative versus quantitative radiographic analysis of foot deformities in children with hemiplegic cerebral palsy. J Pediatr Orthop. 2008;28(3):359–65.
85. LeNoir JL. Congenital idiopathic talipes. Charles C. Thomas: Springfield; 1966.
86. Simons GW. Calcaneocuboid joint deformity in talipes equinovarus: an overview and update. J Pediatr Orthop B. 1995;4(1):25–35.
87. Hardy RH, Clapham JC. Hallux valgus; predisposing anatomical causes. Lancet. 1952;1(6720):1180–3.
88. Hardy RH, Clapham JC. Observations on hallux valgus; based on a controlled series. J Bone Joint Surg Br. 1951;33-B(3):376–91.
89. Piggott H. The natural history of hallux valgus in adolescence and early adult life. J Bone Joint Surg Br. 1960;42(4):749–60.
90. McCluney JG, Tinley P. Radiographic measurements of patients with juvenile hallux valgus compared with age-matched controls: a cohort investigation. J Foot Ankle Surg. 2006;45(3):161–7.
91. Lowery NJ, Wukich DK. Adolescent hallux valgus: evaluation and treatment. Oper Tech Orthop. 2009;19:52–7.
92. Heywood AW. The mechanics of the hind foot in club foot as demonstrated radiographically. J Bone Joint Surg Br. 1964;46:102–7.
93. Coughlin MJ, Mann RA, Saltzman CL. Surgery of the foot and ankle. 8th ed. Philadelphia: Mosby; 2007.
94. Saltzman CL, el-Khoury GY. The hindfoot alignment view. Foot Ankle Int. 1995;16(9):572–6.
95. Nakai T, Takakura Y, Tanaka Y, Sugimoto K, Tamai S, Kurumatani N. Morphologic changes of the ankle in children as assessed by radiography and arthrography. J Orthop Sci. 2000;5(2):134–8.
96. Beals RK, Skyhar M. Growth and development of the tibia, fibula, and ankle joint. Clin Orthop Relat Res. 1984;182:289–92.

3 Neurological Abnormalities of the Pediatric Foot and Ankle

Byron L. Hutchinson

Cerebral Palsy

Cerebral palsy represents the largest group of neuromuscular disorders in the United States. The incidence is 2 per 10,000 live births in the United States [1]. There are approximately 25,000 new cases per year with an economic burden of $921,000.00 per person [2]. Appropriate diagnosis and management of these individuals utilizing the best evidence available is necessary for the foot and ankle surgeon to help contain these costs and be most efficient with the treatment recommendations that are made.

Cerebral palsy is defined as a disorder of posture and movement caused by a non-progressive defect or lesion in the immature brain. Although the condition is considered "non-progressive" from a lesion standpoint, it clearly is clinically progressive from a functional standpoint.

Classic etiology can be broken down into three phases, prenatal, natal, and postnatal (Table 3.1).

The most common prenatal etiologies are erythroblastosis fetalis and fetal anoxia. Premature birth is the most common natal cause, and in the postnatal phase, encephalitis and meningitis are most common. Preterm infants are particularly vulnerable, and delivery prior to 32 weeks of gestation is associated with 33% of cases of cerebral palsy [2]. Magnesium sulfate given prior to delivery has been shown to reduce the risk of preterm infants developing cerebral palsy [3]. In more recent years, MRI has been used to give more specific information about the diagnosis of cerebral palsy [4]. Bax et al. in 2006 demonstrated with MRI that 43% of white matter damage occurred with prematurity and 20% of the cerebral damage was due to obstetric mishap [5].

The clinical evaluation of patients with cerebral palsy involves the understanding of how the condition affects the various extremities involved and the individual as a whole. For example, highly functional patients with CP will improve with surgical intervention where patients with learning disabilities and severe types of CP will need more palliative forms of surgical intervention to improve their quality of life.

There are specific types of cerebral palsy and each has a unique clinical presentation [6]. The most common form is spastic which affects about 65% of patients with this condition. This type is primarily associated with a cerebral lesion and responds extremely well to various types of medical and surgical management. The most common presentation is spastic diplegia or monoplegia (Figs. 3.1 and 3.2).

In rare circumstances patients may present with spastic quadriplegia. The dyskinetic type (athetoid) involves about 25% of cases and is typically confined to the midbrain. Many of these

B. L. Hutchinson (✉)
Franciscan Medical Group: CHIFranciscan Foot & Ankle Associates: Highline Clinic, Seattle, WA, USA
e-mail: byronhutchinson@CHIFranciscan.org

M. L. Butterworth, J. T. Marcoux (eds.), *The Pediatric Foot and Ankle*,
https://doi.org/10.1007/978-3-030-29788-6_3

Table 3.1 Etiology

Prenatal	Natal	Postnatal
Congenital brain defects	Premature birth	Encephalitis
Rubella or viral infections	Asphyxia, trauma Anesthetic complications/over-sedation	Meningitis
Erythroblastosis fetalis, fetal anoxia		Trauma, asphyxia

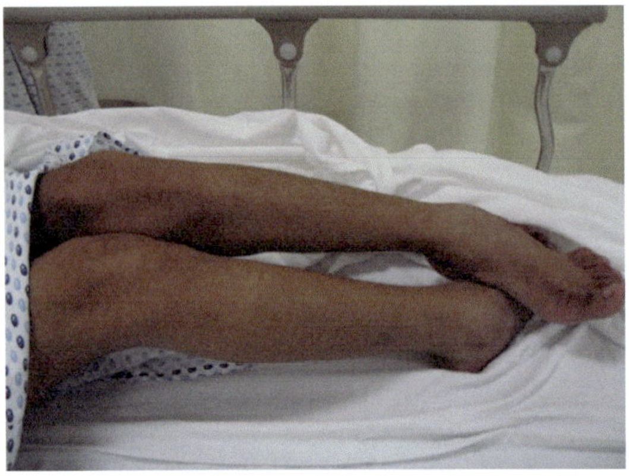

Fig. 3.1 This patient has spastic diplegia. Note the contractures in both lower extremities. There is an equinovarus contracture in the feet and ankles along with contracture of the patient's medial hamstrings

patients have extreme functional disabilities and are often wheelchair or bed bound. Ataxic cerebral palsy represents about 8% of cases and involves the cerebellum. They have difficulty with coordinated movement and often have difficulty ambulating without some form of assistance. The least common form representing 2% of cases is the mixed type. This type has a widespread and variable presentation.

Motor development is another important aspect of cerebral palsy. Early motor developmental reflexes are gone by the time a child is 4–5 years of age. Posturing and asymmetric tonic reflexes can still be present in patients with cerebral palsy (Fig. 3.3). Since there can be a significant delay in motor development in some patients, it is important to consider this when contemplating surgical intervention because the surgical procedure might take much longer for the patient to recover when there has been delayed motor development.

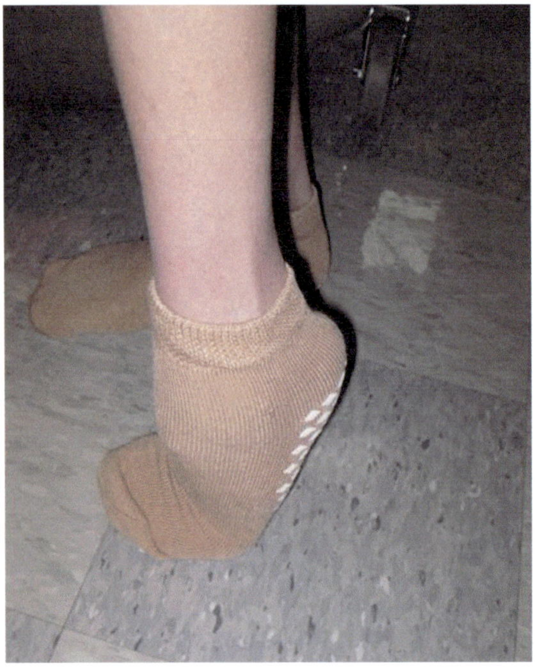

Fig. 3.2 This patient's presentation is spastic monoplegia in the left lower extremity. Note that he has an equinovarus deformity just like Fig. 3.1 but he is clearly more functional

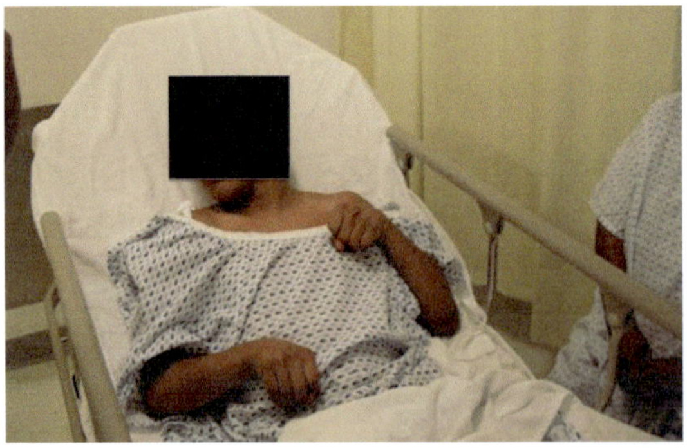

Fig. 3.3 This 9-year-old boy still displays asymmetric tonic reflexes. Note the extension in the left arm toward the chin and flexion of the opposite arm

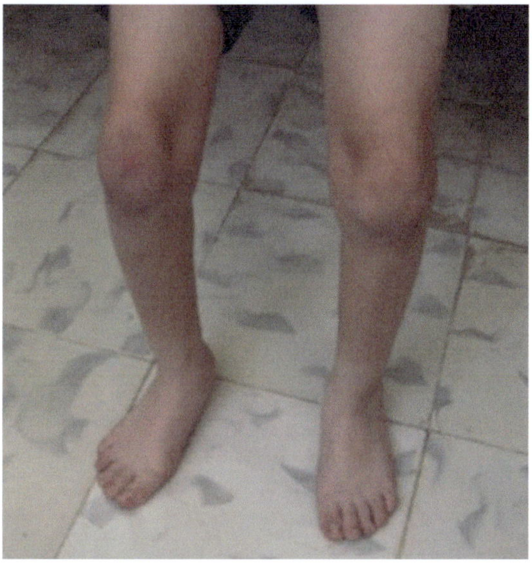

Fig. 3.4 This patient had a TAL procedure bilaterally and developed a crouch gait because of the contractures that are still present with his hamstrings and rectus femoris muscles

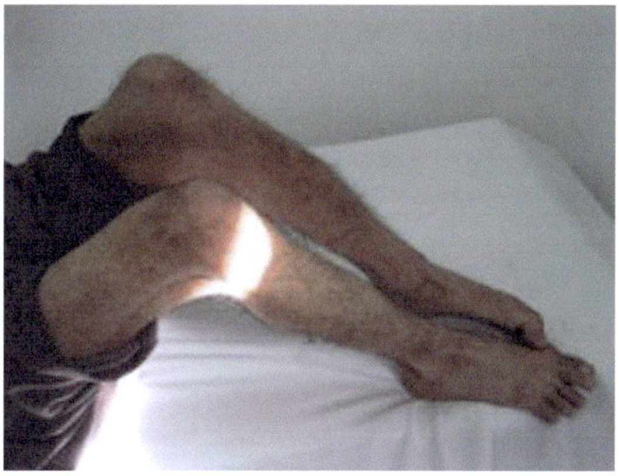

Fig. 3.5 This patient has arthrogryposis and cerebral palsy. Soft tissue procedures in isolation will not help this individual's contractures at the knee

Compensation at all levels must be taken into consideration when evaluating patients with cerebral palsy. Specific lower extremity spasticity can drive and/or mask various modes of compensation, and if one is not aware of this, then surgical management can be less than optimum. Trunk leaning and lordosis are common mechanisms of compensation. The vast majority of patients have equinus, but this might compensate through genu recurvatum as opposed to a lack of dorsiflexion or both. If the surgeon is not aware of this compensation, the surgical plan might place the patient in a postsurgical "Crouch gait" which might be more difficult for the patient to overcome (Fig. 3.4).

The presence of deformity is also extremely important to determine in patients with cerebral palsy. Often, there can be associated conditions such as arthrogryposis or other congenital abnormalities that can impact management decisions (Fig. 3.5). Joint contractures can be supple and due to spasticity, or there might be a rigid contracture of the joint. Certainly, if there are rigid deformities, then conservative management may fail, and if soft tissue procedures are performed in isolation in these circumstances, outcomes will be compromised.

Some patients with cerebral palsy can have learning disabilities and some degree of mental retardation [7]. Seizures occur in a third of patients that have cerebral palsy. Auditory and visual problems can occur as well [8]. Children with learning disabilities may take a long time to learn to ambulate with their particular type of spasticity, and surgery can clearly impact their ability to "learn to ambulate" again after surgery. A strong support network is important for cerebral palsy patients in general but is critically necessary when the patient is suffering any form of mental defect.

Clinical variation in the spastic muscles involved can occur and needs to be evaluated. Patients can present with spastic equinus alone or in combination with tight hamstrings, adductors, or hip flexors (Fig. 3.6). Clinical presentations will vary depending on this involvement, and one might see "toe walking" or scissoring of the gait together or in isolation (Figs. 3.7 and 3.8).

Rotational deformities can also occur in patients with cerebral palsy. One might assume that the adductors are tight when in fact the patient has internal femoral torsion. Torsional evaluation should be routine in these patients and should include hip, knee, and leg evaluations (Fig. 3.9).

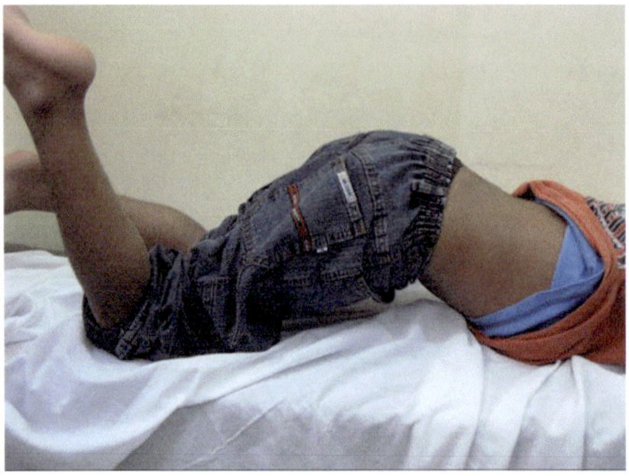

Fig. 3.6 This picture is demonstrating Elly's test which shows contracture of the hip flexors. With the individual prone, the examiner flexes the knee resulting in the hip elevating off of the exam table indicating that the hip flexors are contracted. Normally, with the knee flexed, the hip should stay on the table

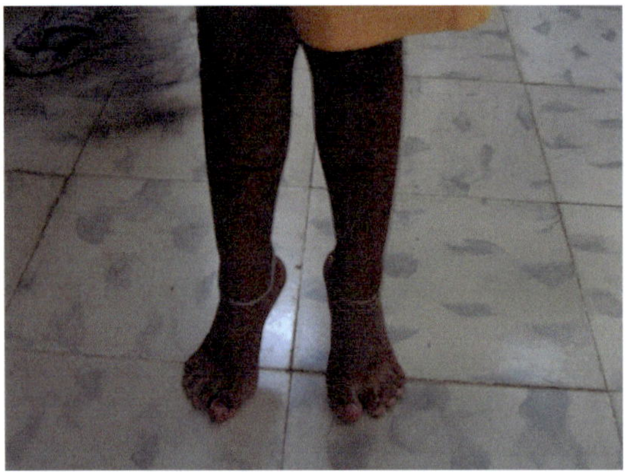

Fig. 3.7 Classic presentation of toe walking with CP

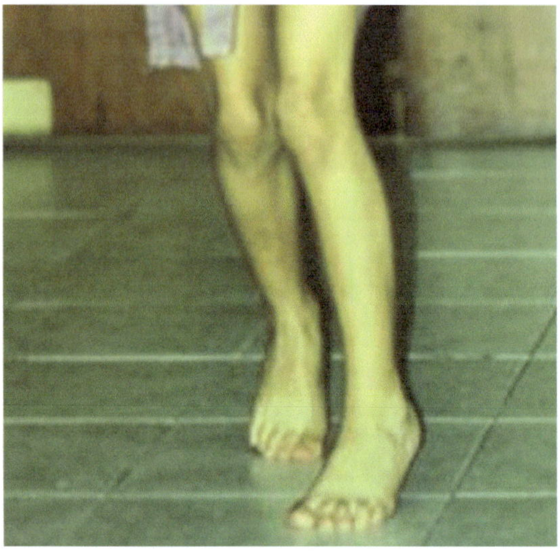

Fig. 3.8 This patient not only is toe walking but one can see the internal position of the knee indicating a scissoring of the gait as well

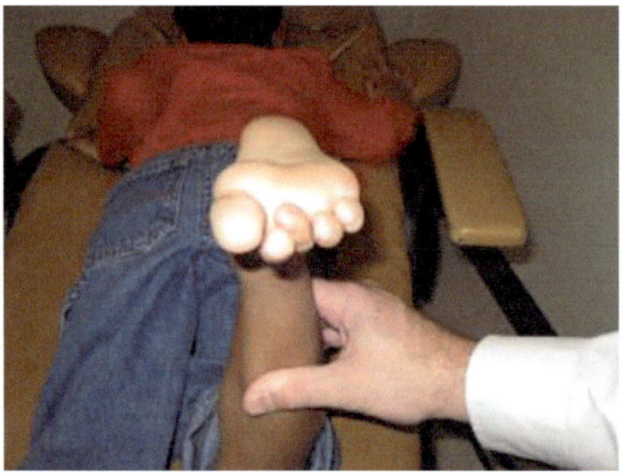

Fig. 3.9 Staheli's foot thigh axis test for torsional deformities of the tibia. This is a normal test with no external rotation of the foot relative to the thigh

Conservative treatment for cerebral palsy centers around physical therapy and the prevention of significant joint contractures. Bracing is the mainstay for maintaining limbs after contractures have been reduced. Reduction of contractures is usually accomplished using botox injections in the vast majority of patients [9]. Chemical neurolysis has been popular in the past but is much more labor intensive and has been replaced by botox in most clinical situations [10]. Palisano et al. in 1997 developed the Gross Motor Function Classification System which helps in determining what treatment modalities will be effective in patients with cerebral palsy [11] (Table 3.2).

The system provides simple, universal language to describe physical function in cerebral palsy. The classification is valid, reliable, and very useful to help guide physicians in recommending conservative modalities vs. surgical procedures.

Surgical intervention occurs in patients from 6 to 12 years of age. Soft tissue releases are the most effective and popular procedures to improve function. With contractures present around the hip, an adductor release is performed (Fig. 3.10). For contracture around the knee, a hamstring

Table 3.2 Gross Motor Function Classification System (GMFCS) from Palisano et al. (1997)

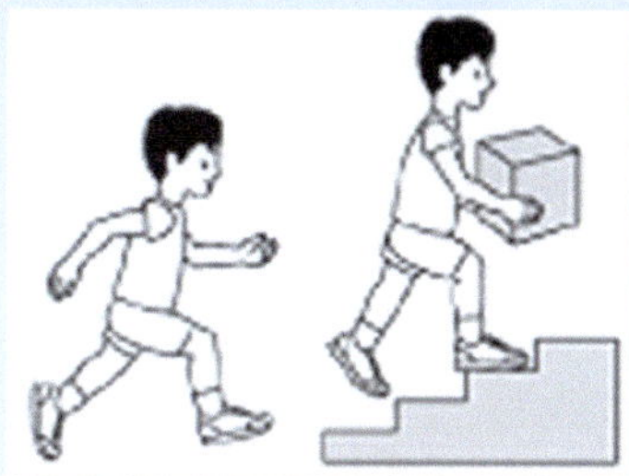	**GMFCS Level I** Children walk indoors and outdoors and climb stairs without limitation. Children perform gross motor skills including running and jumping, but speed, balance, and coordination are impaired
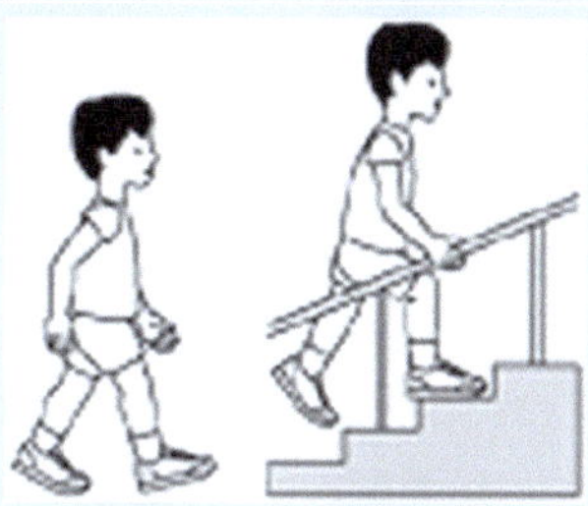	**GMFCS Level II** Children walk indoors and outdoors and climb stairs holding onto a railing but experience limitations walking on uneven surfaces and inclines and walking in crowds or confined spaces
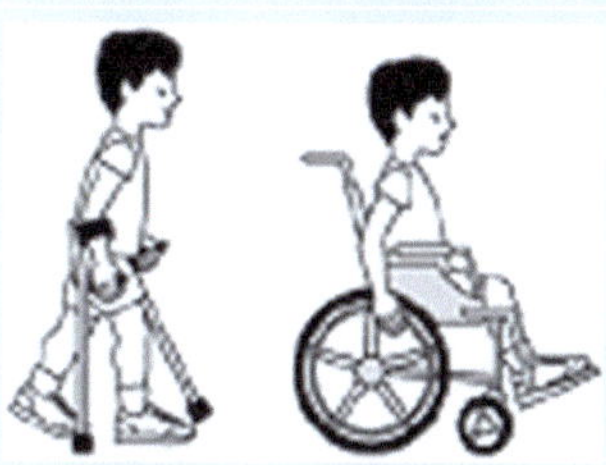	**GMFCS Level III** Children walk indoors or outdoors on a level surface with an assistive mobility device. Children may climb stairs holding onto a railing. Children may propel a wheelchair manually or are transported when traveling for long distances or outdoors on uneven terrain
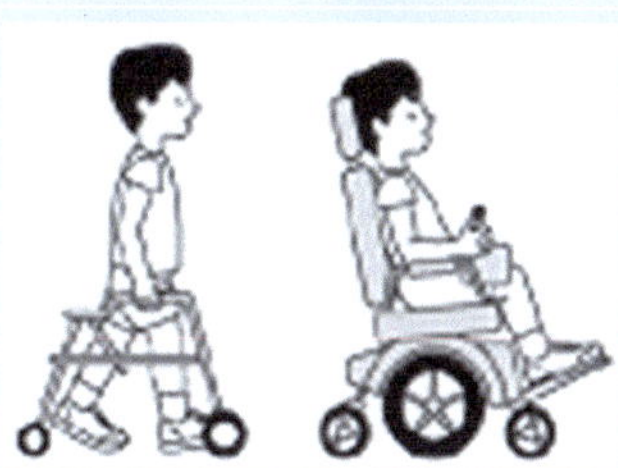	**GMFCS Level IV** Children may continue to walk for short distances on a walker or rely more on wheeled mobility at home and school and in the community
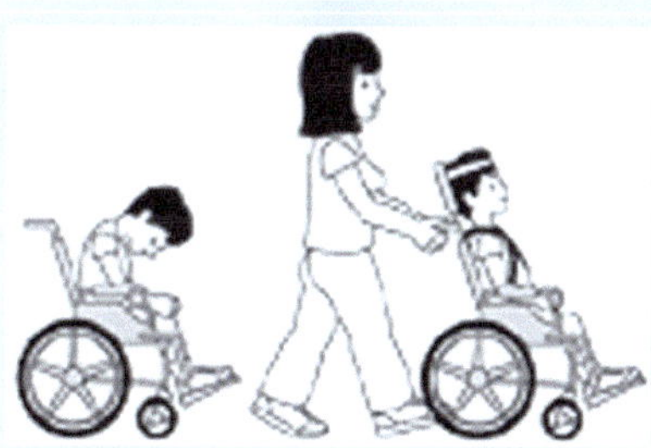	**GMFCS Level V** Physical impairment restricts voluntary control of movement and the ability to maintain antigravity head and trunk postures. All areas of motor function are limited. Children have no means of independent mobility and are transported

release is performed in conjunction with a tendo-Achilles lengthening (TAL) when indicated (Figs. 3.11 and 3.12). Because these contractures can recur, bracing post-operatively is paramount.

A very effective procedure in children is the Murphy-Perrot procedure [12]. The author has utilized this technique for about 15 years with extremely good success rates (Fig. 3.13). There is much less recurrence with this procedure over the traditional TAL, and past concerns about cosmetic appearance have not been seen by the author. In long-standing equinovarus cases, an anterior tibial tendon transfer or posterior tibial tendon transfer can be effective in reducing

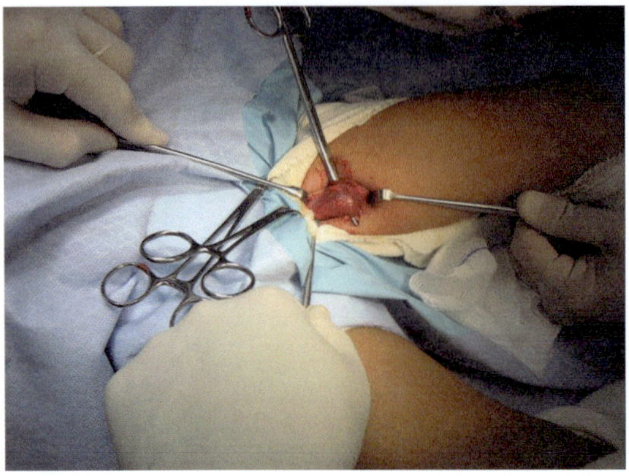

Fig. 3.10 An adductor release is being performed on this patient's left groin

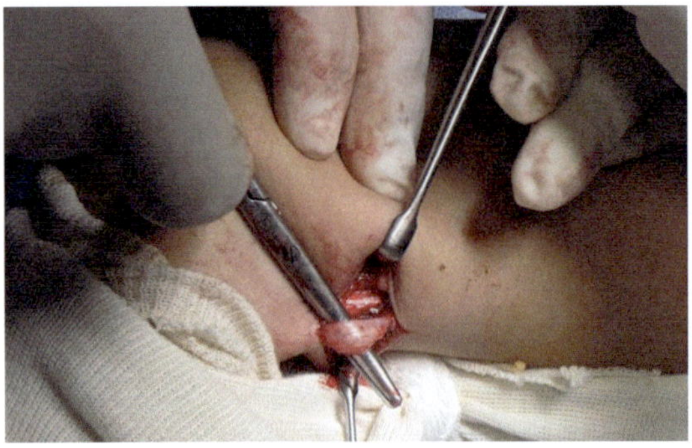

Fig. 3.11 This surgical photo is demonstrating a medial hamstring release being done just behind the knee

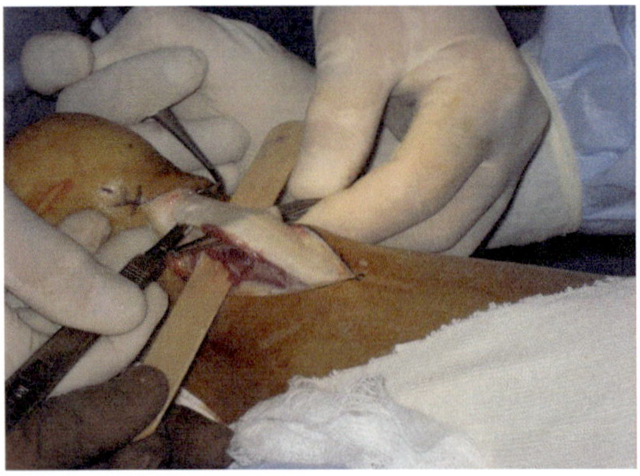

Fig. 3.12 This represents an open frontal plane TAL being performed

recurrence. In adolescence with rigid equinovarus deformities, the author has had great success with gradual correction with percutaneous tenotomies

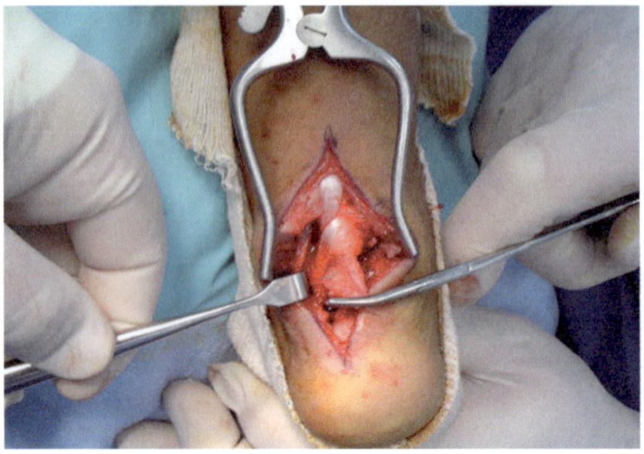

Fig. 3.13 Classic Murphy-Perrot procedure being shown here. Note the advancement of the tendo-Achilles under the FHL tendon

and circular fixation techniques first described by Ilizarov [13]. Lastly, some patients that have significant rigid deformities require arthrodesis procedures of the hindfoot and ankle [14].

Charcot-Marie-Tooth Disease

Charcot-Marie-Tooth (CMT) disease is a hereditary motor and sensory neuropathy characterized by progressive loss of muscle tissue across various parts of the body especially in the lower limbs. It is one of the most common inherited neurological disorders, affecting 1 in 2500 people in the United States [15]. The disease is credited to three physicians, Jean-Martin Charcot and Pierre Marie in Paris and Howard Henry Tooth in England who first identified its characteristics in 1886 [16, 17]. The condition has had numerous names associated with it that have caused confusion in the past. Dyck and Lambert used clinical and electrodiagnostic data to try to classify hereditary motor and sensory neuropathies into specific subtypes [18, 19]. Their work provided a major advance in the understanding of these disorders. More recently, genetic identification and testing for Charcot-Marie-Tooth disease have shed new light on the continuum of types and subtypes that have been characterized in this disease process [20–23].

CMT is caused by certain mutations in several genes that produce proteins involved in the structure and function of either the peripheral nerve axon or its myelin sheath. As a result, these nerves slowly degenerate and lose the ability to communicate with their distal targets. The degeneration of the motor components of the peripheral nerve results in muscle weakness and atrophy in the extremities, and in some cases, the sensory degeneration can result in significant sensory neuropathy.

The gene mutations in CMT disease are inherited as either an autosomal dominant or recessive trait and in certain circumstances can be sex linked on the X chromosome. A detailed discussion of the various mutations is beyond the scope of this chapter. In general, there are many forms of CMT disease based on duplication or depletion of certain genes on various chromosomes. Peripheral myelin protein-22 and protein 0 are two of the most common. Scientists have identified more than 120 different point mutations on the Protein 0 gene alone. Foot and ankle surgeons who treat patients with CMT should be familiar with the most common types of CMT disease and specific characteristics that distinguish each type from a clinical standpoint.

Type 1A Charcot-Marie-Tooth disease (CMT) is an autosomal dominant disease that results from a duplication of the gene on chromosome 17 that carries the instructions for producing the peripheral myelin protein PMP-22. Overexpression of the gene causes the structure and function of the myelin sheath to be abnormal. This causes weakness and atrophy of the lower legs beginning in adolescence initially and later hand weakness and sensory loss. This is the most frequent form of CMT and involves 60–90% of all cases [24–27].

Type 1B is also an autosomal dominant disease caused by mutations in the gene that carries the instructions for manufacturing the myelin protein zero (PO) which is another key component of the myelin sheath. This produces signs and symptoms that are very similar to type 1A. Both subtypes are known as hypertrophic CMT and are characterized by repeated demyelination and remyelination causing the pathognomonic "onion bulb" microscopically.

Type 2 results from abnormalities in the axon of the peripheral nerve cell rather than the myelin sheath. There is typically chronic axonal degeneration and regeneration and no demyelination [18, 19, 28]. This neuronal type differs from type 1 in that the onset of symptoms occurs later without nerve hypertrophy. Hand involvement is less prominent in type 2, but lower extremity weakness and atrophy can be very pronounced.

Type 3 or Dejerine-Sottas disease is a severe demyelinating neuropathy that begins in infancy. Infants have severe muscle atrophy, weakness, and sensory problems. This rare disorder can be caused by a specific point mutation in the P0 gene or a point mutation in the PMP-22 gene. Type 3 is also characterized by hypertrophic nerves, but the early onset in infancy distinguishes type 3 from type 1.

Type 4 comprises several different subtypes of autosomal recessive demyelinating motor and sensory neuropathies. These subtypes are responsible for the most severe disability. Each neuropathic subtype is caused by a different genetic mutation with distinct physiologic and clinical characteristics. Generally, type 4 patients develop symptoms of leg weakness in childhood, and by adolescence, they may not be able to walk. This type may also affect a particular ethnic population.

Sex-linked (CMTX) is caused by a point mutation in the connexin-32 gene on the X chromosome. This protein is expressed in Schwann cells. This protein is thought to be involved in Schwann cell communication with the axon. Most males show moderate to severe symptoms of the disease beginning in late childhood or adolescence, and females typically develop mild symptoms in adolescence or later in life. Some may not develop symptoms of the disease at all.

A thorough history should be taken with particular emphasis on family history. Many families are aware of this condition, and in some cases, they will have detailed records. In some circumstances, discussing the ambulatory difficulties of other family members may give the physician good insight into the possibility that CMT may be the diagnosis. Reports of discomfort, fatigue, and ankle instability are common complaints. There may be complaints of numbness and tingling in the feet and at times the hands. Some patients will be concerned about sensory ataxia and gait abnormalities, and these may be expressed early on in the disease process.

In general, the clinical presentation for types 1 and 2 is very similar, and the vast majority of patients that present to foot and ankle surgeons will be in either of these two groups. Slowly progressive distal weakness and muscle wasting in the legs is a hallmark of the disease. This muscle weakness leads to a pes cavus or equinovarus deformity with contracture of the digits. Initially, the intrinsic muscles are weakened creating clawing of the digits and contributing to the pes cavus deformity [29]. The weakness will eventually involve the peroneus brevis, extensors, and the anterior tibial muscle-tendon unit. The posterior tibial muscle will overpower the anterolateral group of muscles and contribute to the cavus or equinovarus foot type. The peroneus longus is one of the last muscles to weaken. In some cases the gastrosoleal group can become weak, but this is usually a late-stage manifestation. Generally, the thigh muscles are not affected so that when a patient presents with this atrophic pattern in the leg, the appearance can be seen as "stork legs" or inverted champagne bottle (Fig. 3.14). The characteristic steppage gait may be seen along with a foot drop, ankle instability, and shortened stride length.

Weakness of the hands occurs with characteristic thenar and hypothenar eminence wasting resulting in claw hands and dysfunction (Fig. 3.15). Thickening of peripheral nerves may be seen in type 1 but is pathognomonic in type 3 patients around the greater auricular nerve or the common peroneal nerve at the head of the fibular and is often described as Cohen's lamp cord sign.

The cavus deformity may present as flexible or rigid depending upon the length of time the deformity has been present. The muscle imbalance may make the foot seem rigid, but radiographic correlation will provide information about whether the joints are congruous or arthritic. This will impact whether or not closed or open treatment will be indicated and will be discussed later in this chapter. Ankle instability

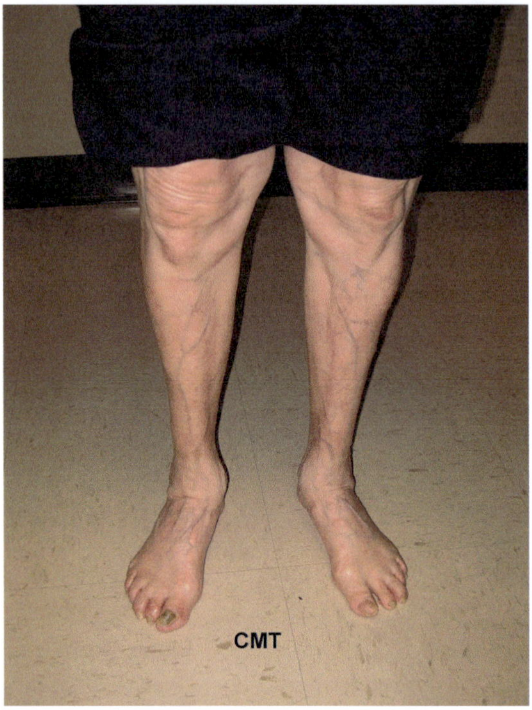

Fig. 3.14 Wasting of the distal musculature in the leg gives the appearance of "stork legs"

is a hallmark of CMT and is due to the muscle weakness pattern. The weakness eventually leads to structural changes in the hindfoot and to a plantarflexed first metatarsal drives the hindfoot varus deformity. This can be assessed with the Coleman Block test (Fig. 3.16). Over time the hindfoot varus deformity can become rigid and not dependent upon the first metatarsal. One should be suspicious of intrinsic ankle varus (Fig. 3.17). This is rarely reported, but the author has found this to be fairly common and if not appreciated can lead to less than optimal results when considering reconstruction.

Plain radiographs of the foot and ankle should be obtained to assess the congruency of the joints and to determine the apex of the deformity (Fig. 3.18). This is important for preoperative planning for deformity correction. The author has not found CT or MRI to be very helpful as a baseline in CMT evaluation. MRI of the spinal

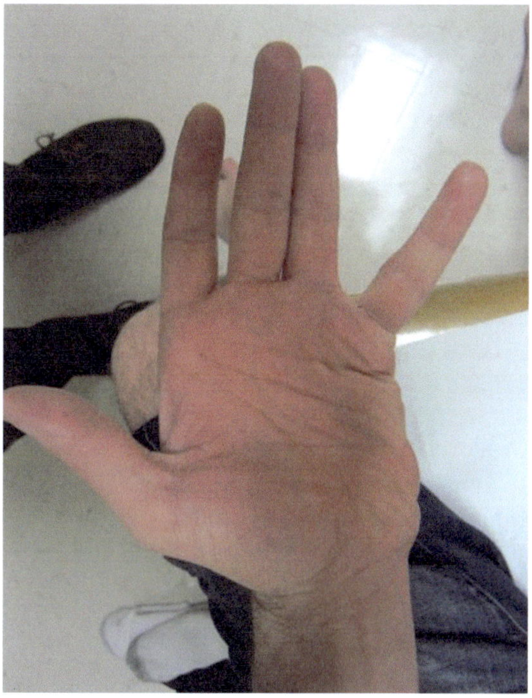

Fig. 3.15 Note the wasting of the thenar and hypothenar eminence resulting in fifth finger drift

cord can be useful if patients display central nervous system involvement such as ataxia or other signs and symptoms of cerebellar involvement [30]. MRI can also be beneficial for rehabilitation planning and future surgical reconstruction in some patients [31].

Electrodiagnostic studies are extremely helpful in patients with CMT [18]. Distal latencies are usually 2–3 times longer than normal in type 1 CMT. In type 2 CMT, there is usually only slight reduction, or in some cases, they can be normal [24].

Genetic testing through DNA analysis is available to determine or aid in the diagnosis of CMT. The testing can be extremely cost prohibitive when a comprehensive test is performed. As a screening technique, algorithms have been developed to obtain information based on the most common gene defects. Recently, Ostern R, Fagerheim T, et al. made recommendations on a simplified algorithm which involved the assessment of age at onset and neurophysiological data followed by testing of four genes: PMP22, MPZ, GJB1 and MFN2 [32]. If patients are negative for

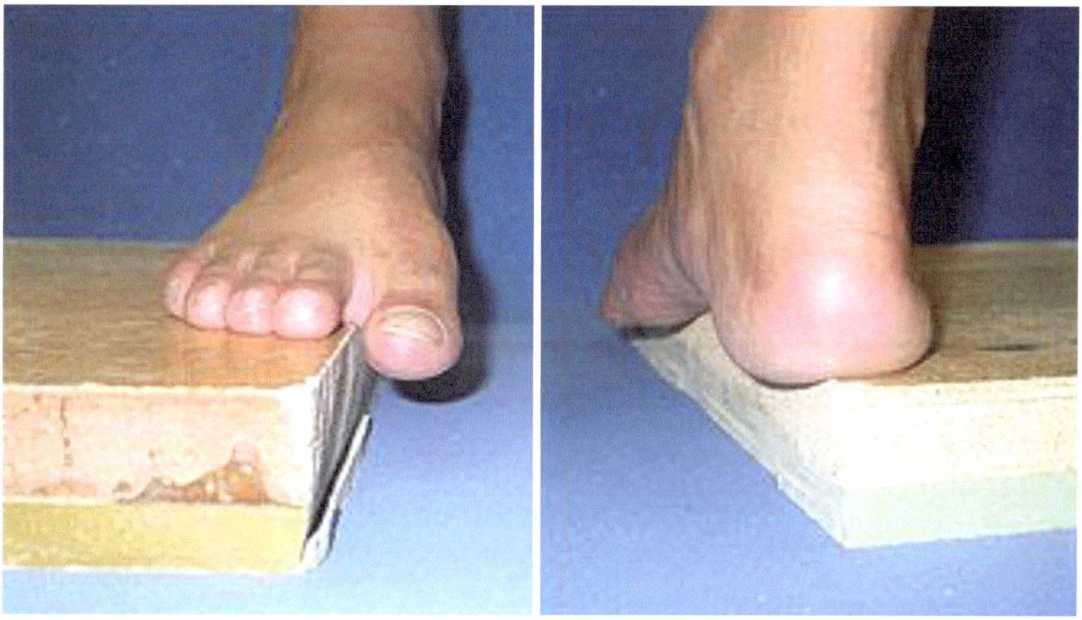

Fig. 3.16 Coleman Block test showing resolution of the hindfoot varus when the first ray is off of the block

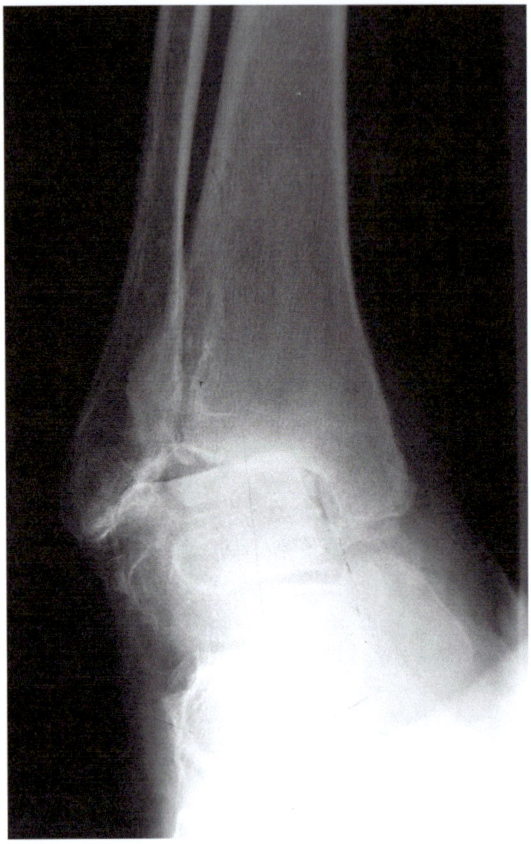

Fig. 3.17 CMT patient with intrinsic ankle varus

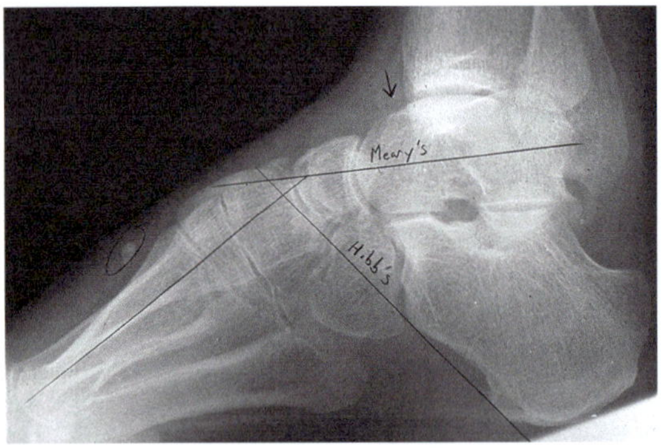

Fig. 3.18 Standard lateral radiograph showing an increase in Meary's and Hibb's angles. Apex of the deformity is at the midfoot

mutations in these four genes, then they should be subjected to a more comprehensive extended molecular genetic analysis.

Conservative therapy for CMT centers on accommodation of the progressive structural deformities. Extra-depth shoes and accommodative orthotics can be used to support the hammertoe contractures and the metatarsalgia seen in these patients. High top boots or shoes can help support the lateral ankle instability seen in CMT. Ultimately, bracing is necessary in many of these patients to assist in ambulation especially as the disease progresses. Various ankle braces can be used for instability, and graphite AFO braces tend to be used for the drop foot and steppage gait that are seen in the later stages of the disease.

Surgical management of CMT must be individualized. The variation and complexity of the clinical presentation make it difficult to formulate specific treatment recommendations. Staging procedures is not uncommon based on the progressive nature of the disease.

As a general rule, the author has found that certain surgical procedures can be performed in many patients with CMT with fairly good success.

Digital deformities are seen in almost all patients with CMT and they are rarely reducible. The author has found that complete sequential release of the digital contractures with PIPJ and DIPJ fusions has the most success. If the contractures are extreme, then metatarsal osteotomies may be employed along with a flexor digitorum longus transfer of the second and third digits [32, 33]. Meticulous soft tissue dissection is important because of the potential for vascular complications due to the long-standing dorsal contracture of the digits (Fig. 3.19). Hallux malleus is common and is often associated with dorsal contracture of the first metatarsal phalangeal joint. A popular surgical combination for this presentation is a hallux IPJ fusion and a Jones teno-suspension of the first metatarsal especially early on in the disease process. Ultimately, the rigidly plantarflexed first metatarsal will require a more proximal fusion and/or dorsiflexory osteotomy (Fig. 3.20).

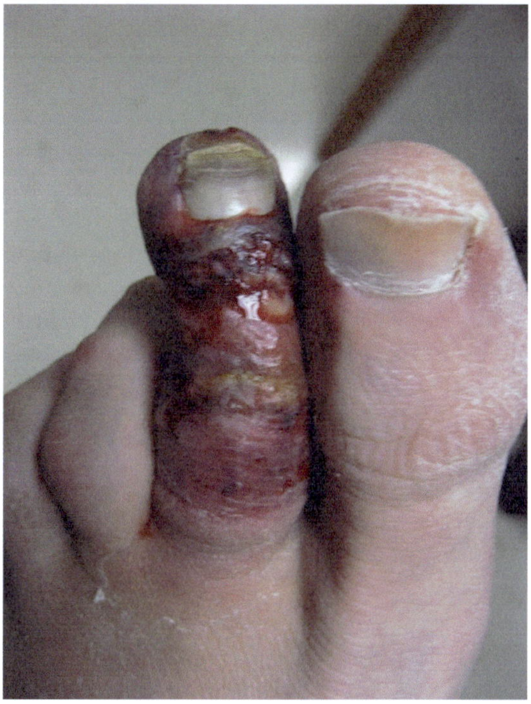

Fig. 3.19 Note vascular compromise from digital surgery

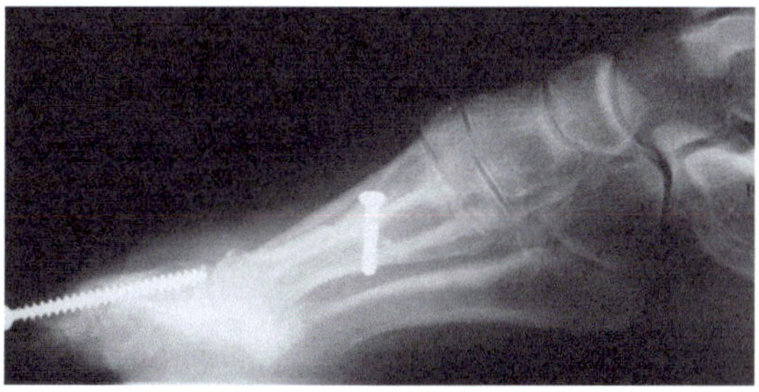

Fig. 3.20 Note reduction of the first metatarsal plantarflexion with a proximal oblique osteotomy

In mild to moderate hindfoot varus, a Dwyer calcaneal osteotomy is often coupled with the first metatarsal osteotomy to establish the tripod effect necessary for even weight distribution. An isolated subtalar joint arthrodesis is much more effective in severe hindfoot varus than a Dwyer. Ultimately, triple arthrodesis is necessary when the deformity is severe and other corrective procedures have failed [34, 35]. The most important consideration in performing triple arthrodesis in these patients is the position of the fusion. Failure to provide a rectus alignment of the hindfoot and forefoot can lead to intrinsic varus ankle deformity.

Tendon transfers and lengthening procedures have been described for patients with CMT [36–39]. In the author's experience, the vast majority of CMT patients eventually have some degree of drop foot with a cavovarus foot deformity. The posterior tibial tendon transfer is an excellent transfer for patients with CMT. The posterior tibial tendon is usually one of the last muscle-tendon units to undergo denervation and atrophy and is a major deforming force for the cavus deformity [40]. The author recommends transfer of the entire muscle-tendon unit through the interosseous membrane and then tenodesis to the lateral cuneiform or cuboid. The Achilles tendon is rarely lengthened because the vast majority of patients with CMT have a pseudoequinus and much of the available hindfoot dorsiflexion is eliminated due to this pseudoequinus in the forefoot. Surgeons should be extremely careful when evaluating equinus in patients with CMT so as not to create a calcaneus gait from lengthening the Achilles tendon.

Spinal Dysraphisms

Spinal dysraphisms are a group of congenital disorders characterized by incomplete closure of the neural tube. This incomplete closure can involve the spinal cord, the meninges, cauda equina, osseous components of the spinal column, and overlying tissues and skin. The most common type of spinal dysraphism is spina bifida or myelomenigocele. The incidence worldwide is 1:1000 live births [41]. The most common location is in the lumbosacral region. Delay in diagnosis can lead to irreversible musculoskeletal, neurologic, and genitourinary effects.

Associated conditions can include hydrocephalus, tethered spinal cord, and latex allergy [42]. Learning disabilities are relatively uncommon unless other congenital abnormalities are present. Latex allergies have been seen in 68% of children with spina bifida [43]. Spinal dysraphisms are believed to be due to a combination of genetic, nutritional, and environmental factors. Not having enough folate in the diet during pregnancy plays a significant role [44]. Generally, these are classified according to the structures that are involved in the incomplete development of the neural tube.

Spina bifida occulta is the mild form of the condition with an incidence of 10–20% [45]. The outer parts of the vertebrae are not completely closed so there is no protrusion of the spinal cord. The skin at the site of the lesion may be normal. It is also common to see a hairy patch, dimpling of the skin, or a birthmark (Fig. 3.21). Women are affected more than men, and often, patients do not even know they have the condition. Because of the insidious nature and slow progressive course, nerve damage occurs before clinical symptoms arise.

Meningocele is the least common form of spina bifida. The vertebrae develop normally, but the meninges are forced into the gaps between the vertebrae. These individuals are unlikely to develop symptoms early on unless they have a tethered cord [46].

In myelomeningocele, the vertebrae do not fuse and the spinal cord protrudes through the opening. This results in the most severe complications including paralysis, loss of sensation, and meningitis. Bladder and bowel tone are typically lost.

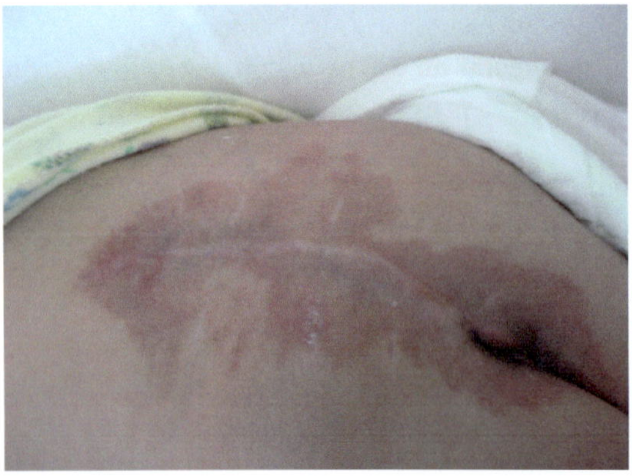

Fig. 3.21 Not the large birthmark on this patient that has had closure of his spina bifida

If the spinal dysraphism is suspected before birth, then amniocentesis can be performed and high levels of alpha-fetoprotein (AFP) may indicate a higher risk of the more severe forms of the condition [47]. AFP is not elevated in spina bifida occulta because the dural lining is maintained. Ultrasound can be useful to detect dysraphisms prior to birth. Medical imaging can confirm the diagnosis after birth.

The initial presentation depends on the extent of the involvement of the spinal cord elements. Bladder and bowel control are daily problems for the vast majority of these patients. Foot and ankle deformities are common and can be severe in nature. Patients may present with cavus or valgus foot deformities. Equinus and gait abnormalities are usually pronounced. Neurotrophic ulcers are common because of the loss of protective threshold. Occult spinal dysraphisms can occur from birth to adulthood. These forms are subtle and are usually covered with skin [48]. Overt forms such as meningocele or myelomenigocele are more common and more obvious clinically and are typically diagnosed at birth.

Surgical intervention to close the neural elements is the most effective initial treatment to prevent further damage to neurological tissue and to prevent infection. In cases where there is hydrocephalus or potential for excess cerebral spinal fluid, shunts can be surgically placed (Fig. 3.22). Success can be difficult if the neurological deficit is severe. Following closure of the neural elements, the most suitable cases for surgical management in the lower extremity are patients that can ambulate with orthopedic appliances and that have simple meningoceles or meningomyeloceles. The goal of surgical intervention in these individuals is to improve ambulation and to create a plantigrade foot. The typical procedures in the lower extremity are tendon transfers and fusions. In severe cases, surgery is typically palliative and includes ostectomies and partial amputations

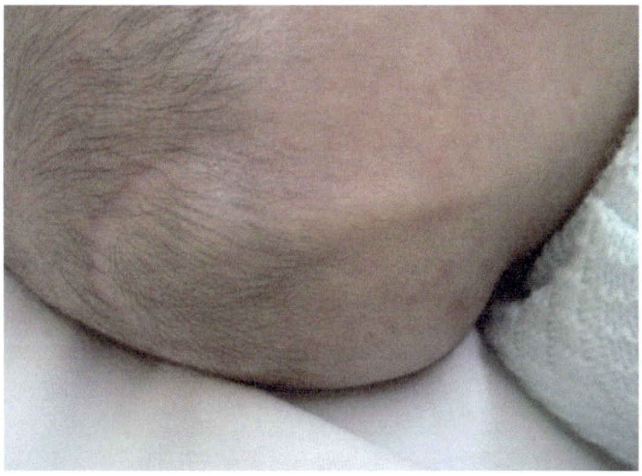

Fig. 3.22 Placement of a shunt is necessary to alleviate any cerebral pressure due to excessive amounts of cerebral spinal fluid

to eradicate osteomyelitis and neurotrophic ulcerations.

Muscular Dystrophy

Muscular dystrophy is a collection of inherited diseases of the muscle that weaken and impede locomotion. These diseases are characterized by progressive skeletal muscle weakness, muscle protein deficits, and ultimately the death of muscle cells and tissue [49]. Some forms of the disease can affect the heart and other organs [50]. The various types of MD affect more than 50,000 Americans [51].

Muscular dystrophy can appear in infancy up to middle age or later, and its form and severity are determined in part by the age at which it occurs. Some types of MD affect only males. Depending on the type and onset, patients afflicted with MD can enjoy a normal lifespan with slowly progressive and mild symptoms or swift and severe muscle weakness and wasting. These individuals may die in their late teens or early 20s.

There are several types of MD and the most common are listed in Table 3.3. Duchenne is by far the most common and was described in the 1860s by Guillaume Duchenne [52].

The diagnosis of MD is based on the results of a muscle biopsy, increased creatine phosphokinase, electromyography, and genetic testing. Clinical presentation depends on the type of MD and the progression of the disease process. All types of muscular dystrophy demonstrate muscle wasting. Duchenne MD shows muscle wasting in the lower extremities with pseudohypertrophy of the calf muscles (Fig. 3.23). Limb-girdle MD will show wasting in both upper and lower extremities. Gower's sign is indicative of progressive weakness making it difficult for the child to get up from a sitting position (Figs. 3.24 and 3.25).

There is no cure for muscular dystrophy and management is palliative. The primary deformities in the foot and ankle that need to be addressed are ankle equinus and equinovarus contractures. Equinus release procedures are used to treat the ankle equinus in ambulatory patients. The use of posterior tibial and anterior tibial transfers can be employed to address any

Table 3.3 Types of Muscular Dystrophy

Type	Gene	Description
Becker	DMD	Less severe variant of Duchenne MD Boys lifespan: Old age
Congenital	Multiple	Birth, general weakness, shortened lifespan
Duchenne distal muscular dystropy	DMD	Most common, boys usually, onset 2 YOA lifespan: 14–45
Emery-Dreyfus	EMD, LMNA	
facioscapulohumeral MD		

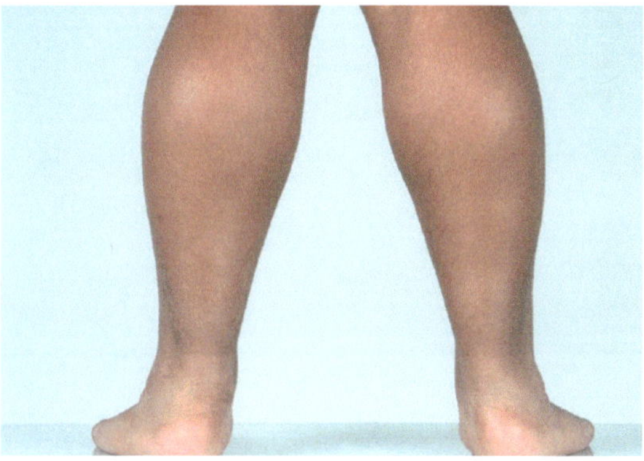

Fig. 3.23 Note the presence of hypertrophy of the calf muscles in this patient with MD

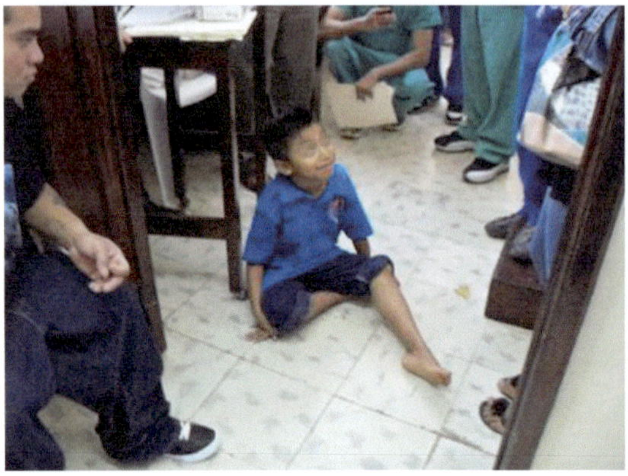

Fig. 3.24 Patient with MD sitting on the floor

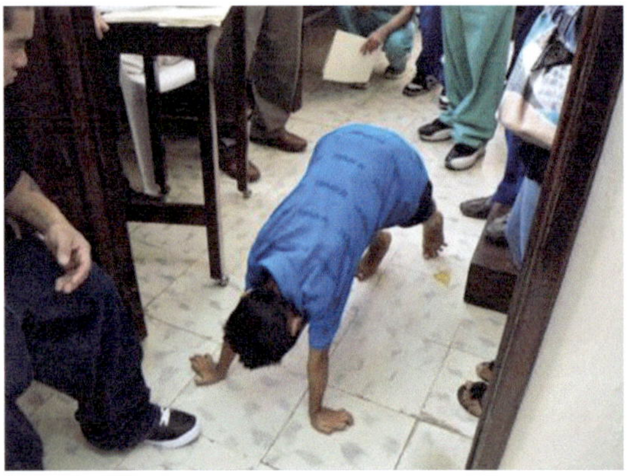

Fig. 3.25 Note this same patient trying to get up off the floor. Gower's sign

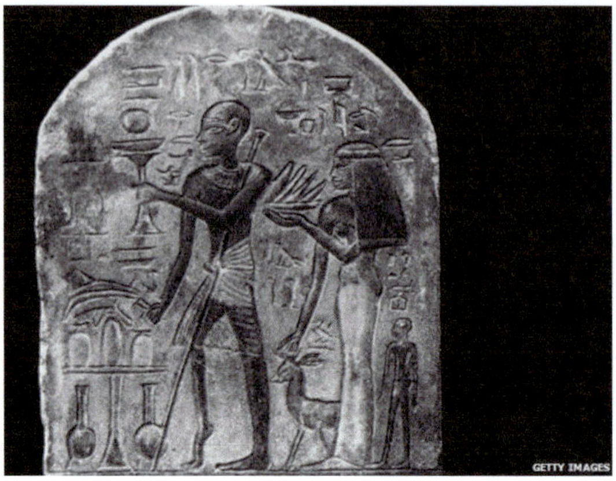

Fig. 3.26 Egyptian Stele from the 18th dynasty showing a polio victim

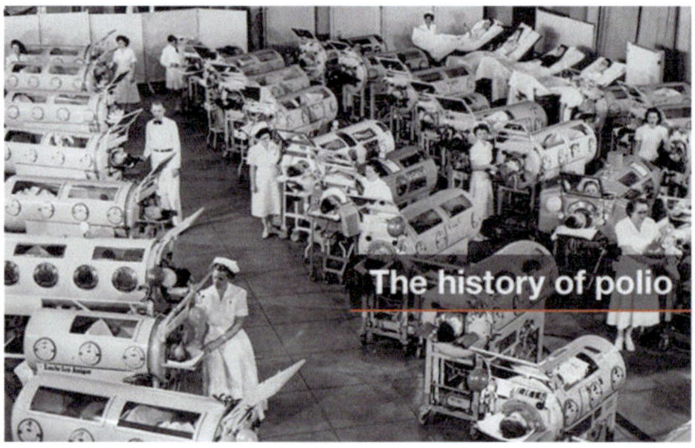

Fig. 3.27 Polio Unit Los Angeles in 1952

equinovarus contractures. Patients experience physical and occupational therapy for a lifetime. Bracing and aerobic exercise are important for maintaining ambulatory abilities as long as possible. Eventually, most patients will be wheelchair bound. Once the wheelchair stage is reached, surgical treatment primarily involves tenotomies to correct the position of feet so that shoes and AFOs can be employed to assist in transfer into the wheelchair or to prevent ulcerations.

Poliomyelitis

Poliomyelitis is an infectious disease caused mainly by the poliovirus. The condition has existed for thousands of years with depictions of the disease in ancient art (Fig. 3.26) [53]. Poliomyelitis was recognized as a distinct condition, by Michael Underwood in 1789 [54]. Karl Landsteiner discovered the virus in 1908 [55]. In the twentieth century, outbreaks of the disease occurred in the United States and Europe making the disease one of the most prevalent childhood diseases at the time, and the polio outbreak in 1952 became the worst in our nation's history [56]. Polio units developed and became the precursors to the modern ICU (Fig. 3.27).

In part due to the epidemics of polio, Jonas Salk developed the first vaccination in the 1950s in hopes of eradicating the disease worldwide. In 1961 the oral form of the vaccination developed by Albert Sabin became commercially available. Unfortunately, the disease has made a comeback with reports in Syria in 2013, and in 2014 the World Health Organization declared a public health emergency of international concern due to outbreaks in Asia, Africa, and the Middle East [57].

Once infected, there is no cure for the disease so prevention is critical. Poliomyelitis is highly contagious, and one can be infected by fecal-oral or oral-oral contamination. The incubation period is 6–20 days in most cases. Following the infection, two clinical presentations occur. Most often, a minor illness can occur that does not involve the central nervous system called abortive poliomyelitis, and this occurs in about 75% of patients infected with the poliovirus. These patients typically are asymptomatic but on occasion will have minor symptoms that are typically upper respiratory in nature with a sore throat and fever. There may be gastrointestinal symptoms such as nausea, vomiting, and abdominal pain.

The major illness, which represents about 1% of the cases, does involve the central nervous system and can be paralytic or non-paralytic. Most of the time, patients will develop non-paralytic aseptic meningitis with symptoms of head and neck ache. They will generally have abdominal and extremity pain, fever, vomiting, lethargy, and irritability. The paralytic form occurs in about 1–4 in 1000 cases characterized by muscle weakness that can eventually progress to complete paralysis. This condition is known as acute flaccid paralysis, and depending on the location of the involvement, patients may need support for respiration. They may have changes in mental status.

The likelihood of developing paralytic polio increases with age, as does the extent of paralysis. In children, non-paralytic meningitis occurs in only 1 in 1000 cases. In adults, paralysis occurs in 1 in 75 cases. In children under 5 years of age, paralysis of one leg is most common and in adults extensive paralysis can lead to quadriplegia and respiratory complications. The spinal form occurs in about 80% of the cases and affects the anterior horn cells. This results in rapid paralysis of the involved muscles especially in the proximal groups in any given limb. The extent of the spinal paralysis depends on the region of the cord affected, which can involve cervical, thoracic, or lumbar regions. Sensation to the affected area is usually not affected.

Treatment for polio is primarily palliative. With skeletal growth, soft tissue contractures, foot deformities, and limb length discrepancies can develop in patients with poliomyelitis [58]. The goal of surgical treatment is to obtain a painless plantigrade foot and a stable lower limb. This is accomplished through conventional corrective osteotomies, arthrodesis, and release of various soft tissue contractures. Open and/or closed treatment with circular external fixation is often used for simultaneous leg lengthening and deformity correction [59].

References

1. Howard J, Soo B, Graham HK, et al. Cerebral palsy in Victoria: motor types, topography, and gross motor function. J Pediatr Child Health. 2005;41:479–83.
2. M.E.N.T.O.R.S. (Methodologies for Experts in Neurotoxin Therapy: Outreach, Resources and Support). Focus on cerebral Palsy. Monograph: a continuing medical education DVD activity. New York: The Institute for Medicaal Studies; 2004.
3. Rouse DJ, Hirtz DG, Thom E, Varner MW, et al. A randomized, controlled trial of magnesium sulfate for the prevention of cerebral palsy. N Engl J Med. 2008;359(9):895–0.
4. Ashwal S, Russman BS, Blasco PA, et al. Practice parameter: diagnostic assessment of the child with cerebral palsy: report of the quality standards subcommittee of the American Academy of Neurology and the practice committee of the Child Neurology Society. Neurology. 2004;62:851–36.
5. Bax M, Tydeman C, Flodmark O. Clinical and MRI correlates in cerebral palsy; the European Cerebral Palsy Study. JAMA. 2006;296:1602–8.
6. Beck EE. Where have all the CP children gone? Dev Med Child Neurol. 1984;26:674.
7. Paneth N, Stark RI. Cerebral palsy and mental retardation in relation to indicators of perinatal asphyxia. An epidemiologic overview. Am J Obstet Gynecol. 1983;147(8):960–6.

8. Knezevic-Pogancev M. Cerebral palsy and epilepsy. Med Pregl. 2010;63(7–8):527–30.
9. Koman AL, Mooney JF, Smith BP, et al. Botulinum toxin type A neuromuscular blockade in the treatment of lower extremity spasticity in cerebral palsy: a randomized, double-blind, placebo-controlled trial. J Pediatr Orthop. 2000;20(1):108–15.
10. Yadav SL, Singh U, Dureja GP, Singh KK, Charturvedi S. Phenol block in the management of spastic cerebral palsy. Indian J Pediatr. 1994;61:249–255.10.
11. Palisano R, Rosenbaum P, Walter S, et al. Development & reliability of a system to classify gross motor function in children with cerebral palsy. Dev Med Child Neurol. 1997;39:214–23.
12. Pierrot AH, Murphy OB. Albert E. Klinkicht Award, 1972. Heel cord advancement. A new approach to the spastic equinus deformity. Orthop Clin North Am. 1974;5(1):117–26.
13. Ilizarov GA. The tension-stress effect on the genisis and growth of tissues: Part II. The influence of the rate and frequency of distraction. Clin Orthop Relat Res. 1989;239:263–85.
14. Julieanne PS, Miller F. Overview of foot deformity management in children with cerebral palsy. J Child Orthop. 2012;7(5):373–7.
15. National Institute of Neurological Disorders and Stroke. Charcot Marie Tooth Fact Sheet.
16. Charcot J, Marie P. Sue une forme particulaire d'atrophie musculaire progressive souvent familial debutant par les pieds et les jamber et atteingnant plus tard les mains. Re Med. 1886;6:97–138.
17. Tooth H. The peroneal type of progressive muscular atrophy. London: Lewis; 1886.
18. Dyck PJ, Lambert EH. Lower motor and primary sensory neuron diseases with peroneal muscular atrophy. I. Neurologic, genetic and electrophysiologic findings in hereditary polyneuropathies. Arch Neurol. 1968;18:603.
19. Dyck PJ, Lambert EH. Lower motor and primary sensory neuron diseases with peroneal muscular atrophy. II. Neurologic, genetic and electrophysiologic findings in various neuronal degenerations. Arch Neurol. 1968;18:61.
20. Saporta AS, Sottile SL, Miller LJ, Feely SM, et al. Charcot Marie Tooth (CMT) subtypes and genetic testing strategies. Ann Neurol. 2011 Jan;69(1):22–33.
21. Harding AE, Thomas PK. Genetic aspects of hereditary motor and sensory neuropathy (types I and II). J Med Genet. 1980;17:329–36.
22. Kijima K, Numakura C, Izumino H, et al. Mitochondrial GTPase mitofusin 2 mutation in Charcot-Marie-Tooth neuropathy type 2A. Hum Genet. 2005;116:23–7.
23. Shy M, Lupski JR, Chance PF, et al. The hereditary motor and sensory neuropathies: an overview of the clinical, genetic, electrophysiologic and pathologic features. In: Dyck PJTP, editor. Peripheral neuropathy, vol. 2. 4th ed. Philadelphia: WB Saunders; 2005. p. 1623–58.
24. Pareyson D. Charcot-Marie-Tooth disease and related neuropathies: molecular basis for distinction and diagnosis. Muscle Nerve. 1999;22:1498–509.
25. Garcia CA. A clinical review of Charcot-Marie-Tooth. Ann N Y Acad Sci. 1999;833:69–76.
26. Hanemann CO, Muller HW. Pathogenesis of Charcot-Marie-Tooth 1A (CMT1a) neuropathy. Trends Neurosci. 1998;21:282–6.
27. Thomas PK. Overview of Charcot-Marie-Tooth disease type IA. Ann N Y Acad Sci. 1999;883:1–5.
28. Vance JM. Charcot-Marie-Tooth disease type 2. Ann N Y Acad Sci. 1999;883:42–6.
29. Sabir M, Lyttle D. Pathogenesis of Charcot-Marie-Tooth disease: gait analysis and electrophysiologic, genetic, histopathologic, and enzyme studies in a kinship. Clin Orthop. 1984;184:223–35.
30. McClusky WP, Lovell WW, Cummings RJ. The cavovarus foot deformity: etiology and management. Clin Orthop. 1989;(247):27–37.
31. Stilwell G, Kilcoyne RF, Sherman JL. Patterns of muscle atrophy in the lower limbs in patients with Charcot-Marie-Tooth disease as measured by magnetic resonance imaging. J Foot Ankle Surg. 1995;34:583–6.
32. Alexander IJ, Johnson KA. Assessment and management of pes cavus in Charcot-Marie-Tooth disease. Clin Orthop. 1989;(246):273–81.
33. Leeuwestejjn AE, de Visser E, Louwerens JW. Flexible cavovarus feet in Charcot-Marrie-Tooth disease treated with first ray proximal dorsiflexion osteotomy combined with soft tissue surgery: a short-term to mid-term outcome study. Foot Ankle Surg. 2010;16(3):142–7.
34. Wukich DK, Bowen JR. A long-term study of triple arthrodesis for correction of pes cavovarus in Charcot-Marie-Tooth disease. J Pediatr Orthop. 1989;9: 433–7.
35. Saltzman CL, Fehrle MJ, Cooper RR, et al. Triple arthrodesis: twenty-five and forty-four year follow-up of the same patients. J Bone Joint Surg Am. 1999;81:1391–402.
36. Ward CM, Dolan LA, Bennett DL, et al. Long-term results of reconstruction for treatment of a flexible cavovarus foot in Charcot-Marie-Tooth disease. J Bone Joint Surg Am. 2008;(12):2631–42.
37. Holmes JR, Hansen ST. Foot and ankle manifestations of Charcot-Marie-Tooth disease. Foot Ankle. 1993;14(8):476–86.
38. Roper BA, Tibrewal SB. Soft tissue surgery in Charcot-Marie-Tooth disease. J Bone Joint Surg Br. 1989;71(1):17–20.
39. Boffeli TJ, Tabatt JA. Minimally invasive early operative treatment of progressive foot and ankle deformity associated with Charcot-Marie-Tooth disease. J Foot Ankle Surg. 2015;54(4):701–8.
40. Fenton CF III, Schlefman BS, McGlamry ED. Surgical considerations in the presence of Charcot-Marie-Tooth disease. J Am Podiatry Assoc. 1984;74: 490–8.

41. Memet Ozek M. Spina bifida: management and outcome. Milan: Springer; 2008. p. 58.
42. Centers for Disease Control and Prevention. Spina bifida: health issues and treatments. 2011. Retrieved March 30, 2012.
43. Boettcher M, Goettler S, Eschenburg G, et al. Prenatal latex sensitization in patients with spina bifida: a pilot study. J Neurosurg Pediatr. 2014;13(3):291–4.
44. Cawley S, Mullaney L, McKeating A, et al. Knowledge about folic acid supplementation in women presenting for antenatal care. Eur J Clin Nutr. 2016; https://doi.org/10.1038/ejcn.2016.104.
45. Sandler AD. Children with spina bifida: key clinical issues. Pediatr Clin North Am. 2010;57(4):879–92.
46. Herman JM, McLone DG, Storrs BB, Dauser RC. Analysis of 153 patients with myelomeningocele or spinal lipoma reoperated upon for a tethered cord. Presentation, management and outcome. Pediatr Neursurg. 1993;19(5):243–9.
47. Shoro AA. Estimation of the levels of amniotic fluid alpha fetoprotein (AFP) for the prenatal diagnosis of spina bifida and anencephaly. Methods Find Exp Clin Pharmocol. 1981;3(6):391–5.
48. Anderson FM. Occult spinal dysraphism. J Pediatr. 1968;73:163–77.
49. Emery AE. The muscular dystrophies. Lancet. 2002;359(9307):687–95.
50. Turakhia P, Barrick B, Berman J. Patients with neuromuscular disorder. Med Clin North Am. 2013;97(6):1015–32.
51. Ciafaloni E, Fox DJ, Pandya S, Westfield CP, Puzhankara S, et al. Delayed diagnosis in Duchenne muscular dystrophy: data from the Muscular Dystrophy Surveillance, Tracking, and Research Network (MDStarnet). J Pediatr. 2009;155(3):380–5.
52. Duchenne GBA. Recherches sur la paralysie pseudo-hypertophique au paralysie myo-sclerosique. Arch Gen Med. 1868;11:5–25.
53. Paul JR. A history of poliomyelitis. Yale studies in the history of science and medicine. New Haven: Yale University Press; 1971. p. 16–8.
54. Underwood M. Debility of the lower extremities. A treatise on the diseases of children, with general directions for the management of infants from the birth. 2nd ed. London: J. Mathews; 1789. p. 88–91.
55. Skem T. 100 years poliovirus: from discovery to eradication. A meeting report. Arch Virol. 2010;155(9):137–81.
56. Wheeler DS, Wong HR, Shanley TP. Science and practice of pediatric critical care medicine. London: Springer; 2009. p. 10–1.
57. Sharara SL, Kanj SS. War and infectious diseases: challenges of the Syrian Civil War. PLoS Pathog. 2014;(11):e1004438.
58. Tachdjian MO. The neuromuscular system. In: Tachdjian MO, editor. Pediatric orthopedics. 3rd ed. Philadelphia: WB Saunders Co; 1990. p. 1605–770.
59. Kirienko A, Peccati A, Abdellatif I, et al. Correction of poliomyelitis foot deformities with Ilizarov method. Strategies Trauma Limb Reconstr. 2011;6(3):107–20.

Digital Deformities of the Pediatric Foot

4

Irina Bazarov and Mitzi L. Williams

Polydactyly

Polydactyly is a common congenital digital deformity characterized by formation of supernumerary digits. It is the most common congenital deformity of the hand and foot, with incidence in the foot of approximately 1 per 1000 live births [1]. Bilateral involvement is seen in 25–50% of patients [2]. No gender predilection is observed. Prevalence appears to be higher in black and Asian populations [3]. Polydactyly of the hand or foot can be associated with genetic syndromes, such as Pallister-Hall, Lawrence-Moon-Bardet-Biedl, and Ellis-Van Creveld [2], or may occur as an isolated trait with an autosomal-dominant pattern of inheritance [4]. Up to 30% of subjects report positive family history of this trait [2].

Many classification systems for polydactyly have been described. Anatomic classification has been proposed by Temtamy and McKusick [5]. It divides the deformity into preaxial, postaxial, and mixed based on the location of the supernumerary digit relative to the line bisecting the second ray. In this classification, preaxial polydactyly refers to duplication of the first or second digit, while postaxial polydactyly refers to duplication of the third, fourth, or fifth digits (Fig. 4.1).

Each category is further subdivided into types, based on the morphology of the supernumerary digit. Preaxial polydactyly is subdivided into four types: duplication of the hallux (type 1), duplication of the triphalangeal hallux (type 2), duplication of the second digit (type 3), and polysyndactyly (type 4). Postaxial polydactyly is subdivided into two types: a fully developed extra digit (Type A) and a rudimentary extra digit (Type B).

Temtamy's and McKusick's classification system doesn't account for all types of polydactyly, so several other classification systems followed in an attempt to provide the most comprehensive approach to describing the condition. Venn-Watson has proposed a scheme based on morphological configuration of the metatarsal [6]. He subdivided preaxial polydactyly into two groups: short block first metatarsal and wide first metatarsal. Postaxial polydactyly was subdivided into five categories, from least differentiated to more differentiated: soft tissue duplication, wide metatarsal head, T metatarsal, Y metatarsal, and complete duplication (Figs. 4.2 and 4.3).

I. Bazarov
Department of Podiatry, Kaiser Permanente, San Jose, CA, USA
e-mail: Irina.bazarov@kp.org

M. L. Williams (✉)
Kaiser San Francisco Bay Area Foot and Ankle Residency Program, Department of Orthopedics and Podiatric Surgery, Kaiser Permanente, Oakland, CA, USA

Pediatry Institute Faculty Member, American Academy of Foot and Ankle, Osteosynthesis, Oakland, CA, USA
e-mail: mitzi.l.williams@kp.org

M. L. Butterworth, J. T. Marcoux (eds.), *The Pediatric Foot and Ankle*,
https://doi.org/10.1007/978-3-030-29788-6_4

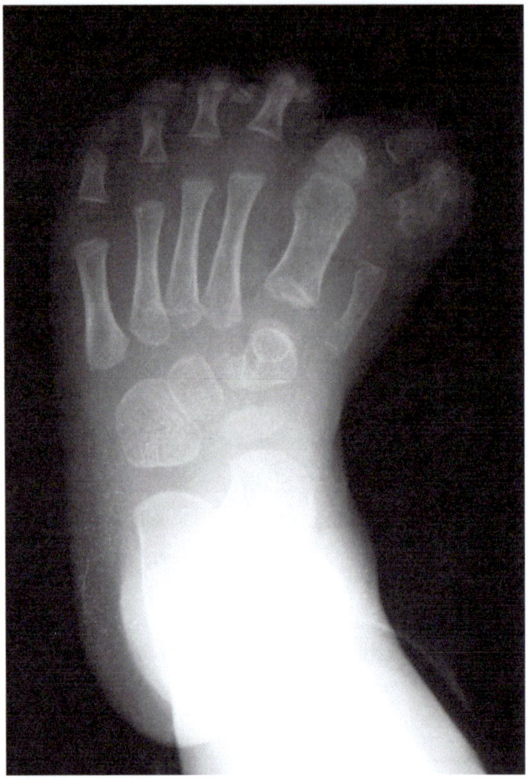

Fig. 4.1 Preaxial polydactyly

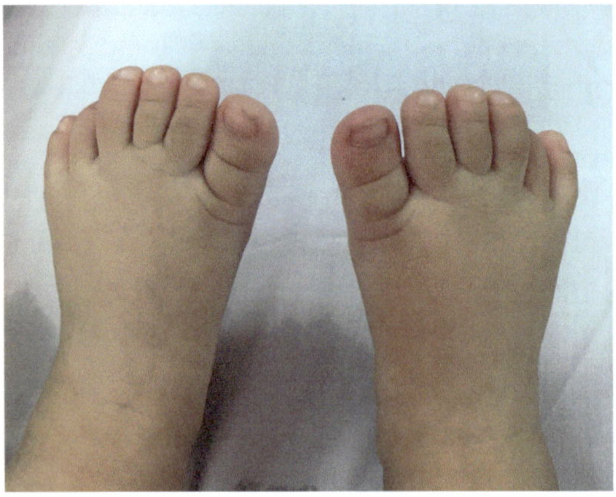

Fig. 4.2 Postaxial polydactyly

Watanabe and colleagues [7] based their classification system on the ray involvement and the level of duplication. They subdivided medial ray polydactyly into tarsal, metatarsal, proximal, and distal phalangeal types and central and lateral ray polydactyly into metatarsal, proximal, intermediate, and distal phalangeal types.

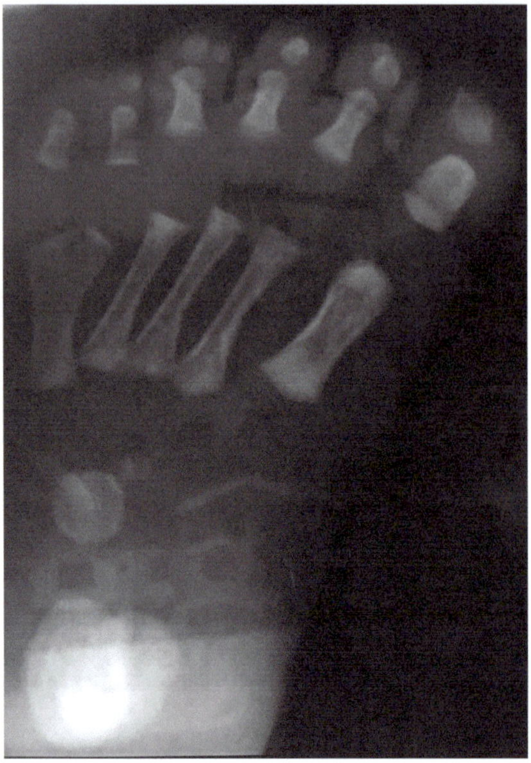

Fig. 4.3 Postaxial polydactyly, Y metatarsal

Lee and colleagues have proposed a classification system of postaxial polydactyly based on the site of origin of extra digit [8]. They divided accessory digits into five types: a floating type, middle phalangeal (MP) type, proximal phalangeal type, fifth metatarsal type, and fourth metatarsal type. The proximal phalangeal type is further subdivided into proximal phalangeal lateral (PPL), proximal phalangeal medial, and proximal phalangeal head (PPH) types. The fourth metatarsal type involves an abnormal-appearing extra digit syndactylized with the fifth digit. The authors reported that the supernumerary toes that were more distal in origin demonstrated higher degree of osseous fusion with the normal toes and were thus more difficult to manage.

Seok and Kwon have devised a classification system for polydactyly of the foot based on the key anatomic features of the deformity affecting surgical planning. This classification aimed to provide guidelines for surgical decision-making and predict outcomes. Their classification system, entitled SAM, categorizes each deformity based on the presence and the extent of syndactylism, axis deviation, and metatarsal extension. Three types were described within each category, from least severe to most severe, with each deformity designated by a combination of three letters (S, A, M, with numbers 0–2). For instance, $S_0A_0M_2$ describes a deformity with no syndactylism, less than 15 degrees of axis deviation, and metatarsal shaft duplication. The combination of letters and numbers for each deformity would also serve to guide surgical treatments, with S0 requiring simple excision versus S1 and S2 necessitating a skin graft, A1 and A2 warranting a closing wedge osteotomy and possible collateral ligament reconstruction, and M 1 and 2 potentially dictating a need for proximal extension of the dissection and excision of redundant parts of the metatarsal.

One may also consider utilizing the terms tibial polydactyly and fibular polydactyly for the location of the duplicated digit. The authors prefer this terminology as patients can have a congenital dysmorphic feature of the tibial or fibular aspects of the entire lower limb in association with polydactyly.

Treatment indications for foot polydactyly include shoe-fitting problems, pain and cosmesis, or social anxiety. Conservative treatment options are limited to accommodative shoe gear with widened toe box to prevent impingement and orthotics or metatarsal pads to relieve transfer metatarsalgia [4]. Surgical treatment is pursued if conservative treatment options fail to alleviate pain and for social concerns. Surgical approach and procedure choice are guided by the anatomic location of the deformity and the morphology of the supernumerary digit.

While there is not an absolute age in which to surgically intervene, many tend to wait until at least the second or third year of life to operate. Surgery should be delayed until at least the second year of life to reduce the risk of anesthesia-related complications [4]. With concerns for general anesthesia effects on cognitive development in children under 3 years of age, one may delay if patient is stable. Delaying surgical intervention can facilitate improved identification of the hypoplastic digit and the redundant tissue [4]. Unfortunately, in the presence of persistent skin problems and/or infections, some patients may require intervention sooner.

Postaxial (fibular) polydactyly is the most common form of polydactyly in the foot, accounting for roughly 80% of all cases [1]. Typically, it is also the simplest one to treat. Most studies advocate removal of either the most lateral or the most underdeveloped digit [1, 9, 10]. In the cases involving duplication or widening of the metatarsal head, excision of the redundant bone, capsular repair, and possible stabilization of the joint with a K-wire are recommended. Amputation of the most lateral digit is typically performed through a racquet incision [11]. The incision is extended proximally in a linear fashion in the cases necessitating removal of a redundant metatarsal. Long-term postoperative follow-up demonstrates that surgical treatment of postaxial polydactyly is generally very successful, with low rate of recurrences or complications [1, 9]. Osseous recurrence rates and duplicated nail regrowth rates tend to be higher in younger surgical patients.

Preaxial polydactyly is seen in 11 to 16% of all polydactyly cases [4]. Surgical treatment of preaxial polydactyly consists of removal of the most medial or the most rudimentary hallux. Careful soft tissue rebalancing with reattachment of abductor and adductor halluces tendons and intermetatarsal ligament repair is recommended to prevent hallux varus, which is a frequent complication of this surgery. In his series of 16 preaxial polydactyly cases, Phelps reported an 88% incidence of hallux varus [1]. The prevalence of hallux varus was noted to be higher in block metatarsal deformities.

Central polydactyly is the least common form of polydactyly, occurring in 6% of cases [1]. Its treatment involves excision of the supernumerary digit, which is traditionally performed through a dorsal racquet incision [12]. Persistent forefoot widening is one of the most frequent complications of this procedure [1, 7]. To improve esthetic and functional outcomes, Allen introduced a novel approach for central ray excision using plantar and dorsal advancement flaps. This technique was shown to result in improved cosmetic and functional outcomes, with forefoot narrowing maintained with growth after a mean follow-up of 8 years [12]. Due to extensive soft tissue dissection associated with this approach, special attention needs to be paid to preservation of blood supply to the adjacent digits to avoid vascular compromise.

Primary complications of surgery for the treatment of polydactyly include recurrence, infection, wound healing problems, nail bed problems, persistent swelling, and pain. Recurrence rates can be reduced by delaying surgery to allow for osseous growth. Care should be taken to minimize tension on surgical incisions. Dehiscence rates are higher when tension is increased or when hemostasis is not maintained. A running subcuticular closure or absorbable sutures in a simple fashion may be utilized to avoid office suture removal. Nylon skin closure may also be beneficial especially in areas of mobility or additional tension. The authors do not promote suture ligation in an infant given risks of infection, wound complications, and an amputation neuroma.

Syndactyly

Syndactyly is a common congenital deformity characterized by the presence of webbing between the toes. It is seen in 1 per 2000 people and usually involves 2nd and 3rd toes [4]. Syndactyly is caused by the rapid arrest in embryologic development of the limb buds between 6th and 8th weeks IU, which can be caused by genetic factors or an intrauterine assault [13]. It occurs either as an isolated deformity or as a part of a genetic syndrome. Syndactyly is seen more commonly in whites compared to blacks and exhibits no gender predilection (Fig. 4.4) [13].

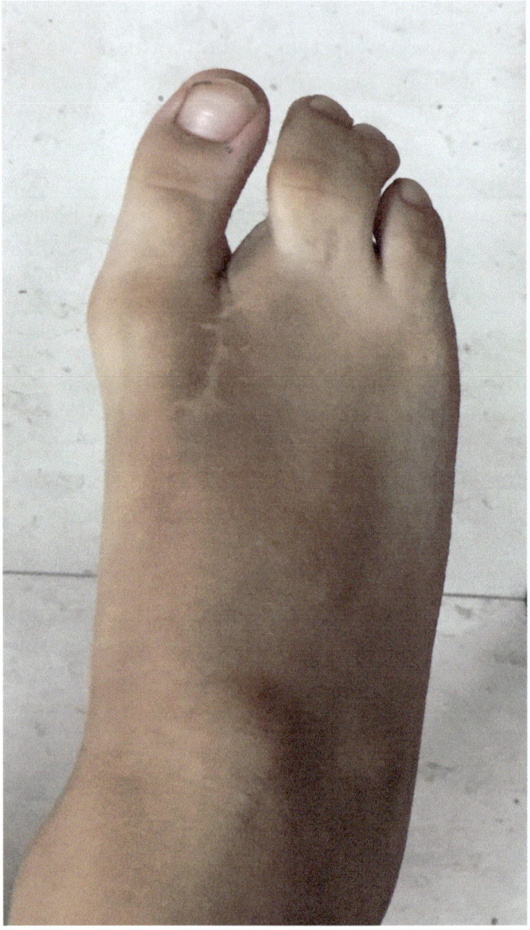

Fig. 4.4 Complex digital abnormality demonstrating syndactyly

Davis and German have classified syndactyly as incomplete or partial (the webbing doesn't extend to the distal aspect of the digits), complete (the webbing extends to the distal aspect of the digits), simple (no phalangeal involvement), and complicated (abnormal phalangeal bones) [14]. Temtamy and McKusick proposed an alternative classification based on the presence of associated deformities [5]. They divided the syndactyly into five types, zygodactyly (type 1), synpolydactyly (type 2), ring finger-small finger syndactyly (type 3), Hass type (type 4), and syndactyly with metatacarpal fusion (type 5). Zygodactyly refers to presence of webbing between the toes without duplication of the digits. Synpolydactyly refers to syndactyly of the 4th and 5th toes with associated polydactyly of the 5th toe included in the web between the 4th and 5th digits. Types 3–5 refer to syndactyly of the hand and will not be discussed here.

Definitive treatment of syndactyly consists of surgical reconstruction of the webspace. Due to high incidence of postoperative complications seen with this procedure, treatment is typically not indicated for syndactyly without associated bony deformities [15]. Synpolydactyly, on the other hand, is commonly associated with functional problems, such as difficulty with shoe gear fitting, and may be addressed surgically.

Studies recommend delaying surgery until at least 3 years of age to minimize the risk of anesthesia-related complications. Although waiting until the fifth year of life may facilitate a more complete radiographic assessment of the problem, prolonged waiting period may cause distress.

Surgical options for desyndactylization include skin flaps, grafts, and tissue expansion. Various combinations of Z-plasties have been described [15–17]. Careful planning of the flap placement is necessary to avoid excessive tension on the desyndactylized digits and skin necrosis. Hypertrophic scar formation may lead to severe digital contracture and is one of the most common causes of failure of the procedure [15]. The use of full-thickness skin grafts obtained from the dorsum of the foot, groin, and abdomen has been described. Possible concerns associated with this procedure include donor site morbidity and pigmentation mismatch [4].

Macrodactyly

Macrodactyly is a rare congenital deformity of the hands and feet characterized by the enlargement of soft tissue and osseous elements of the digit [18]. The condition may occur as a part of a syndrome, such as Klippel-Trenaunay-Weber, proteus, or neurofibromatosis, or as an isolated phenomenon [19]. The etiology of the deformity is unknown, though some studies implicate hyperinduction of a neurotrophic mechanism responsible for normal pedal growth [20]. Slight male predilection has been noted [21]. Second and third digits are affected most often [21]. The deformity is manifested by the enlargement of the bony phalanges and accumulation of the fibrofatty tissue (Fig. 4.5).

Concomitant metatarsal enlargement is seen in over 50% of the patients [4]. Tendons and nerves are often spared in the foot [21]. The condition is described as static, when the enlargement of the digit is present at birth, and its growth is proportional to the growth of the normal digits, or progressive, when the involved digit grows faster than the normal digits [19].

Clinically and radiographically, the affected foot appears wider and longer compared to the unaffected one. The enlarged digit tends to sublux

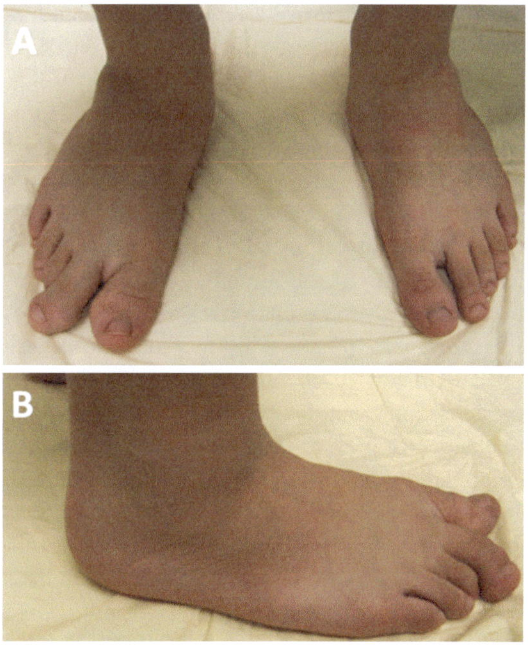

Fig. 4.5 (**a**) Macrodactyly. (**b**) Second toe demonstrates asymmetrical growth of soft tissue and bone

dorsally and deviate laterally or medially due to asymmetrical growth of the soft tissue and bone. Finding a shoe to accommodate the deformity can be challenging. Due to abnormal biomechanics and pain, patients with macrodactyly frequently exhibit apropulsive gait.

Treatment options include shoe gear modifications for mild deformity and surgical correction for moderate or severe deformity. The goal of surgical treatment is to produce a painless cosmetically acceptable foot that can be accommodated in regular shoe gear.

Optimal timing of surgical intervention is controversial. Most authors recommend performing the surgery before or around the walking age (12–13 months) in order to minimize the effect on the adjacent digits and prevent gait abnormalities [21, 22]. Some authors, however, advocate waiting anywhere from 4 years of age to skeletal maturity, to facilitate proper assessment of the growth potential of the hypertrophic tissues [23].

Pre-operative evaluation should include clinical examination and weight-bearing X-rays of the affected foot. Procedure selection should be guided by the anatomic location and the level of the deformity. Macrodactyly limited to phalanges can be treated with isolated digital procedures, which include soft tissue debulking, phalangectomy, arthroplasty or arthrodesis, epiphysiodesis, and amputations. Isolated soft tissue debulking is usually not recommended, as it carries a risk of wound healing complications and high recurrence rate [22]. Procedures for shortening of the digit include arthrodesis [19], excision of the distal phalanx and soft tissue reconstruction with a dorsal flap [24], phalangectomy of the middle phalanx [25], and epiphysiodesis of the proximal phalanx [26]. Indications for digit-sparing procedures, however, may be limited to mild cases of static macrodactyly, since these surgeries don't address increased girth of the digit, and are associated with high recurrence rates especially in cases of progressive deformity. Studies suggest that in cases of moderate or severe deformity, and progressive form of macrodactyly, digital amputations may be more successful [18].

Options for treatment of macrodactyly of the forefoot include epiphysiodesis with soft tissue debulking and ray resection. Chang and colleagues have proposed a simple protocol for treatment of forefoot macrodactyly based on the ratio of metatarsal spread angles (MSA) between the affected and unaffected foot [22]. The MSA is measured on anteroposterior weight-bearing radiographs and represents an angle formed by the medial border of the first metatarsal and lateral border of the fifth metatarsal. The authors suggested that MSA can be reduced by an average of 10 degrees following a ray resection. Based on this finding, they suggested that macrodactyly with MSA of less than 10 degrees can be treated with a combination of metatarsal epiphysiodesis and soft tissue debulking, while deformities with MSA greater than 10 should be addressed with ray resection.

Treatment of hallux and first ray macrodactyly is especially challenging due to the important role of the first ray in weight bearing and normal gait. Studies recommend avoiding resection whenever possible and performing shortening and debulking procedures instead [22].

Curly Toes (Fig. 4.6)

Curly or underlapping toe is a common congenital digital deformity characterized by plantarflexion, medial deviation, and varus rotation of the toe at the distal interphalangeal (DIP) or both DIP and proximal interphalangeal (PIP) joints. The condition is often hereditary, with positive family history and autosomal-dominant pattern of inheritance [13]. Bilateral involvement is common. Third, fourth, and fifth digits are most frequently affected [27]. The etiology of the deformity is not completely understood. Curly toes are seen more frequently in patients with flexible pes planus and metatarsal adductus

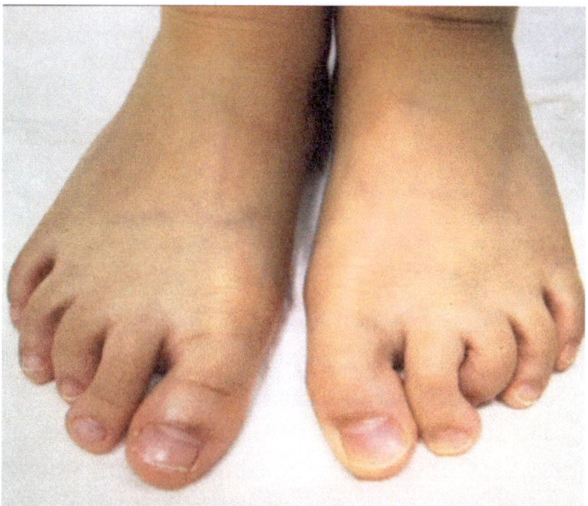

Fig. 4.6 Curly toe

[28], which may suggest that the flexor stabilization mechanism is an important driving force in this deformity.

Curly toes are usually noticed in early infancy. At this stage, they are rarely symptomatic but may cause parental anxiety. Parental reassurance and education are the main goals of that initial visit. Spontaneous self-correction of the deformity before the age of 6 occurs in up to 25% of the patients [29]. Therefore, delaying surgical intervention until the age of 6 is usually recommended.

Toe strapping is one of the available non-operative treatment modalities, which can be attempted at any age. Its effectiveness, however, is controversial. In a study by Turner, toe strapping was performed daily on 28 children over 5 months of age for an average of 13 months [30]. No statistically significant difference was noted in the improvement rates between the study group and a control group, consisting of children, who received no treatment. In another study, Smith and colleagues performed daily toe strapping for 3 months on 68 children with underlapping and overlapping toes, all of whom were no older than 10 days [29]. The authors observed a 94% improvement rate, which led them to suggest that toe strapping may be more successful in younger children.

Surgical treatment is reserved for patients with persistent deformity that is symptomatic. The patients may present with blisters or calluses at the tip of the underlapping toe or the plantar aspect of the adjacent toe. Others may present with nail deformities or pain in shoes [31]. Waiting until the child is at least 6 years old is recommended to allow a toe sufficient time to self-correct. If condition is becoming more semi rigid intervention may take place sooner to minimize the need for osseous procedures to come.Likwise if the child is undergoing another procedure under general anesthesia it may be performed to minimize subsequent anesthesia events. Tendon transfers and tenotomies are recommended for the patients with reducible curly toe deformity, while arthroplasties, arthrodesis procedures, and phalangectomies are reserved for patients with semi-rigid or rigid contractures.

Flexor-to-extensor tendon transfer has been popularized by Girdlestone and Taylor for treatment of claw toes in 1951 [32]. The procedure allows to recreate the dynamic pull of the intrinsic muscles and provides triplanar correction [33]. This procedure was shown to be effective for correction of central curly toes, 2, 3, and 4. The procedure is performed through a dorsolateral incision made over the extensor expansion. The long flexor is divided close to its insertion and transferred dorsolaterally, slightly distal to the extensor expansion, where it is attached under tension. Toe stiffness is a common side effect following this procedure [27].

Open or percutaneous flexor tenotomy may be preferred to flexor-to-extensor tendon transfer to avoid postoperative toe stiffness. The procedure is performed through a small transverse stab incision on the plantar aspect of the toe or a more extensive longitudinal incision [34]. The long and short flexor tendons are released, and the toe is pinned with a K-wire or taped in the corrected position. Studies comparing flexor-to-extensor transfer and flexor tenotomy procedures suggest similar success rates with both procedures, with patient satisfaction being higher with flexor tenotomy [27, 35]. This procedure is also preferred for treatment of the underlapping fifth toe, for which flexor-to-extensor tendon transfer is not indicated [31].

Treatment of a rigid or semi-rigid overlapping toe involves proximal interphalangeal joint arthroplasty or fusion with concomitant flexor tenotomy or transfer [31]. Dorsolateral closing wedge arthroplasty may be performed to shorten and derotate the digit [36]. The procedure may be supplemented with capsular releases and phalangeal osteotomies for corrections of severe deformities. Postoperatively, the toe is usually held reduced with a K-wire for 6 weeks to prevent loss of correction. Treatment of a rigid underlapping fifth toe represents a surgical challenge. No satisfactory solutions for this problem have been described as of yet.

Overlapping Toes

Overlapping toe is a congenital deformity characterized by adduction and hyperextension of the toe at metatarsophalangeal joint, which results in the toe overriding the adjacent digit. Fourth and fifth toes are most commonly involved [13]. The condition is seen bilaterally in about 25% of patients [37] and may be a source of considerable discomfort. The etiology of the deformity is not completely understood. Strong familial component has been implied. Tightness of dorsomedial capsule, ligaments, extensor tendon, and skin at the medial aspect of the digit is frequently noted [37].

As with curly toes, parents' education and reassurance are essential in treating small children. Depending on the severity of the deformity, crossover toes may remain asymptomatic, which is the case in about 50% of the patients [38]. Spontaneous resolution of the deformity when the child begins to walk occurs in about 15% of the cases [37].

Symptomatic patients complain of painful corns on both the overriding and the underriding digits, pain on the ball of the foot, footwear-related discomfort, and activity limitations. Non-operative treatment options include toe strapping, shoe gear accommodations, callus debridement, orthotics, and activity modification. The effectiveness of toe strapping is controversial [29, 30], but it may provide temporary relief by holding the toe in the reduced position while the patient is wearing shoes.

Surgical treatment options include soft tissue procedures, osseous corrections, and amputations. Soft tissue procedures are indicated for treatment of reducible deformities in younger patients and consist of skin plasties, soft tissue releases, and tendon transfers.

Dorsomedial skin contracture at the base of the overlapping toe can be addressed with V-to-Y skin plasty [39, 40], double-racquet incision [38], or syndactylization of the overlapping toe to the adjacent digit [41]. When performing a V-to-Y plasty, a V-shaped incision is placed over the dorsomedial base of the affected toe [40]. The apex of the incision is extended proximally to form a "Y" and is closed without tension. No high-quality outcome data on this technique is available, but in his small case series of 10 patients with overlapping 5th toes treated with a combination of V-to-Y skin plasty, capsulotomy, and extensor tenotomy, Paton reported deformity recurrence in 60% of the patients at 2 years mostly due to formation of the hypertrophic scar [40]. Double-racquet incision was described by Butler and consists of a circumferential incision around the base of the digit with plantar and dorsal handles, which allow for contracture release and skin closure [38]. In his retrospective case series of 36 pediatric patients with overriding 5th toe, Black reported excellent results in 78% of the patients. Potential complication of this procedure is neurovascular compromise, which can be avoided by employing meticulous dissection. Syndactylization of the overlapping toe with an adjacent toe (usually 4th and 5th toes) has been advocated for young children as a technically simple technique for permanent splinting of the overlapping toe. Good functional outcomes have been reported by Marek et al. [42]. In older children and adults with a more rigid deformity, concomitant phalangectomy is recommended [13]. Abnormal cosmetic appearance of the toe following the procedure may be a cause of dissatisfaction for the parents and the patient. Therefore, thorough pre-operative discussion with the parents and patient is recommended.

Extensor tendon lengthening or release, along with release of dorsomedial metatarsophalangeal joint capsule, is an important part of soft tissue correction for treatment of the overlapping toe. Lapidus reported excellent results with extensor stabilization consisting of transfer of the long extensor tendon to the abductor digiti minimi [43]. The drawbacks of the procedure are extensive dissection and postoperative toe stiffness.

Osteotomy or arthroplasty is indicated for treatment of the rigid overlapping toe deformity, which is usually seen in older patients. Complete proximal phalangectomy of the 5th toe has been described with mixed outcomes due to high incidence of overshortening of the toe leading to hammertoe deformity of the adjacent digit [13].

Amputation of the overlapping toe was popularized in the 1940s but subsequently drifted out of favor mostly due to cosmetic concerns. Amputation remains, however, a simple procedure with rapid functional recovery and effective pain relief [31]. Occasional complaints of prominent 5th metatarsal head leading to plantar lateral callus formation can be addressed with padding or possible osseous procedure of the metatarsal.

Digital Deformities and Genetic Syndromes

Congenital digital deformities may occur as an isolated condition or as a part of a known genetic syndrome. In some cases, digital deformities may be the most easily recognizable manifestations of a generalized genetic disorder. A foot and ankle surgeon may, therefore, be the first clinician to make the diagnosis and refer the patient for further evaluation. For this reason, general knowledge of genetic syndromes associated with digital pathology and understanding of the elements of history and clinical exam that may provide the necessary clues are very important. Below, we provide a brief review of the genetic syndromes associated with digital deformities.

Polydactyly is encountered in over 300 of well-characterized genetic syndromes [44, 45]. When it is a part of a generalized genetic condition, polydactyly can be seen in several generations and be bilateral and symmetrical [44]. Ellis-Van Creveld syndrome is an autosomal recessive condition characterized by postaxial polydactyly; dwarfism; dysplasia of nails, teeth, and gums; and congenital heart disease. About half of the patients die in early childhood due to cardiopulmonary complications. The rest of the patients may live well into the adulthood and be functional members of the society occupying variety of jobs despite their significant orthopedic malformations. Weiner reported on a large community of Amish patients with Ellis-Van Creveld living in rural Pennsylvania, who successfully participated in a variety of manual labor jobs [46].

Polydactyly is a commonly seen feature of Down syndrome, or Trisomy 21. Patients with this disorder suffer from intellectual and physical disability, generalized joint laxity, and hypotonia. Foot problems are very prevalent in this patient population, with up to 66% of patients experiencing foot pain daily [47]. Besides polydactyly, patients with Down syndrome often present with severe pes planus and hallux valgus [48]. The clinical exam of these patients is notable for reduced lower extremity muscle strength, apropulsive gait pattern, and postural instability [49]. Treatment approach to these patients should be focused on reducing pain and providing a stable weight-bearing platform. Multiple deformities may need to be addressed simultaneously instead of focusing on correcting just one specific deformity or one area of the foot.

Multiple syndactylies of the hands and feet are the hallmark of Apert's syndrome. The condition is very rare, with incidence of 1 case per 65,000 live births [50]. It is characterized by craniosynostosis, midfacial hypoplasia, syndactyly of all digits, and a broad thumb or hallux. Other common features seen in patients with Apert's are fusions between metatarsals and tarsal coalitions (Fig. 4.7) [51].

The extent and severity of a limb deformity dictates treatment approach. As is the case in patients with Down syndrome, the surgical goal for patients with Apert's syndrome is to provide

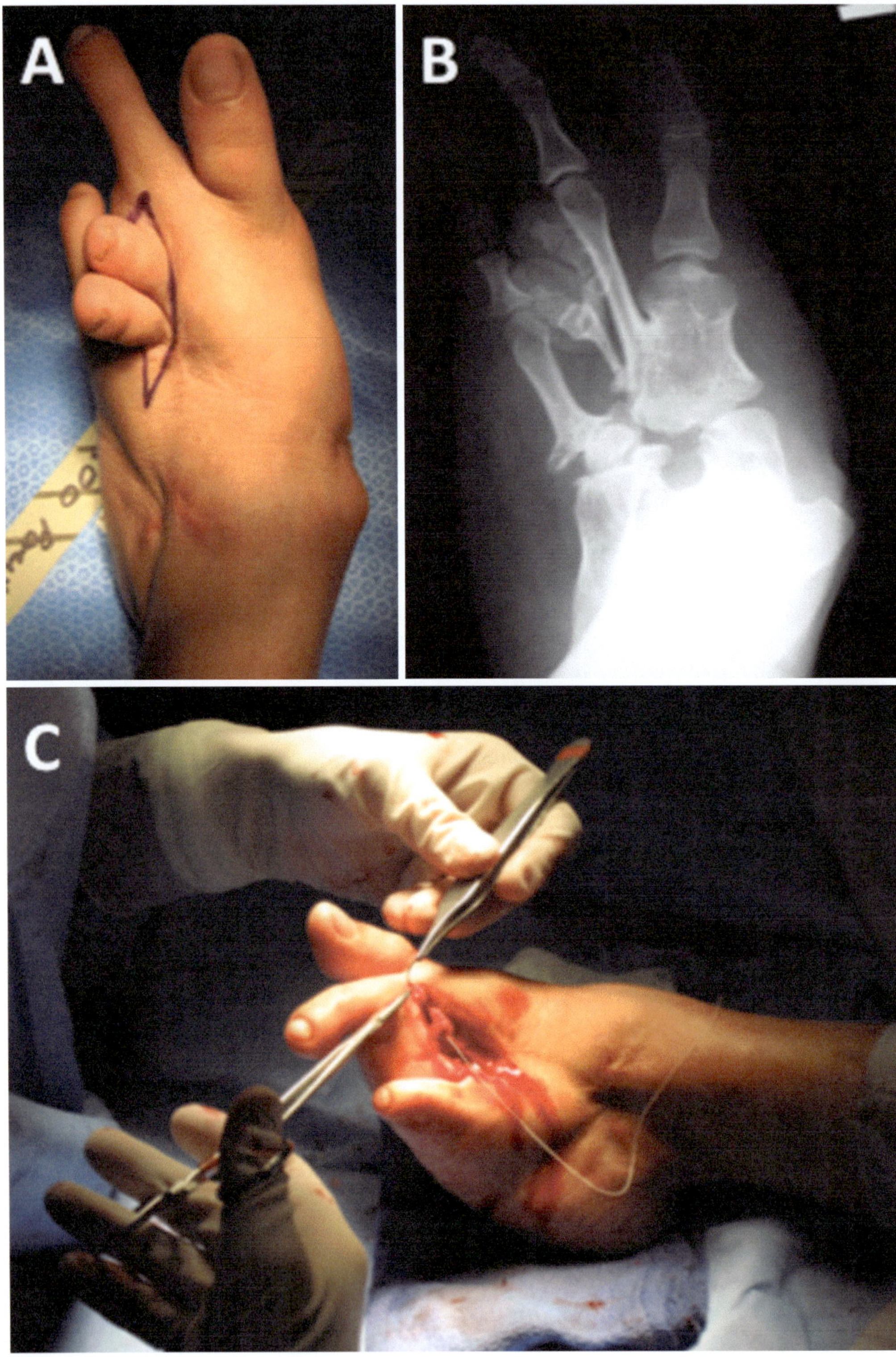

Fig. 4.7 (**a**) Clinical presentation of Apert's syndrome. (**b**) Abnormal configuration of forefoot and tarsal bones. (**c**) Amputation of digits

a stable pain-free platform for walking. Release of syndactylies is not recommended unless the syndactyly is associated with polydactyly [50]. Osteotomies and amputations are used to address a fixed deformity. As with majority of syndromes, addressing the whole foot instead of its specific parts is recommended to provide more functional results and avoid additional surgery.

Premature birth and low birth weight is associated with cerebral palsy. With increased survival rates of premature infants among neonatal intensive care units, clinicians may see more digital deformities linked to cerebral palsy and the equinus, equinovarus, or valgus deformities which can arise. Early intervention is key to assist with developmental delays while deformities of the foot and digits require individual evaluation.

References

1. Phelps DA, Grogan DP. Polydactyly of the foot. J Pediatr Orthop. 1985;5(4):446–51.
2. Fahim R, Thomas Z, DiDomenico LA. Pediatric forefoot pathology. Clin Podiatr Med Surg. 2013;30(4):479–90.
3. Frazier TM. A note on race-specific congenital malformation rates. Am J Obstet Gynecol. 1960;80:184–5.
4. Lee HS, Lee WC. Congenital lesser toe abnormalities. Foot Ankle Clin. 2011;16(4):659–78.
5. Temtamy S, McKusIcK V. Synopsis of hand malformations with particular emphasis on genetic factors. Birth Defects Orig Artic Ser. 1969;5(3):125–84.
6. Venn-Watson EA. Problems in polydactyly of the foot. Orthop Clin North Am. 1976;7(4):909–27.
7. Watanabe H, Fujita S, Oka I. Polydactyly of the foot: an analysis of 265 cases and a morphological classification. Plast Reconstr Surg. 1992;89(5):856–77.
8. Lee HS, Park SS, Yoon JO, Kim JS, Youm YS. Classification of postaxial polydactyly of the foot. Foot Ankle Int. 2006;27(5):356–62.
9. Morley SE, Smith PJ. Polydactyly of the feet in children: suggestions for surgical management. Br J Plast Surg. 2001;54(1):34–8.
10. Galois L, Mainard D, Delagoutte JP. Polydactyly of the foot. Literature review and case presentations. Acta Orthop Belg. 2002;68(4):376–80.
11. Christensen JC, Leff FB, Lepow GM, Schwartz RI, Colon PA, Arminio ST, et al. Congenital polydactyly and polymetatarsalia: classification, genetics, and surgical correction. 1981. J Foot Ankle Surg. 2011;50(3):336–9.
12. Osborn EJ, Davids JR, Leffler LC, Gibson TW, Pugh LI. Central polydactyly of the foot: surgical management with plantar and dorsal advancement flaps. J Pediatr Orthop. 2014;34(3):346–51.
13. Wagreich C. Congenital deformities. Banks A, Downey MS, Martin DE, Miller SJ, editor. Baltimore: Williams & Wilkins; 2001.
14. Davis JG, Syndactylism WJ. Arch Surg. 1930;21(1):32–75.
15. Lim YJ, Teoh LC, Lee EH. Reconstruction of syndactyly and polysyndactyly of the toes with a dorsal pentagonal island flap: a technique that allows primary skin closure without the use of skin grafting. J Foot Ankle Surg. 2007;46(2):86–92.
16. Itoh Y, Arai K. A new operation for syndactyly and polysyndactyly of the foot without skin grafts. Br J Plast Surg. 1995;48(5):306–11.
17. Kajikawa A, Ueda K, Katsuragi Y, Momiyama M, Horikiri M. Aesthetic repair for syndactyly of the toes using a plantar rectangular flap. Plast Reconstr Surg. 2010;126(1):156–62.
18. Hop MJ, van der Biezen JJ. Ray reduction of the foot in the treatment of macrodactyly and review of the literature. J Foot Ankle Surg. 2011;50(4):434–8.
19. Barsky AJ. Macrodactyly. J Bone Joint Surg Am. 1967;49(7):1255–66.
20. Inglis K. Local gigantism (a manifestation of neurofibromatosis): its relation to general gigantism and to acromegaly; illustrating the influence of intrinsic factors in disease when development of the body is abnormal. Am J Pathol. 1950;26(6):1059–83.
21. Kalen V, Burwell DS, Omer GE. Macrodactyly of the hands and feet. J Pediatr Orthop. 1988;8(3):311–5.
22. Chang CH, Kumar SJ, Riddle EC, Glutting J. Macrodactyly of the foot. J Bone Joint Surg Am. 2002;84-A(7):1189–94.
23. Krengel S, Fustes-Morales A, Carrasco D, Vazquez M, Duran-McKinster C, Ruiz-Maldonado R. Macrodactyly: report of eight cases and review of the literature. Pediatr Dermatol. 2000;17(4):270–6.
24. Tsuge K. Treatment of macrodactyly. Plast Reconstr Surg. 1967;39(6):590–9.
25. Kotwal PP, Farooque M. Macrodactyly. J Bone Joint Surg. 1998;80(4):651–3.
26. Topoleski TA, Ganel A, Grogan DP. Effect of proximal phalangeal epiphysiodesis in the treatment of macrodactyly. Foot Ankle Int. 1997;18(8):500–3.
27. Pollard JP, Morrison PJ. Flexor tenotomy in the treatment of curly toes. Proc R Soc Med. 1975;68(8):480–1.
28. Downey MRL. Common pediatric digital deformities. In: DV S, editor. Foot and ankle disorders in children. St. Louis: Mosby; 1992.
29. Smith WG, Seki J, Smith RW. Prospective study of a noninvasive treatment for two common congenital toe abnormalities (curly/varus/underlapping toes and overlapping toes). Paediatr Child Health. 2007;12(9):755–9.

30. Turner PL. Strapping of curly toes in children. Aust N Z J Surg. 1987;57(7):467–70.
31. Talusan PG, Milewski MD, Reach JS Jr. Fifth toe deformities: overlapping and underlapping toe. Foot Ankle Spec. 2013;6(2):145–9.
32. Taylor RG. The treatment of claw toes by multiple transfers of flexor into extensor tendons. J Bone Joint Surg. 1951;33-B(4):539–42.
33. Biyani A, Jones DA, Murray JM. Flexor to extensor tendon transfer for curly toes. 43 children reviewed after 8 (1-25) years. Acta Orthop Scand. 1992;63(4):451–4.
34. Ross ER, Menelaus MB. Open flexor tenotomy for hammer toes and curly toes in childhood. J Bone Joint Surg. 1984;66(5):770–1.
35. Hamer AJ, Stanley D, Smith TW. Surgery for curly toe deformity: a double-blind, randomised, prospective trial. J Bone Joint Surg. 1993;75(4):662–3.
36. Choi JY, Park HJ, Suh JS. Operative treatment for fourth curly toe deformity in adults. Foot Ankle Int. 2015;36(9):1089–94
37. Murgier J, Knorr J, Soldado F, Bayle-iniguez X, Sales de Gauzy J. Percutaneous correction of congenital overlapping fifth toe in paediatric patients. Orthop Traumatol Surg Res. 2013;99(6):737–40.
38. Black GB, Grogan DP, Bobechko WP. Butler arthroplasty for correction of the adducted fifth toe: a retrospective study of 36 operations between 1968 and 1982. J Pediatr Orthop. 1985;5(4):439–41.
39. Wilson JN. V-Y correction for varus deformity of the fifth toe. Br J Surg. 1953;41(166):133–5.
40. Paton RW. V-Y plasty for correction of varus fifth toe. J Pediatr Orthop. 1990;10(2):248–9.
41. Leonard MH, Rising EE. Syndactylization to maintain correction of overlapping 5th toe. Clin Orthop Relat Res. 1965;43:241–3.
42. Marek L, Giacopelli J, Granoff D. Syndactylization for the treatment of fifth toe deformities. J Am Podiatr Med Assoc. 1991;81(5):248–52.
43. Lapidus PW. Transplantation of the extensor tendon for correction of the overlapping fifth toe. J Bone Joint Surg. 1942;25:555–9.
44. Malik S. Polydactyly: phenotypes, genetics and classification. Clin Genet. 2014;85(3):203–12.
45. Biesecker LG. Polydactyly: how many disorders and how many genes? 2010 update. Dev Dyn. 2011;240(5):931–42.
46. Weiner DS, Jonah D, Leighley B, Dicintio MS, Holmes Morton D, Kopits S. Orthopaedic manifestations of chondroectodermal dysplasia: the Ellis-van Creveld syndrome. J Child Orthop. 2013;7(6):465–76.
47. Pikora TJ, Bourke J, Bathgate K, Foley KR, Lennox N, Leonard H. Health conditions and their impact among adolescents and young adults with Down syndrome. PLoS One. 2014;9(5):e96868.
48. Lim PQ, Shields N, Nikolopoulos N, Barrett JT, Evans AM, Taylor NF, et al. The association of foot structure and footwear fit with disability in children and adolescents with Down syndrome. Journal of foot and ankle research. 2015;8:4.
49. Galli M, Cimolin V, Pau M, Costici P, Albertini G. Relationship between flat foot condition and gait pattern alterations in children with Down syndrome. J Intellect Disabil Res. 2014;58(3):269–76.
50. Fearon JA. Treatment of the hands and feet in Apert syndrome: an evolution in management. Plast Reconstr Surg. 2003;112(1):1–12; discussion 3–9.
51. Collins ED, Marsh JL, Vannier MW, Gilula LA. Spatial dysmorphology of the foot in Apert syndrome: three-dimensional computed tomography. Cleft Palate Craniofac J. 1995;32(3):255–61; discussion 62.

Pediatric Brachymetatarsia

5

Bradley M. Lamm, Emily D. Pugh, and Jessica M. Knight

Introduction

Brachymetatarsia is a condition that occurs when the epiphyseal growth plate in one or more metatarsals closes prematurely, causing anatomic shortening. The fourth metatarsal is most commonly affected, and when more than one metatarsal is involved, the condition is termed brachymetapody. The fourth digit tends to sit elevated on the dorsum of the foot causing pain, calluses, and irritation along with other associated clinical concerns (Fig. 5.1). Acute and gradual lengthening are both employed in surgical correction of brachymetatarsia, and when length of 1 cm or more is desired, gradual lengthening with external fixation, termed distraction osteogenesis, is preferred [1].

The condition arises from congenital, acquired, or idiopathic origin. Acquired short metatarsals are caused by trauma, infection, tumor, Freiberg's disease, radiation, or surgery, which can be associated with skeletal and systemic abnormalities such as sickle cell anemia, multiple epiphyseal dysplasia, multiple hereditary exostosis, and juvenile rheumatoid arthritis. Acquired brachymetatarsia is mainly unilateral in presentation, whereas congenital brachymetatarsia is more often bilateral and associated with other skeletal abnormalities [1, 2].

Brachymetatarsia brought about through iatrogenic means during surgery may be due to osteotomies of the metatarsals, traversing the physis during fixation, and internal or external fixation inducing either premature growth arrest or synostosis between metatarsals. A malpositioned first metatarsal following bunion surgery or an overly aggressive first metatarsal medial cuneiform arthrodesis can also result in an iatrogenically short first metatarsal [1, 2].

Treatment of brachymetatarsia involves managing the symptomatic biomechanical issues as well as cosmetic and psychological concerns. Clinical issues include dorsal displacement of the affected toe, painful corns and calluses, toe dysplasia including a short phalanx, and transfer metatarsalgia. Shoeing can pose difficulty due to the high riding toe on the dorsum of the foot, which produces plantar metatarsal head calluses and dorsal digital corns [1, 3]. The adjacent digits tend to deviate into the position of the short toe, creating deformities of these digits. Windswept deformity of the digits with resulting bunion deformity is seen in cases of long-standing

B. M. Lamm (✉)
Foot and Ankle Deformity Center and Fellowship, Paley Orthopedic and Spine Institute at St. Mary's Medical Center and Palm Beach Childerns Hospital, West Palm Beach, FL, USA

E. D. Pugh
Foot and Ankle Surgeon, Harvard Vanguard Medical Associates, Wellesley, MA, USA

J. M. Knight
Weil Foot and Ankle Institute, Northwest Community Hospital Medical Group, Arlington Heights, IL, USA

M. L. Butterworth, J. T. Marcoux (eds.), *The Pediatric Foot and Ankle*,
https://doi.org/10.1007/978-3-030-29788-6_5

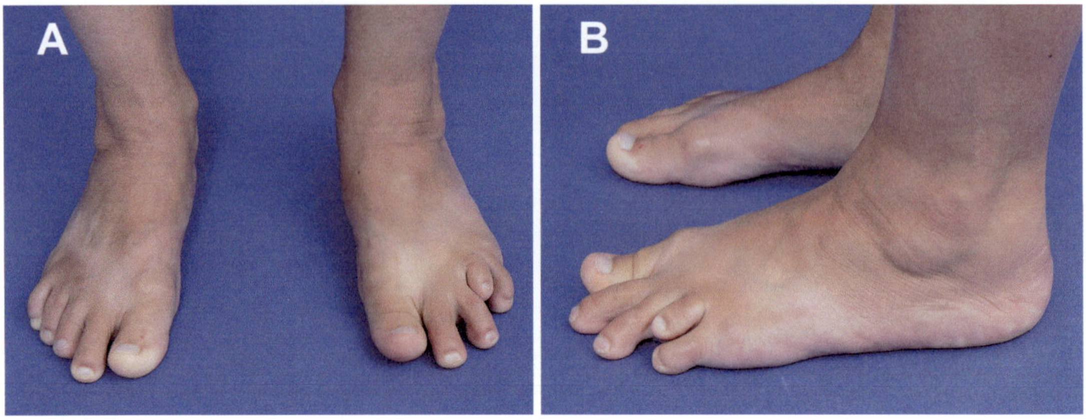

Fig. 5.1 Clinical preoperative photograph of a congenital short fourth metatarsal on the left. Note the elevation and dorsal displacement of the fourth digit. (**a**) Front view. (**b**) Side view

brachymetatarsia as the digits assume a global transverse deviation. Surgery to lengthen the metatarsal can address the root of these deformities while also thus improving cosmesis and decreasing associated pain; once lengthening has been adequately achieved, further operative fine-tuning can rebalance the foot by addressing accompanying deformities [4].

Incidence

The prevalence has been reported to be anywhere from 1 in 1820 to 1 in 4586 [5, 6] in the lesser metatarsals and 1 in 10,000 in the first metatarsal [7]. Females are affected more frequently with a female-to-male ratio of 25:1 [6], and the condition occurs bilaterally in 72% of patients [8]. Brachymetatarsia is either isolated or associated with systemic syndromes, endocrinopathies, or dysplasias including polydactyly and syndactyly.

Clinical Evaluation

Because brachymetatarsia often coexists with other skeletal or systemic abnormalities, obtaining a detailed patient history is critical. In the absence of a concomitant systemic diagnosis, the patient should undergo a complete medical evaluation prior to surgical intervention. Performing a comprehensive clinical examination of the lower extremity is crucial in evaluating the affected metatarsals and identifying potential coexisting deformities.

Specific maneuvers in the clinical evaluation are employed in both weightbearing and nonweightbearing exams. In weightbearing stance, the affected digit's elevation is observed with the foot flat and again with the foot in the propulsive phase of gait in order to determine its purchase (or lack thereof) on the weightbearing surface (Fig. 5.2). With the foot nonweightbearing, plantarflexing the MTPJ's simultaneously renders the metatarsal heads prominent through the dorsal skin, thereby displaying the metatarsal heads in their natural parabola. Thorough examination of the skin should also be performed for the assessment of callus patterns, which provide useful information regarding load distribution.

A dorsally displaced digit typically accompanies the congenitally short metatarsal; this occurs as the child develops, and the shortened metatarsal attempts to contact the ground at the same level as the adjacent metatarsal heads. This increased declination of the metatarsal head results in retrograde buckling at the MTPJ, producing dorsal displacement of the associated digit. The abnormal digital alignment causes calluses at the dorsal PIPJ of the elevated digit. When the first metatarsal is involved, the increased metatarsal declination also produces more plantar pressure beneath the metatarsal head, resulting in a plantar callus and cavus foot.

Compensatory soft tissue contracture at the MTPJ should be evaluated by manually plan-

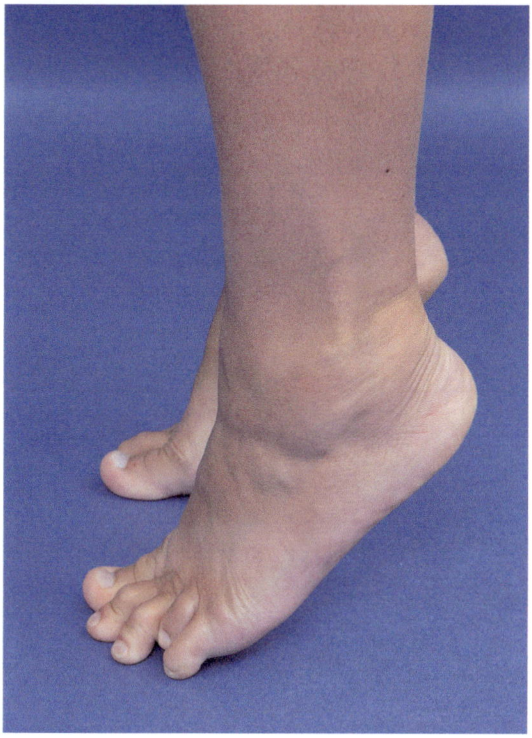

Fig. 5.2 Clinical preoperative photograph of a congenital short fourth metatarsal with the foot positioned in the propulsive phase of gait; note the fourth digit's lack of purchase during propulsion

tarflexing the joint to assess its reducibility and potential for realignment. The Kelikian push-up test is performed to simulate weightbearing by loading the lateral column of a non-weightbearing foot. Only when simulated weightbearing is achieved can the digital reducibility be tested. Just as isolated hammertoe deformities have varying levels of reducibility, the stiffness of hammertoe deformities occurring concomitantly with brachymetatarsia ranges from flexible to semirigid to non-reducible. Reducible digits allow for plantarflexion at the proximal phalanx, which brings the toe plantigrade. Semi-reducible deformities prohibit plantarflexion at the MTPJ, which prevent the digit from being plantigrade. Non-reducible deformities also prohibit plantarflexion at the MTPJ with the difference being that the digit is entirely dislocated. In these cases, a complete MTPJ release including dorsal capsulotomy, medial and lateral collateral ligament release, extensor tendon lengthening, and plantar plate release is recommended. A partial MTPJ release with a dorsal capsulotomy should be performed for reducible deformities. Arthroplasty and arthrodesis are counterproductive as these will shorten an already shortened toe. Typically it is not necessary to lengthen the combined extensor tendon of the toe when the fixator is placed. In some cases, this may be done after lengthening. The placement of digital half-pins to bridge the external fixator across the MTPJ allows the digit to remain in its anatomic position during and after lengthening [9].

Radiographic Evaluation

A key component in the preoperative workup of any brachymetatarsia correction is a thorough radiographic evaluation. The affected metatarsals typically exhibit slight deviation in both the sagittal and transverse planes; therefore, obtaining standard weightbearing views for bilateral feet allows for multiplanar analysis of the short metatarsals, which is critical for preoperative planning of external fixation placement and osteotomy level.

The anteroposterior (AP) radiograph is ideal for the evaluation of the metatarsal parabola, which is the angle formed by connecting the distal articular surfaces of the first, second, and fifth metatarsals (Fig. 5.3a). The parabola is quantitatively measured as an angle formed between a line connecting the distal ends of the first and second metatarsals and a line connecting the distal ends of the second and fifth metatarsals. The angle between these two lines is defined as the metatarsal parabola angle (normal = 142.5°). Deviation from this normal value indicates that one or more elongated or shortened metatarsals are present. Bilateral radiographs are helpful when assessing patients with multiple short metatarsals. Additionally, the AP view is used to measure first metatarsal protrusion distance (normal = 2 mm plus or minus), which is defined as the distance between the most distal points of the second and first metatarsals. Finally, the transverse plane deviation of the short metatarsal is also important to assess. While brachymetatarsia of the first and second metatarsals usually lacks

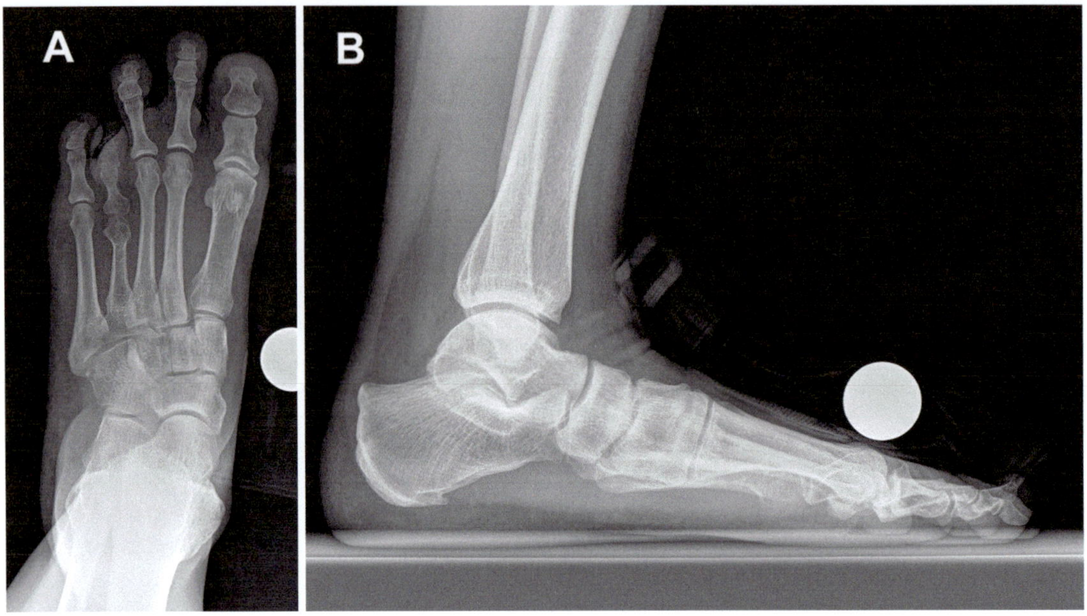

Fig. 5.3 Preoperative left foot radiographs of a congenitally short fourth metatarsal. (**a**) AP view. (**b**) Lateral view

any transverse plan deformity, affected third and fourth metatarsals typically have a slight medial bow. To assess for this bowing, the fourth intermetatarsal angle (normal = 8–10°) is employed. When lengthening a metatarsal with a slight medial bow, an accurate vector of lengthening is critical. Not taking this bowing into account may result in encroachment of the metatarsal heads and transverse deviation of the digit with subsequent pain.

On the lateral radiograph, increased declination of the affected metatarsal is appreciated at the distal metaphyseal diaphyseal junction (region of the previous growth plate), which can result in a flexion deformity of the distal metatarsal (Fig. 5.3b). The corresponding proximal phalanx of the short metatarsal is therefore dorsally displaced secondary to the soft tissue adaptation to a shorten metatarsal [3]. The short metatarsal declination defines the plane of lengthening as the half-pins of the external fixation device are mounted perpendicular to the longitudinal bisection of the metatarsal in the sagittal plane.

Preoperative planning is important to identify the amount of metatarsal length necessary to reestablish the metatarsal parabola. Predication of the metatarsal length discrepancy also provides an accurate calculation of the number of days required for lengthening. Measuring the length discrepancy is accomplished by drawing the metatarsal parabola angle and measuring the longitudinal distance between the most distal point on the affected metatarsal head to the metatarsal parabola line. The amount of length needed is then doubled to determine the approximate number of days required for the lengthening phase of the treatment (0.5 mm/day). For example, if the amount of metatarsal length needed to reestablish the metatarsal parabola is 20 mm, the amount of time required to obtain this length would be approximately 40 days based on the desired distraction rate of 0.5 mm per day. The latency phase (5 days) is then added to this to calculate the total duration of the lengthening phase (45 days).

The rate of distraction may need to be adjusted, however, during the postoperative period depending on the course of the lengthening phase, and therefore patient education is paramount. The consolidation period typically takes at least the same amount of time as the lengthening phase or longer. Consolidation time is variable but typically ranges from 2 to 4 months [9].

Lamm Classification of Brachymetatarsia

Throughout the author's vast experience in surgical correction of brachymetatarsia, there have been discrete types of deformity noted within the affected ray. These deformities range from purely shortened length of the metatarsal to irregularities of specific regions of the bone, including the shaft, joint and head. Three broad categories exist: type A includes those metatarsals that are normal in all respects aside from their shortened length; type B involves angulation of the shaft of the affected metatarsal; and type C, congruency of MTP joint which is associated with MTPJ imbalances and metatarsal head and phalangeal base irregularity. The classification system provides one number (1, 2, 3, 4, 5) and 3 letters (A, B, C). The number indicates which metatarsal is short or hypoplastic. For example, 1 would indicate the first metatarsal, and 4 would indicate the fourth metatarsal.

Treatment Options

Procedures to treat brachymetatarsia attempt not only to lengthen the metatarsal but to restore the metatarsal parabola and maintain or improve foot and digital function, thereby decreasing pain [9–15]. Two primary surgical techniques have been devised for the correction of brachymetatarsia: acute and gradual lengthening. Acute metatarsal lengthening (one-stage) is performed with or without insertion of bone graft and can be employed in cases where less than 1 cm of length is desired. Gradual lengthening involves placement of an external fixator with distraction osteogenesis. Other techniques include lengthening the short metatarsals and shortening the long metatarsal with or without bone graft, insertion of synthetic implant, slide osteotomy with or without bone graft, and amputation of the digit [12].

The distraction osteogenesis method of metatarsal lengthening (callus distraction), while preferred for lengthening of 1 cm or more [1], may offer distinct advantages over acute lengthening regardless of the desired length [16]. Callus distraction reduces the risk of neurovascular compromise due to the simultaneous gradual stretch on the tendons, nerves, and vessels compared with acute lengthening, which can cause severe acute soft tissue stretch [1, 2]. Bone grafting and donor site morbidity are completely avoided since distraction osteogenesis allows for natural regenerate bone formation.

Patients may prefer distraction osteogenesis for multiple reasons, one of which may include the ability to have input regarding the final length obtained. Another primary advantage of having an external fixator device is the means to be weightbearing as tolerated in a surgical shoe and shower throughout the entire course of treatment, additionally, due to the minimally invasive nature of the procedure and absence of a large surgical incision.

Gradual distraction has been shown to have the lowest incidence of complications when compared to acute lengthening [17, 18] and is the preferred technique in cases where previous reconstructive procedures have failed due to its relatively predictable nature [19]. The technique can be performed in a minimally invasive fashion via percutaneous metatarsal osteotomy, which preserves the periosteum and decreases adjacent soft tissue disruption, thereby maximizing the healing potential and minimizing scarring [4]. Gradual lengthening has been undertaken by multiple forms of external fixators, including mini-Hoffman, Ilizarov semicircular, and monolateral devices [20–23].

Postoperative stiffness of the MTPJ is one inherent risk accompanying distraction osteogenesis, which commonly results from compression to the joint during the lengthening phase [24, 25]. As the amount of metatarsal lengthening increases, so does the risk for subluxation and stiffness to the MTPJ. To decrease the risk of postoperative stiffness, the forces exerted on the joint must be lessened; this can be accomplished by spanning the MTPJ with a second external fixator as first described by Lamm in 2010 and outlined in the following section.

Surgical Technique

The patient is positioned supine on a radiolucent table with a bump under the hemisacrum, obtaining a foot forward position. Preoperative planning with a four-pin small external fixator determines the initial spread and locations of the pins. The half-pins are placed in a bicortical fashion percutaneously under fluoroscopy, perpendicular to the shaft of the metatarsal.

The first half-pin is placed at the metaphyseal-diaphyseal junction as distal as possible. Under fluoroscopic guidance on a lateral view, a 1.8 mm wire is inserted percutaneously to predrill the hole concentrically, perpendicular to the metatarsal. Then a stab incision is made adjacent to the wire with subsequent replacement of the wire with a 2.5 mm half-pin, usually measuring 70 mm in total length and 20 mm of thread length. This first pin determines the plane of lengthening because the fixator is then mounted in a perpendicular fashion. Care is taken to ensure that metatarsal head's final position is located at the appropriate level in the sagittal plane. On a lateral view radiograph, the dorsal cortex of the short metatarsal is parallel to the adjacent metatarsals, and therefore placing perpendicular half-pins accurately positions the metatarsal head. When closely evaluating the lateral radiograph, an increased fourth metatarsal declination is noted at the level of the distal metaphyseal-diaphyseal junction (region of the growth plate). This distal flexion deformity of the metatarsal head produces an extension contracture of the toe.

To ensure sufficient lengthening potential, the external fixator is set so that the lengthening bar is long enough to accommodate the desired metatarsal length. In cases where the affected metatarsal is excessively short, spanning the Lisfranc joint may be necessary by placing the most proximal half-pin proximal to the metatarsal base.

The second half-pin that is inserted into the base of the metatarsal is the most proximal of all four half-pins. It is just distal to the Lisfranc joint and situated so that it is parallel to the first pin in both the sagittal and transverse planes. Insertion occurs in a similar fashion as the first half-pin, with a percutaneous 1.8 mm wire used as a predrill for half-pin placement. This second half-pin is critical in establishing the direction of metatarsal lengthening as two fixed points determine a line and is important because it determines the final position of the metatarsal head in the transverse plan. Thus, bending the wire distally and superimposing the wire on the distal half-pin determines the direction of planned lengthening. This placement is important to ensure the metatarsal is not lengthened into an adjacent metatarsal. The proximal half-pin is moved slightly medially or laterally in the base of the metatarsal to adjust the alignment prior to completing the predrill hole. Also, this second half-pin (25 mm thread length and 70 mm pin length) determines the position of the most proximal half-pin duo and thus indirectly determines the osteotomy level. Therefore, the more proximal this second pin is placed, the closer the level of the osteotomy will be to the metaphysis; this is preferable, as a diaphyseal osteotomy requires a longer consolidation phase.

The third pin is placed just distal to the second pin at the base of the fourth metatarsal, and the fourth and final pin placed is placed just proximal to the first pin in the shaft. The third and fourth half-pins are placed in the same fashion as the previous two half-pins, utilizing a 1.8 mm wire as a predrill. The third and fourth predrill holes are performed through the pin guide provided in the small external fixator set. This ensure accurate and parallel placement of the remaining half-pins.

Two threaded pins 1.6 mm in diameter are then placed into the base of the proximal phalanx through two small percutaneous dorsal stab incisions. These two pins are inserted through the second external fixation pin clamp mounted distally on the distraction bar. The proximal phalanx pins are mounted in approximately 15° of flexion as compared to the metatarsal declination. A maximum dorsiflexion lateral digital fluoroscopic view is obtained to determine proper pin placement. The two phalangeal threaded pins are connected to the external fixator after the osteotomy is performed.

A 5 mm incision is made using a number 15 blade between the two metatarsal half-pin clusters, just distal to the most proximal set of pins and lateral to the affected metatarsal at the level of the proximal metaphyseal-diaphyseal junction. A straight hemostat is used to dissect down to the metatarsal, avoiding periosteal disruption. To begin the osteotomy, a 1.8 mm wire is used to drill multiple orthogonal holes into the metatarsal under fluoroscopic control. A small Hoke osteotome is then used to complete the osteotomy without producing excessive osteotomy displacement, which can tear the periosteum. Application of the preset external fixator with subsequent tightening of the device reduces the osteotomy and positions the metatarsal in both sagittal and AP view upon checking with fluoroscopy.

Two 1.6 mm threaded pins in the proximal phalanx are attached to a fixation block on a second small external fixator, which is piggybacked onto the primary fixator. The toe is then manually reduced, and the distal pin block is attached to the distraction bar. This is utilized to maintain a neutral toe position and to protect the MTPJ from subluxation and compression during lengthening. About 3 mm of acute distraction at MTPJ is then executed. While manually loading the foot (push-up test), the toe is reduced into a rectus position and the pin clamp is tightened. By incorporating distraction of the MTPJ into the construct, postoperative stiffness is decreased. Additionally, performing the osteotomy at the proximal metaphyseal-diaphyseal junction decreases the forces directly exerted onto the MTPJ.

Once both fixators are applied and final position checked via fluoroscopic imaging on both AP and lateral views, the incision is closed and a compressive wrap dressing is applied around all six pins. Postoperatively, the patient is allowed immediate weightbearing as tolerated in a wooden bottom surgical shoe. Bilateral brachymetatarsia is addressed in one surgical setting, and immediate weightbearing as tolerated in wooden bottom surgical shoes is permitted.

Distraction is begun after a latency period of 5–7 days. Once distraction begins, it should typically occur at a rate of 0.25 mm twice per day, although this rate and the duration of the latency period are adjusted according to multiple factors, including age and health of patient, technique, and location of osteotomy. Follow-up should occur every 2 weeks during the lengthening phase of treatment, with serial radiographs taken to assess progress. Once adequate length has been achieved, the consolidation period commences and its duration depends on multiple factors; these include location of osteotomy, age of the patient, medical health status, medications, tobacco use, and the rate and amount of lengthening. The typical consolidation period ranges from 2 to 4 months. Once the fixator is removed, weightbearing as tolerated in a surgical shoe ensues for an additional 4 weeks to ensure healing of the pin sites.

It should be noted that the first and second consecutive half-pins each determine an important aspect of alignment. The first pin is placed into the neck of the metatarsal, perpendicular to the metatarsal axis; therefore, this pin is the primary determining factor in sagittal plane lengthening. Since the half-pin is perpendicular to the metatarsal shaft and the short metatarsal declination angle is normal, the final position of the metatarsal head will become level with the adjacent metatarsals. The second half-pin determines the direction or vector of metatarsal lengthening, as it takes two points to define a line. It is important that the vector of metatarsal lengthening be such that the final position of the metatarsal head is located at the appropriate level between the third and fifth metatarsals [4]. Figures 5.4, 5.5, 5.6, and 5.7 shows the postoperative clinical and radiographic results.

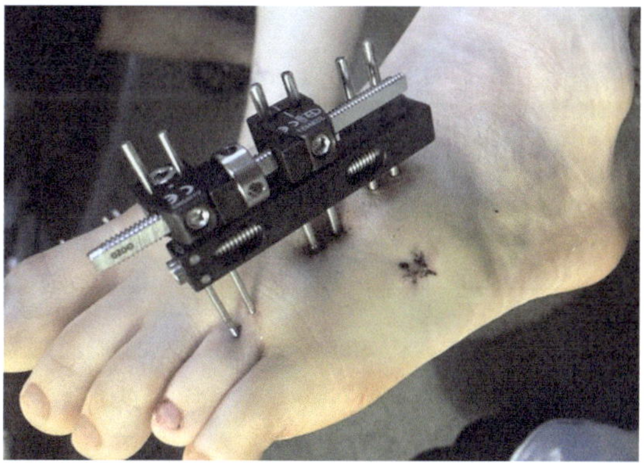

Fig. 5.4 Postoperative clinical photograph showing a fixator applied to the fourth metatarsal and fourth toe. Note spanning of the fourth metatarsal phangeal joint provides toe realignment and protection

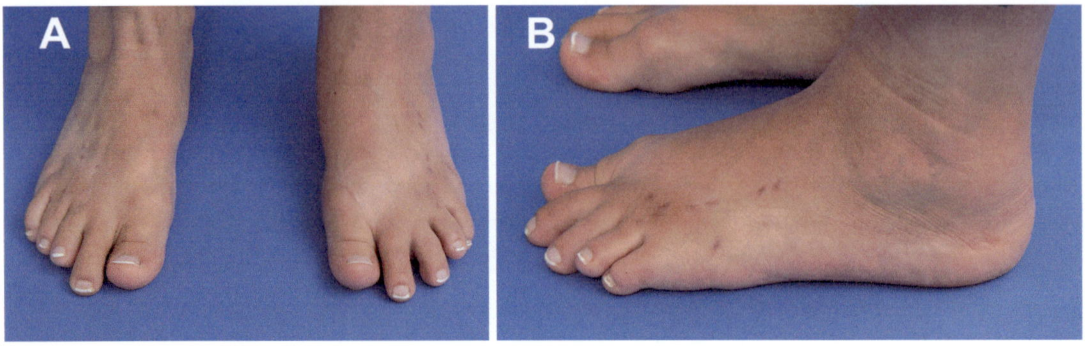

Fig. 5.5 Postoperative clinical photographs showing reduction of the previously elevated and dorsally displaced fourth digit. (**a**) Front view. (**b**) Side view

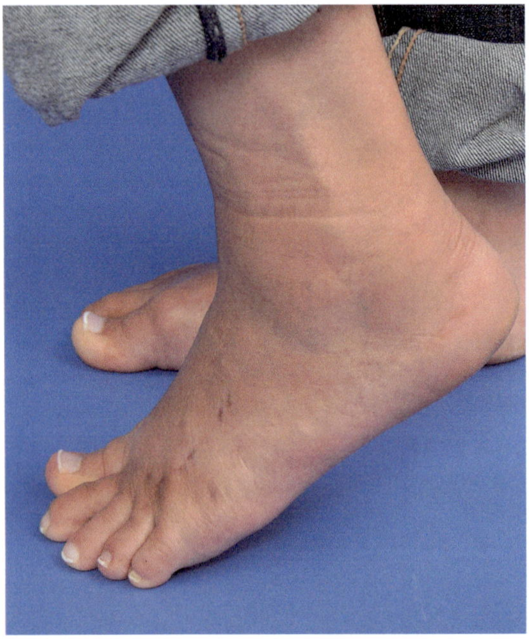

Fig. 5.6 Clinical postoperative photograph of a congenital short fourth metatarsal with the foot positioned in the propulsive phase of gait; note increased purchase of the fourth digit during propulsion as well as the degree of motion at the MTPJ

Complications

Callus distraction with external fixation is successful in restoring the length of the metatarsal as well as achieving adequate toe position and maintaining function at the MTPJ. Despite continual advances in this technique, complications inherent to the use of external fixation and those unique to brachymetatarsia can arise. These include digital contractures, malalignment in the transverse and sagittal planes, over- or under-lengthening, nonunion/malunion or delayed union, premature consolidation, metatarsalgia, MTPJ stiffness, and pin site infection [9, 26].

Digital Contractures

During the process of bone lengthening, the adjacent musculature generates tension, which can lead to joint contractures. The intrinsic plantar muscles of the foot when under tension during the distraction process can cause the digit to become plantarflexed at the MTPJ. As the amount of metatarsal lengthening increases, the amount of muscular tension also increases, which produces a greater influence on the toe. Patients with brachymetatarsia initially present with a dorsally displaced toe and dorsal contracture of the MTPJ. By bridging the MTPJ, joint alignment and position of the digit are controlled [9, 26].

Malalignment

Failure to achieve accurate placement of the first half-pin (most distal) or the second half-pin (most proximal) may result in malalignment in either the transverse or sagittal plane. Transverse plane deformity occurs when the head of the lengthened bone is not spaced equally between the adjacent

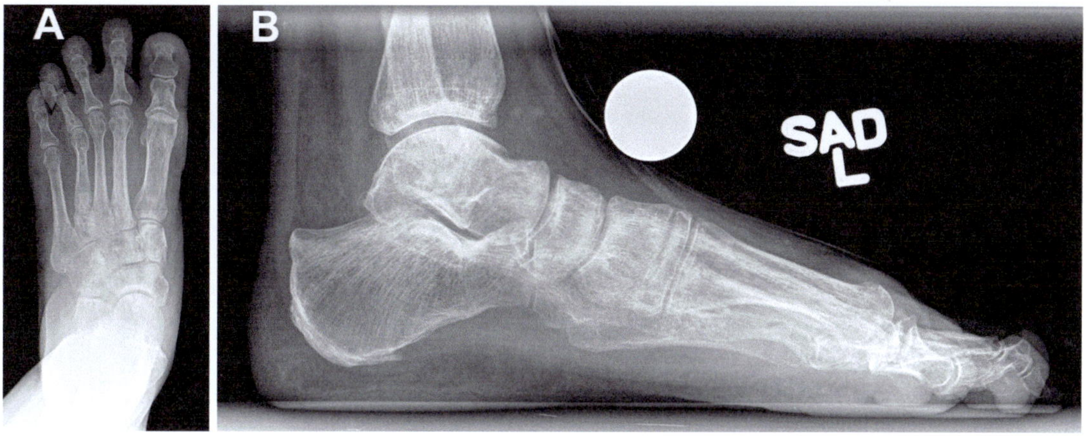

Fig. 5.7 Postoperative left foot radiographs of a congenitally short fourth metatarsal after callus distraction. (**a**) AP view. (**b**) Lateral view

metatarsals, which results in capsular or collateral ligament instability. This can induce soft tissue impingement as well as transverse plane deviation of the corresponding digit. More commonly, the deviation in the transverse plane occurs secondary to overlengthening of the metatarsal.

In the sagittal plane dorsiflexion or plantarflexion at the MPTJ may incite metatarsalgia and digital deformity. Creating a plantigrade metatarsal head in the sagittal plane provides the necessary realignment for normal pedal function [26].

Overlengthening/Underlengthening

Maintaining adequate postoperative follow-up is critical to avoid over- or underlengthening of the metatarsal. The recommended interval between appointments and serial x-rays is 2 weeks to properly assess progress. Inadequate restoration of the metatarsal parabola may cause pain and secondary digital deformities. Lengthening of the first metatarsal more than 40% of its original length has been reported to create a cavus deformity after distraction osteogenesis [10, 26].

Nonunion/Malunion

Nonunion, malunion, or delayed union of the metatarsal may occur despite the minimally invasive nature of percutaneous osteotomy technique and its known benefits for bone regenerate. Delayed consolidation may result from intraoperative events including traumatic corticotomy, excessively rapid distraction, and unstable external fixation configuration. Minimizing damage to the periosteum and endosteum during surgery decreases the risk of delayed consolidation. Additionally, factors intrinsic to the patient should be addressed preoperatively, including nutritional status, smoking, and hypoparathyroidism. Postoperative incidents such as infection and trauma to the construct may also produce delayed consolidation. Treatment entails the use of an external bone stimulator with concomitant use of nutritional supplements containing calcium and vitamin D [26].

Premature Consolidation

Without correct external fixation adjustments, premature consolidation may occur; typically, this happens when the rate of distraction is too slow. Other causes may include incomplete osteotomy during surgery as well as prolonged latency following application of the external fixator [27].

Repeat osteotomy may be necessary to correct premature consolidation, and this should take place at a separate location from the original osteotomy site. Alternatively, increasing the distraction phase of treatment may also resolve the issue [26].

Metatarsalgia

If proper length of the metatarsal is not achieved, the resulting underlengthening or overlengthening may result in metatarsalgia or MTPJ stiffness [25, 28]. The final sagittal plane position of the metatarsal can feel prominent to the patient and create pain, which occurs in overlengthening. Deformity and stiffness at the MTPJ can arise from overlengthening; although pinning the digit prevents MTPJ subluxation, it may also lead to stiffness [9].

Pin Site Infection

A known complication of any external fixation device is a pin site infection, and these usually resolve with a course of oral antibiotics [2]. Infections generally develop from the outside to inside [27] and can be minimized by ensuring maintaining sufficient pin stability. Dressings including sterile gauze and Ilizarov sponges function as protective barriers between the skin and the outside environment. Tightly dressing the pin sites with sterile gauze prevents pistoning of the skin on the pin, which happens with transient edema, thereby inhibiting inflammation at the pin site. Educating patients in the preoperative setting on proper pin care techniques is critical to decrease the risk of infection. When a pin site infection goes untreated, spread of the infection from soft tissues to the bone may occur and treatment with IV antibiotics or operative debridement and pin removal may become necessary [26].

Conclusion

Future directions in the surgical correction of brachymetatarsia through distraction osteogenesis may involve internal lengthening methods that have been developed for the femur and tibia. Until such time occurs, the callus distraction method of gradual correction has been shown to reliably and safely lengthen the metatarsal while maintaining adequate position of the adjacent digit by spanning the MTPJ with external fixation. Provided a stable fixation construct is applied and regular follow-up scheduled, patients can successfully achieve restoration of a normal metatarsal parabola and proper digital alignment and function.

References

1. Davidson RS. Metatarsal lengthening. Foot Ankle Clin. 2001;6(3):499–518.
2. Levine SE, Davidson RS, Dormans JP, Drummond DS. Distraction osteogenesis for congenitally short lesser metatarsals. Foot Ankle Int. 1995;16(4):196–200.
3. Root ML, Orien WP, Weed JH. Normal and abnormal function of the foot. Clinical biomechanics, vol. 2. Los Angeles: Clinical Biomechanics Corporation; 1977. p. 455.
4. Lamm BM. Percutaneous distraction osteogenesis for treatment of brachymetatarsia. J Foot Ankle Surg. 2010;49(2):197–204.
5. Mah KK, Beegle TR, Falknor DW. A correction for short fourth metatarsal. J Am Podiatr Med Assoc. 1983;73(4):196–200.
6. Urano Y, Kobayashi A. Bone lengthening for shortness of the fourth toe. J Bone Joint Surg. 1978;60A:91–3.
7. Takakura Y, Tanaka Y, Fujii T, et al. Lengthening of short great toes by callus distraction. J Bone Joint Surg. 1997;79B:955–8.
8. Handelman RB, Perlman MD, Coleman WB. Brachymetatarsia: a review of the literature and case report. J Am Podiatr Med Assoc. 1986;76(7):413–2416.
9. Lamm BM. Metatarsal lengthening. In: Rozbruch RS, Ilizarov S, editors. Limb lengthening and reconstruction surgery. New York: Informa Healthcare; 2007. p. 291–302.
10. Oh CW, Satish BR, Lee ST, et al. Complications of distraction osteogenesis in short first metatarsals. J Pediatr Orthop. 2004;24(6):711–5.
11. Wilusz PM, Van P, Pupp GR. Complications associated with distraction osteogenesis for the correction of brachymetatarsia: a review of five procedures. J Am Podiatr Med Assoc. 2007;97(3):189–94.
12. Schimizzi A, Brage M. Brachymetatarsia. Foot Ankle Clin. 2004;9(3):555–70, ix.
13. Lee KB, Yang HK, Chung JY, et al. How to avoid complications of distraction osteogenesis for first brachymetatarsia. Acta Orthop. 2009;80(2):220–5.

14. Lelievre J. Pathology of the foot [in French]. Paris: Masson; 1971.
15. Harris RI, Bearth T. The short first metatarsal: its incidence and clinical significance. J Bone Joint Surg Am. 1949;31(3):553–65.
16. Fox IM. Treatment of brachymetatarsia by the callus distraction method. J Foot Ankle Surg. 1998;37(5):391–5.
17. Magnan B, Bragantini A, Regis D, et al. Metatarsal lengthening by callotasis during the growth phase. J Bone Joint Surg Br. 1995;77(4):602–7.
18. Gilbody J, Nayagam S. Lengthening of the first metatarsal through an arthrodesis site for treatment of brachymetatarsia: a case report. J Foot Ankle Surg. 2008;47(6):559–64.
19. Choi IH, Chung MS, Baek GH, et al. Metatarsal lengthening in congenital brachymetatarsia: one-stage lengthening versus lengthening by callotasis. J Pediatr Orthop. 1999;19(5):660–4.
20. Herzenberg JE, Paley D. Ilizarov applications in foot and ankle surgery. Adv Orthop Surg. 1992;16:162–74.
21. Masuda K, Fujita S, Fuji T, Ohno H. Complications following metatarsal lengthening by callus distraction for brachymetatarsia. J Pediatr Orthop. 1999;19(3):394–7.
22. Skirving AP, Newman JH. Elongation of the first metatarsal. J Pediatr Orthop. 1983;3:508–10.
23. Steedman JT, Peterson HA. Brachymetatarsia of the first metatarsal treated by surgical lengthening. J Pediatr Orthop. 1992;12:780–5.
24. Paley D, Kovelman HF, Herzenberg JE. Ilizarov technology. In: Stauffer R, editor. Advances in operative orthopaedics, vol. 1. St. Louis: Mosby-Year Book; 1993. p. 243–87.
25. Baek GH, Chung MS. The treatment of congenital brachymetatarsia by one-stage lengthening. J Bone Joint Surg Br. 1998;80-B:1040–4.
26. Lamm BM, Gourdine-Shaw MC. Problems, obstacles, and complications of metatarsal lengthening for the treatment of brachymetatarsia. Clin Podiatr Med Surg. 2010;27:561–82.
27. Paley D. Problems, obstacles, and complications of limb lengthening by the Ilizarov technique. Clin Orthop Relat Res. 1990;(250):81–104.
28. Choudhury SN, Kitaoka HB, Peterson HA. Metatarsal lengthening: case report and review of the literature. Foot Ankle Int. 1997;18(11):739–45.

Pediatric Metatarsus Adductus

6

Patrick Stephen Agnew

The Trouble with Kids

The trouble with kids in foot and ankle medicine and surgery is multifaceted. This is likely true for many other disciplines also. In no particular order, the following issues arise.

Nobody wants their child to be in a control group. If there is a chance that a particular treatment might help a particular parent's child, the odds are that the parents will elect to try the treatment even in the event that a certain amount of risk exists. This leaves families vulnerable to coercion; and researchers are at a loss for recruiting a control group.

The consequences of treatment are often not appreciated for long periods of time, stretching out into decades. The procedure that seems to help a young child may over time be later recognized to be detrimental. Examples include treatment of metatarsus adductus via midfoot soft tissue releases and the use of reversed last shoes to improve the appearance of the same entity.

Nobody wants to hurt a child. Even many lower life form animals are very protective of their young. Only the worst sort of human is unmoved by the suffering of a child. The fact is that some treatments hurt and that pain can be felt by the child's parents, the provider, the technicians administering the treatment, the siblings of the child, and the civilized societies at large.

These and other factors can make decision-making in this special population difficult. Furthermore, providers and researchers can be equally vulnerable to the emotional trap of feeling that once they have arrived at a decision it must be defended (right or wrong) valiantly.

Whenever we develop new treatments or institute already, "accepted treatments," we must bear in mind these pitfalls. We must try, wherever possible, to follow standard scientific methods. When that is not possible, we must admit the shortcomings of the products of our research.

Incidence

The incidence of midfoot adduction, or at least reporting, has increased [1]. One case per one thousand live births is widely accepted.

Etiology (Fig. 6.1)

Midfoot adduction may be a result of malformation ("manufacturing defects") and/or deformation ("packaging defects") [2]. The left foot is more commonly involved, possibly because that foot is more commonly positioned against the mother's spine in utero [3]. The condition is also more common

P. S. Agnew (✉)
Family and Community Medicine, Eastern Virginia Medical School, Norfolk, VA, USA

M. L. Butterworth, J. T. Marcoux (eds.), *The Pediatric Foot and Ankle*,
https://doi.org/10.1007/978-3-030-29788-6_6

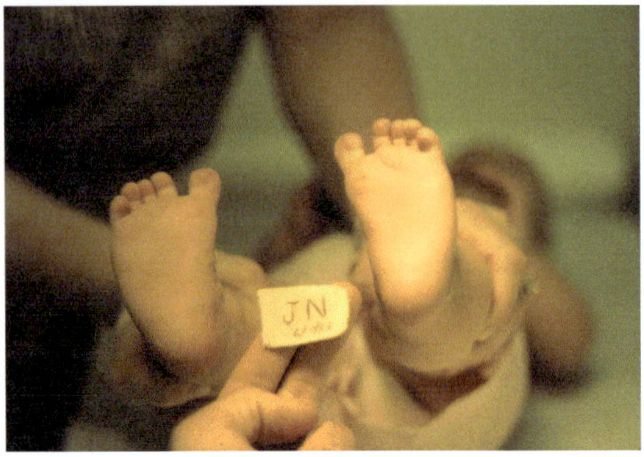

Fig. 6.1 Common pediatric presentation

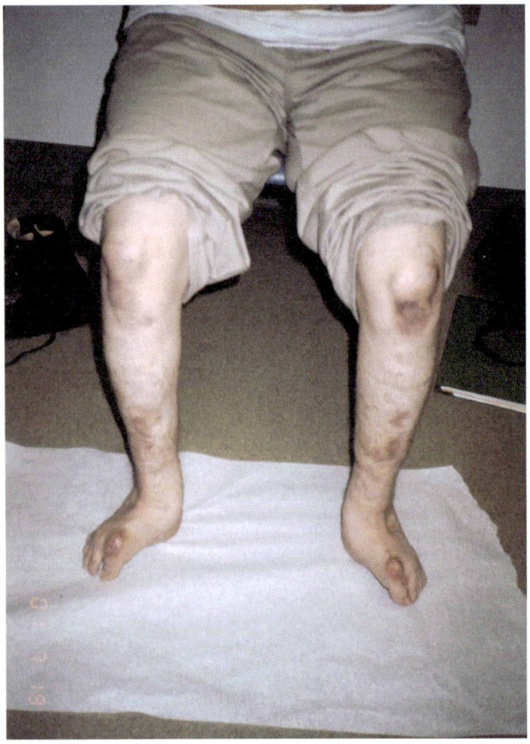

Fig. 6.2 Metatarsus adducto varus in an adult with Ehlers-Danlos syndrome

in first pregnancies, possibly because the uterus is usually tighter than in later pregnancies. Connective tissue diseases may make the fetus more vulnerable to these deforming forces because the ligaments that would normally be stronger than the immature bone fail to protect them [4, 5] (Figs. 6.2, 6.3 and 6.4). Whether midfoot adduction is more common in siblings has been debated [6, 7].

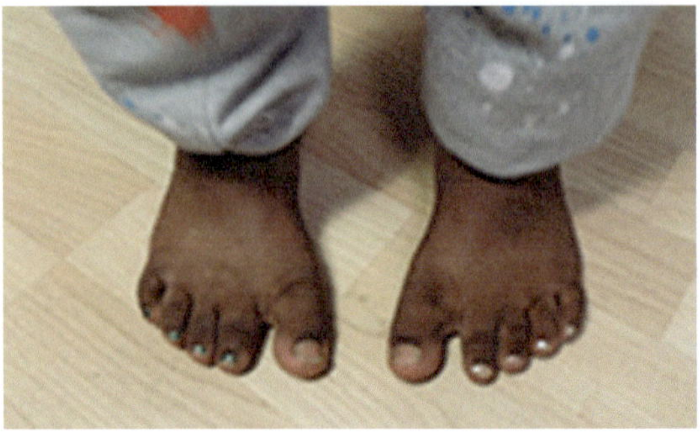

Fig. 6.3 Metatarsus primus varus. Special athlete with trisomy 21 and difficult shoe fitting

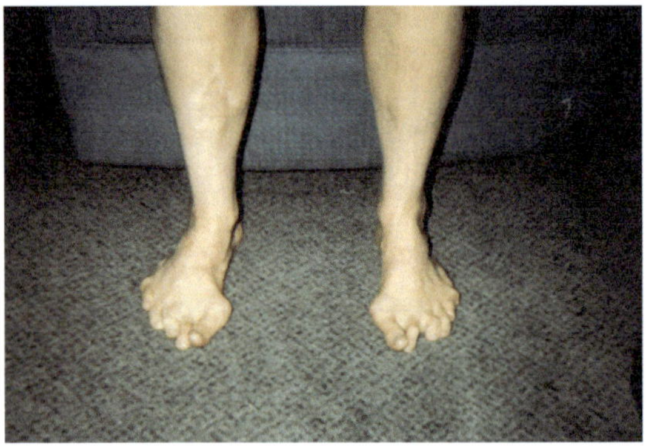

Fig. 6.4 Adult with Z foot and Ehlers-Danlos syndrome

Abnormality of the medial cuneiform has been demonstrated in some cases [8]. This further supports the use of the term midfoot adduction. Abnormal insertion of the abductor hallucis has been reported as a possible cause of midfoot adduction [9].

Nosology

The term metatarsus varus never really was a useful descriptive term [1]. First off, it is a throwback to the time during which anatomy was described in cadavers hanging from gallows. In weight-bearing bipedal humans, the position of the foot is more accurately described as adducted. In fact, in most cases, it may not even be the metatarsals themselves that are adducted, but more on that later. This author cannot believe that they actually want me to start communicating differently at the age of 56; however, the introduction of ICD 10 may actually present an opportunity to more accurately describe the deformity or malformation. Then again the added complexity might only muddle communications beyond utility. This author for one tends to be a "lumper" not a "splitter." One thing that all of the variations of metatarsus "varus" share in common is midfoot adduction. This is a descriptive term that I hope will be adopted in the education of individuals who attempt to diagnose and manage these conditions. The term metatarsus adductus attributed to Ganley and Ganley is interchangeable [10].

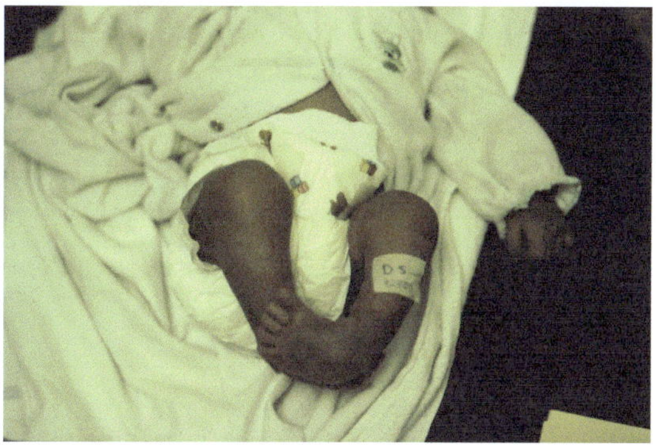

Fig. 6.5 Midfoot adduction in a patient with talipes equinovarus

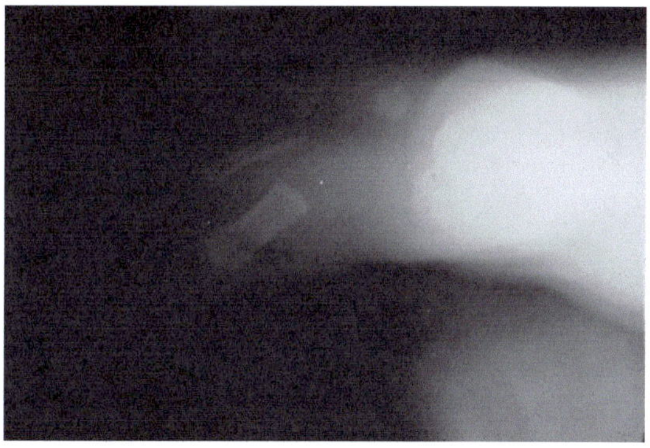

Fig. 6.6 Obviously abnormal forefoot to rear foot relationship despite the absence of ossified midfoot bones

Diagnosis

Diagnosis of midfoot adduction may appear obvious. Using the term midfoot adduction alone actually makes this true to a certain extent. However, specific identification of the involved bones and joints can be difficult. Confounding factors include the age of presentation, the patient's relative connective tissue integrity, muscle strength, nerve control (upper and lower motor neurons), patient cooperation, parent anxiety, examiner's skill and experience, and other factors.

Fortunately, our management recommendations may not be altered in young, skeletally immature patients. However, older children, especially surgery candidates, must undergo more detailed diagnosis including bone imaging. The apex of deformity should be identified and, ideally, corrected. Radiographic angle measurements may be helpful but are notoriously vulnerable to technique variation and evaluator inconsistency [11] (Figs. 6.5 and 6.6). Furthermore, ideally, patients should be identified prior to midfoot bone ossification. Simple recognition of a deformity in the midtarsal bones, as opposed to the metatarsals, may yield better decision-making results. Ganley and Ganley did propose a reproducible radiograph technique using the calcaneus as a reference point [10]. A normal relationship between the bisections of the calcaneus and the second metatarsal is about 15° on a dorsal plantar view. Meta-analysis of papers was published on the angle formed by the frontal plane bisection of the tarsal bones and the bisection of the second metatarsal average 15° and higher in skeletally mature individuals who have midfoot adduction [12–15].

It is also necessary to recognize relatively common variations such as:

- Metatarsal or midfoot adduction with (true) forefoot varus (metatarsus adducto varus) [16].
- Metatarsal adduction with midfoot translation (complex metatarsus adductus) [17]
- Metatarsal adduction or midfoot adduction with rear foot varus (cavo adductovarus) [18]
- Metatarsal adduction with rear foot valgus (skew foot) [17]

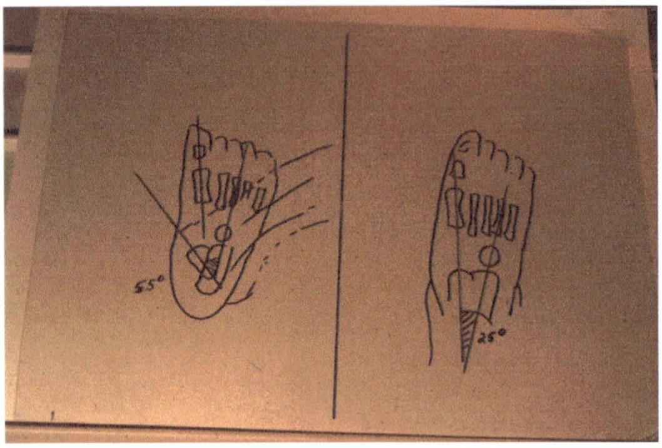

Fig. 6.7 Drawings donated by Dr. Ganley's family detailing the forefoot to rear foot relationship in a patient with clubfoot pre- and post-casting

- Metatarsal adduction with midfoot translation and rear foot valgus (complex skew foot) [17]
- Metatarsal adduction or midfoot adduction with equinus and forefoot varus (talipes equinovarus) (Fig 6.7)

An almost infinite spectrum of severity and combinations of deformity of all of the involved bones, connective tissues, and anatomical segments can exist also. Terms such as c foot, ding foot, hooked foot, parrot foot, and pigeon toed are encountered but should be discouraged being inadequate to describe the deformities and conceivably insensitive [16].

Recognizing possibly related/adjacent/comorbid issues is essential. Developmental and/or congenital hip dislocation or dislocate ability are possible examples, although controversy exists regarding this assertion [6]. Unresolved femoral retroversion or accelerated femoral anteversion may coexist with midfoot adduction. Excess medial and lateral tibial torsion may also be present, conceivably for the same reasons as midfoot adduction is thought to occur [19]. Congenital and/or developmental equinus or pseudoequinus should be recognized and appropriately addressed.

Digital deformity, primary or secondary to inadequately managed midfoot adduction, is often present. Hallux valgus and/or lesser digit contractions are progressive and often eventually disabling [20–22]. These may be addressed in a variety of ways at any age and with any comorbidities but with varying degrees of potential success. As with any pediatric deformity or malformation, early recognition and management may be expected to provide better results.

Identification of systemic and/or regional comorbidities is highly desirable. Many congenital syndromes include midfoot adduction. Foot and ankle care providers should also consider treatment and/or referral of patients with these issues to appropriate providers.

Physical Examination

A proper environment for the examination may yield optimal data. This may include avoiding nap time for restless children, or targeting nap time in sound sleepers. A hungry child may be distracted by feeding during the examination, or may be inconsolable. Planning along with parents is essential to success. Specially decorated pediatric examination rooms with popular character images may help to relax a child. It has been said that about one of the only cultural similarities that Americans have in common is a few Disney characters. Setting aside the examiner's white coat may avoid a lot of noise, tears, and combat.

We recommend the A.R.M. method devised by James V. Ganley, DPM [23]. "A" refers to attitude. The resting attitude of the lower extremities during physical examination is evaluated. Sometimes the patient's anxiety can cause confusing postures. However, a patient-repeated assessment will reveal that in the majority of times some particular attitude such as midfoot adduction is demonstrated. "R" refers to relationships of segments of the lower extremities. The forefoot is angled toward the midline of the body in all variations of midfoot adduction. This may or may not be easily appreciated if other segments including the rear foot and ankle are also deformed. Conditions such as tibial torsion may mask or complicate the assessment [24].

The "M" refers to movement. The range of motion of the relevant structures is evaluated. Is the deformity fixed or reducible? Can overcorrection in the midfoot abduction be induced? Again these movements may be influenced by the patient's emotional and physical state (Fig. 6.8).

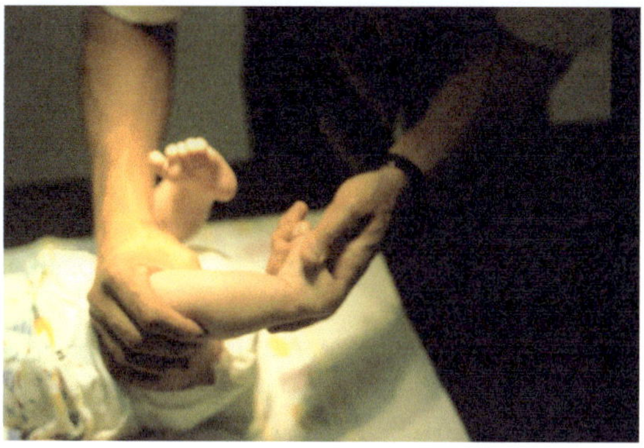

Fig. 6.8 Examination of an infant with excessive medial tibial movement. Photo of the author by Dr. Ganley

Conservative Management

Anyone who comprehensively treats adult foot and ankle issues cannot ignore the persistent presence of midfoot adduction in a large percentage of patients seeking help. The theory that the vast majority of midfoot adduction is spontaneously resolving is not supportable from this perspective [10]. Based on some authors' data, it has been shown that pediatricians and pediatric orthopedists trend toward a nihilistic hands-off, wait-and-see approach and orthopedic surgeons and podiatrists tend to be more inclined to treat infants who have congenital abnormalities [2]. The innuendo seems to be that the pediatricians and pediatric orthopedists are better trained or more knowledgeable in their decision-making; but while maintaining that stereotyping is not ever reliable, orthopedic surgeons and podiatrists have the advantaged perspective of seeing countless adults in whom this condition did not go away, but instead contributed to adult-onset problems.

A variety of methods of treatment have been suggested. A confounding factor in deciding on treatment techniques and appropriateness include the highly variable age of presentation. Usually, midfoot adduction is recognized at birth. All too often an unsupportable prognosis for spontaneous recovery is made. A simple but knowledgeable examination of relatives of the infant will often reveal persistent deformity/malformation and related pathology. This may be masked to the inadequately educated eye by compensatory secondary deformities such as overpronation. Overpronation creates a relatively rectus-appearing adult foot that still maintains midfoot adduction. However, now that foot also has subtalar and the tarsal joint dysfunction. Secondary forefoot deformities may have also emerged such as hallux valgus and fifth metatarsal splaying. This overpronation may have occurred spontaneously or through irrational iatrogenic intervention such as reverse last shoes and/or stretching.

Optimally, a several decades long, adequately powered, study with appropriate blinding and controls would reveal the true incidence of persistence of midfoot adduction and its contribution to related pathology. I doubt that such a study will ever be conducted (see "The Trouble with Kids" above). In the absence then of adequate evidence-based decision-making, the individual provider must at least be completely honest with the patient and the patient's caregiver(s) on what is not known. Then they share decision-making and can go forward with adequate informed consent.

Management decisions are often predicated on age of onset and will be discussed in that structure as follows.

Neonates (Fig. 6.9)

When midfoot adduction is identified in a neonate, a sincere and a thorough effort to decide whether or not to treat is appropriate.

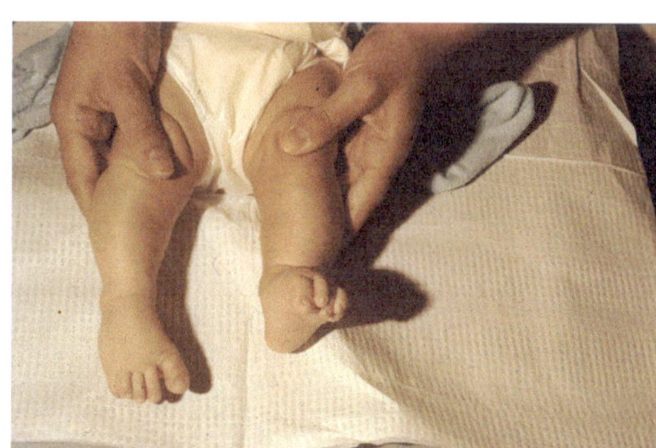

Fig. 6.9 Infant attitude with midfoot adduction right and calcaneal valgus left

Diagnosing severity based on the "flexibility" of the deformity has been advocated [10]. Very little is available to define what constitutes a reproducible evaluation of this supposed characteristic and prognostic significance. Nothing has been proposed to factor in highly variable contributing issues such as collagen abnormalities, neuromuscular developmental anomalies, examiner's capabilities, and other variables (Fig. 6.10). We are also not aware of any validated predictive capacity of these nebulous assessments. We therefore consider the classification of these deformities as mild, moderate, and severe to be a clinically irrelevant. We do consider comorbidities and family histories to be extremely relevant. Relatives may be unaware of possible related pathology. These related pathologies may, again, include (Fig. 6.11):

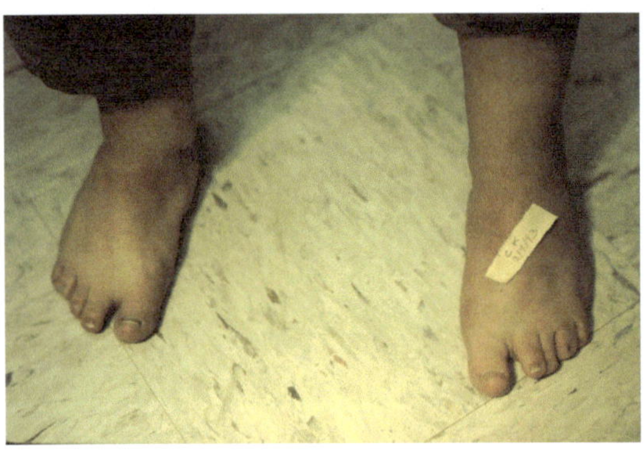

Fig. 6.10 Patient with a syndrome that includes midfoot adduction and brachy digital

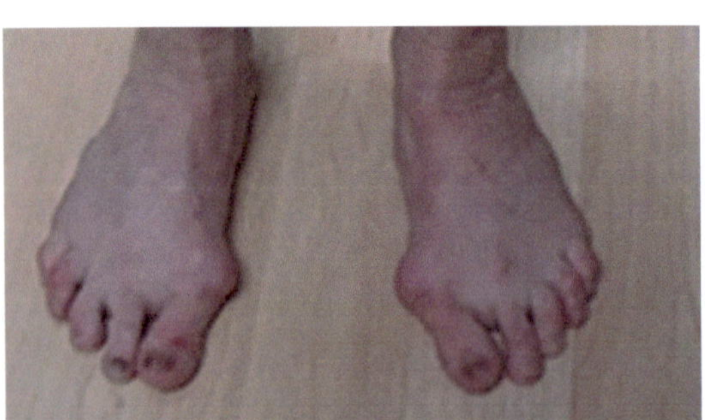

Fig. 6.11 Common adult presentation, notice the easily overlooked 5th metatarsal base prominence

1. Hallux valgus with or without overpronation
2. Lesser digit contraction via flexor stabilization failure (with overpronation) or extension substitution (in the uncompensated adducted midfoot)
3. Fifth metatarsal adductus with or without bunionettes (influence of MA on plantar pressures)
4. Fifth metatarsal base pain (Fig. 6.12a, b)
5. Increased incidence of lateral foot and ankle sprains and fractures
6. Poor shock absorption throughout the weight-bearing skeleton
7. Rapid foot wear deterioration
8. Clumsiness

Even with neuromuscular and connective tissue and other contributing variabilities or disease ruled out, treatment is still usually recommended by this author. Again, there is no validated prognostic evaluation currently available. The golden opportunity in the rapidly growing plastic non-weight-bearing infant should not be squandered. Treatment in this age group may be highly effective and carries very minimal risk.

Young Children

In a preschool and early school age child, again, deformity will have been "baked into" maturing bone to some degree. Some correction of deformity conservatively by bracing, splinting, or even casting may be achievable. However, the theory that the deformity must be treated by casting or splinting for as long as it has been present makes conservative treatment at this time extraordinarily unpalatable. That having been said, the likelihood of stigmatization is less likely in the preschool child than the school age child where greater peer interaction occurs. Treatment may therefore at least be attempted cautiously. Again, a thorough informed consent is indicated.

Surgery in this age has met with relatively disappointing results. Midfoot capsulotomies have been followed longitudinally by some authors and have revealed a stiff dysfunctional foot later in life. One minimally invasive technique to attempt some soft

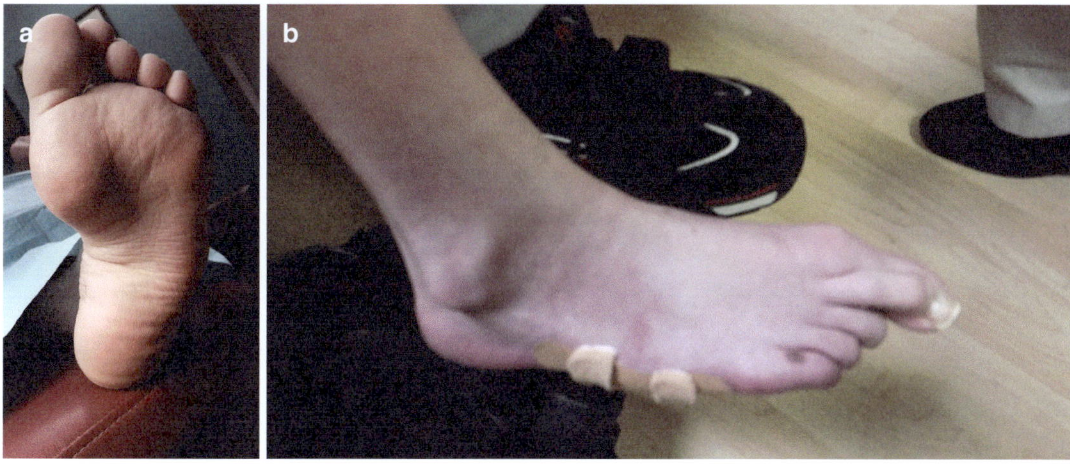

Fig. 6.12 (**a**) Adolescent patient with Charcot-Marie-Tooth disease. Figure (**b**) depicts a special needs of nonambulatory adolescent with cross under hallux valgus and fifth metatarsal base lesion from difficult shoe fitting

tissue rebalancing in the hopes of allowing some bone remodeling might be the Lichtblau procedure. In selected cases where the majority of deformity involves the first metatarsal and the first toe, release of the abductor hallucis tendon near its insertion or lengthening of that structure may be appropriate. The procedure does permit a surgical approach with only a small risk of neurologic or vascular injury. Injury to growth plates in the adjacent bones also seems unlikely with even reasonable skill.

School Age Children

Although otherwise normal patients in this age group may have achieved the ability to reason and cooperate with treatment of some level, their willingness to do so may be highly limited. Whether they are consciously aware of that or not, the emergence of self-awareness may result in self-consciousness over any visible treatment. Treatment while sleeping may provide some degree of success, but will undoubtedly prolong the duration of treatment. Fully reversing deformity in this age group may not be a realistic goal any longer. Treatment in this age group may include splinting and bracing or even casting. Again, a very limited soft tissue balancing procedure with release of the abductor halluces tendon may be appropriate.

Cautious use of a foot orthosis may help to reduce the risk of compensatory deformation of the hind foot. Some cosmetic improvement in the angle of gait may also be achieved through the use of "gait plate"-type extensions. These however should also be used with caution to avoid derangement of more proximal structures including the ankle, the knee, and the hip.

It is sometimes pointed out that a number of sprinters and other athletes exhibit some degree of in toeing as adults. It is implied that this may provide a better propulsive structure for a short distance acceleration. I am not aware of any author advocating the creation or inducement of in toeing. One might also surmise that the majority of people who maintain metatarsus adductus into adulthood will not be competitive athletes and instead will have to find shoes that can comfortably fit their deformed feet.

Adolescent Patients

Figure 6.13 depicts common preadolescent presentation. This is undoubtedly the most vulnerable age group for unintended psychological harm through treatment. Self-awareness has by this point in many cases become self-absorption, and our current culture inarguably overemphasizes physical appearance. That having

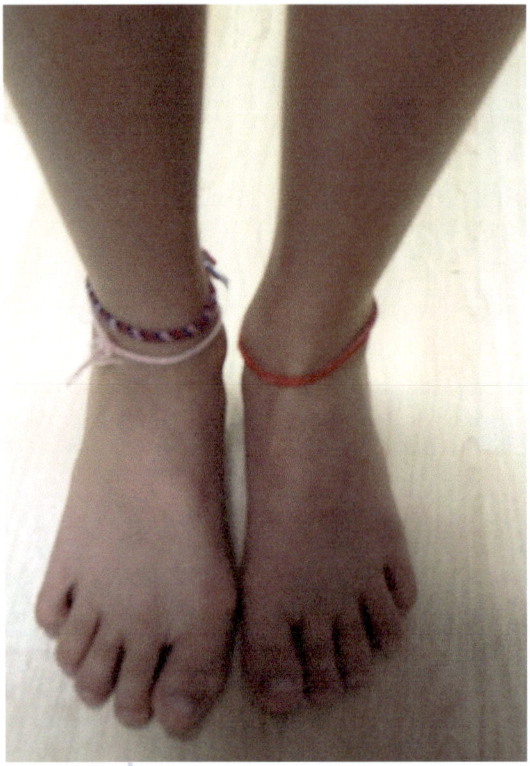

Fig. 6.13 Common adolescent presentation

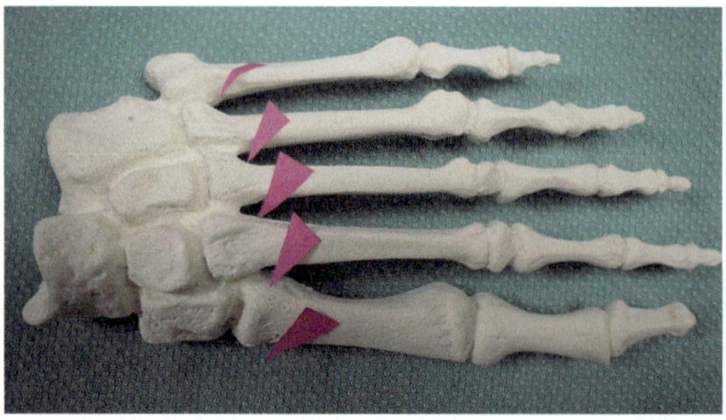

Fig. 6.14 Closing wedge osteotomies

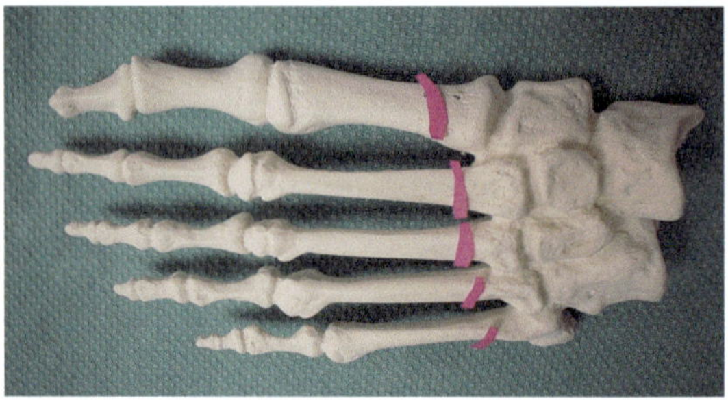

Fig. 6.15 Transverse plane osteotomies

been said, the failure to have treated the patient earlier in life may already have caused irreparable harm. At this point accommodation of the deformity is appropriate for the majority of the patients. Appropriate shoe selection more often than not with protective orthotic arch support to prevent compensatory overpronation of the hind foot seems appropriate. In rare recalcitrant painful cases, surgical intervention may be appropriate. Various surgical approaches have been proposed and have generally met with relatively satisfactory results. These may include multiple metatarsal osteotomies as well as tarsal osteotomies. Examples include closing base wedge osteotomies and oblique multiple metatarsal osteotomies (Figs. 6.14 and 6.15). Although capable of achieving satisfactory results, these procedures are somewhat technically challenging. The risk of complications with the single metatarsal osteotomy is well known. This risk is additive with each additional metatarsal osteotomy. Overcorrection, under correction, nonunion, and malunion all are realistic concerns as well as general surgical concerns such as infection, wound healing, deep vein thrombophlebitis, etc.

Furthermore, Dr. James V. Ganley famously illustrated that if one would look at the radiographic outline of a "normal metatarsal" when compared to a metatarsal in many patients with a clinical metatarsus adductus, the metatarsals will in most cases appear identical. This implies that the actual deformity in many cases is more proximally placed. Wherever possible, surgical intervention at the actual site of deformity is geometrically preferable. Therefore, osteotomy of the tarsals may be more appropriate in many cases. Added advantages to intervention at this level include the greater cancellous bone content for bone healing and the smaller number of osteotomies necessary. Therefore, osteotomies at this level are, in this surgeon's experience, preferable. Figure 6.16a–c depicts radiographs of a 9-year-old patient with syndromic clubfoot treated as an infant recovering from recent residual midfoot adduction correction.

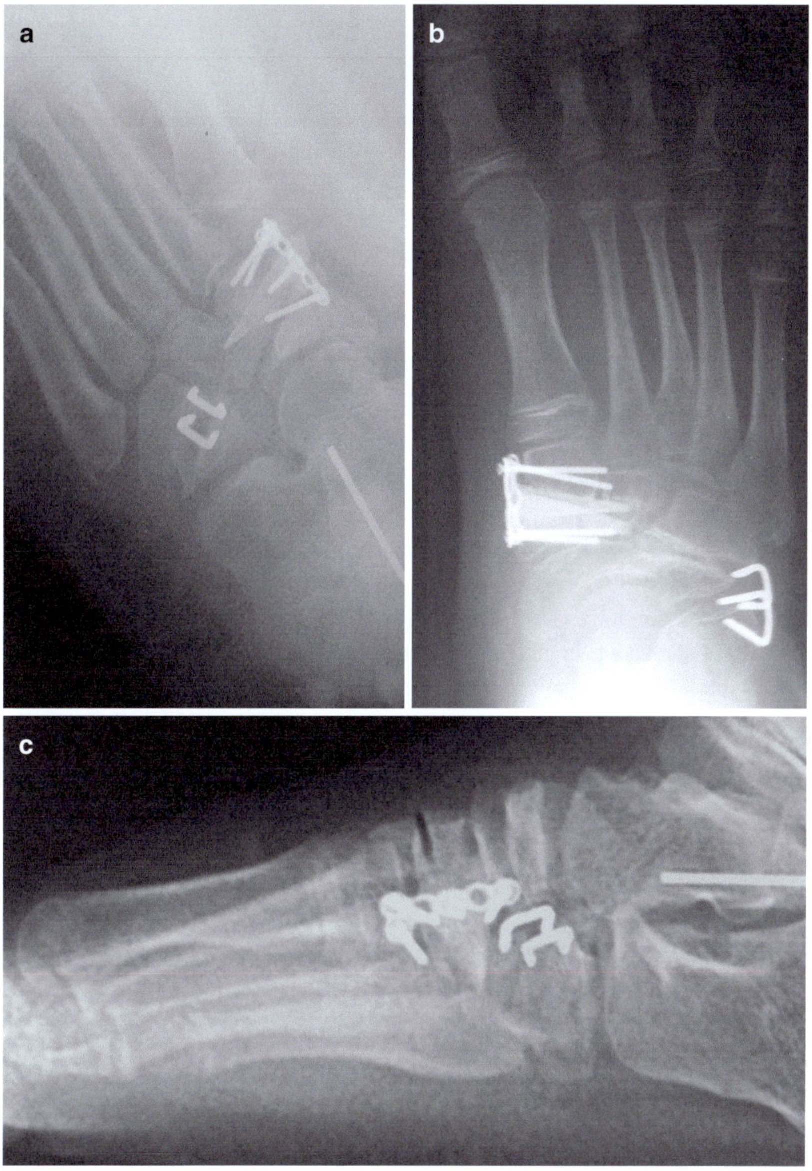

Fig. 6.16 (**a**–**c**) 9-year-old syndromic clubfoot treated as an infant recovering from recent residual midfoot adduction correction

The avoidance of growth plates also increases the appeal of the surgery at this level. The greatest drawback is the likely need for an opening osteotomy medially and the necessity of bone or appropriate substitute grafting. These procedures of course carry some limited predictability regarding a final outcome, added cost, and potentially additional surgery for bone graft harvesting. The lateral closing osteotomy carries with it some technical challenges not the least of which is the limited amount of bone available for removal and then stabilization. The greater ability to correct deformity in multiple planes however (when compared to metatarsal osteotomies) may add to the appeal of midfoot osteotomies for the correction of improvement in mid- or hind foot deformities brought on through an ill conceived iatrogenic compensation.

Young Adults

Young adults who have achieved skeletal maturity and up through the age of older adults who may be in a skeletal decline are probably the most severely affected individuals by unresolved or untreated midfoot adduction. Ironically, these patients more often than not are totally unaware of their birth defect. They may present with a clinically common hallux valgus and/or tailor's bunion deformities. They may also present with fifth metatarsal styloid process bursitis; peroneal (also known as fibularis) tendon injuries, both chronic and acute; as well as lateral foot and/or ankle sprain and fractures [25, 26]. Unfortunately, these patients did not benefit from what could have been a few weeks of casting as infants. Many of these conditions are difficult to correct requiring aggressive surgical procedures, and some such as peroneal tendon injuries and lateral ankle ligament injuries are prone to very poor healing. Details of treatment of these consequences are beyond the scope of this textbook, but any provider who offers comprehensive foot and ankle care should look at these adults as strong motivation to correct deformities in infants.

Older Adults

Neglected patients in this category may suffer from all of the consequences discussed in the younger adult. Older patients may also carry the added burden of multisystem disease, deconditioning of the bone and muscle, and deteriorating perfusion making a successful intervention even more challenging.

Treatments

"Benign" Neglect

Watchful waiting (wasting?) or active surveillance is often advocated. This is often recommended by the same authors that advocate in some cases casting of not yet ambulatory infants. The obvious contradiction in these two approaches is irrational to the extreme. How long do you watch? How long do you wait? Why would you wait until it is much more difficult to correct the problem?

Any healthcare provider with any experience whatsoever would agree that it would be much easier to cast splint or in any other way interact with an infant than it is with a toddler of two or three. A school age child may be in some cases cooperative, but already the skeleton has matured enough to make successful treatment to take much longer and be much less likely to result in complete correction. Furthermore, some practitioners who recommend neglect of the deformity also point out that treatment with bracing and splinting may affect the patient's self-esteem at that time or later in life. They actually use this rationale to imply that treatment in childhood is inappropriate while failing to delineate any stratification regarding age of treatment or type of treatment. Of course, it is obvious that a school age child wearing a visible brace or splint might possibly be stigmatized and may suffer psychological injury as a result. It seems extraordinarily unlikely that an infant wearing a well-molded cast for a few weeks early in life would be similarly harmed. Again, we ask, why then would anyone decide to postpone treatment of an obvious deformity?

Stretching

Telling caregivers to "stretch" at every diaper change is sometimes recommended by some authors [27]. This may be an excellent example of Voltaire's assessment that medicine is the art of entertaining the patient while the condition gets better by itself. The exception in this case being that the condition may in many cases not get better by itself. The act of "stretching" is not supportable. In the otherwise normal child, the ligaments of the lower extremity are likely stronger than the developing bone. The belief that one can stretch the ligaments in order to allow the bones to develop normally is therefore irrational. The expectation that primary caregivers will have the clinical skill to perform manipulations appropriately seems in this author's estimation to be unrealistic [1]. Infant casting and manipulation of midfoot adduction or of other deformities requires specific training experience and knowledge. Casting techniques are however effective when appropriately applied by knowledgeable providers [28].

Casting

Manipulation followed by casting is the basis of pediatric deformity treatment. Use of this technique has been documented as far back in time as ancient Egypt. Successful treatment of difficult and complex deformities such as talipes equinovarus has been proven again and again [12]. Detailed treatises have been published extensively on casting techniques [29].

Splinting

The use of various splints and braces to "correct" midfoot adduction is a mixed bag. Some well-thought-out apparatus that help protect the hind foot from iatrogenic deformation by overpronation may be entirely appropriate [30]. Cosmetically, effective techniques such as reverse last shoes undoubtedly failed to redirect the growth of deformed bones and instead overpronate the rear foot causing iatrogenic deformity [31]. The foot may appear rectus as a result of this intervention, but now has two or more deformities instead of correction of the initial deformity.

It is necessary for any device to at least stabilize the calcaneus in a neutral or an even slightly inverted position to prevent overpronation. Proper fit is obviously essential. Complete discussion of proper application and potential negative effects with the parents is necessary. Application instructions usually accompany new braces, and printed patient instructions are desirable.

Negative events/effects are very rare in our experience, and reports are absent from the literature. Concerns may include skin irritation. A little baby powder in the brace and/or the use of socks can keep moisture from accumulating under the brace. Ill-fitting braces may, of course, irritate or even in the worst cases damage the skin and deeper structures. Periodic confirmation of proper fit and use of splints or braces is recommended. Specific frequency of these examinations may be recommended by manufacturers. We recommend examination soon after fitting and dispensing. We also recommend use during naps first to unveil issues in the light of day and over shorter time periods (Fig. 6.17).

Surgery

Detailed surgery descriptions are beyond the scope of this text, but are thoroughly published and studied. Categories of intervention may include soft tissue releases, forefoot osteotomies, midfoot osteotomies, and rear foot osteotomies.

Soft tissue procedures include the abductor hallucis release [32] and the Heyman-Herndon and Strong procedure [33]. We no longer recommend the latter since stiffness has been reported later in life [34]. We still perform the Lichtblau procedure sometimes as a standalone intervention. Any tendency for the patient to have hallux valgus still remains to be a concern. Many metatarsal osteotomies including closing base wedge osteotomies and transverse plane osteotomies such as the Lepird osteotomy have been devised [35].

Midfoot osteotomies are the most common form of surgical intervention that we use [36, 37]. We often prefer these procedures for several reasons as pointed out by Ganley and Ganley [10].

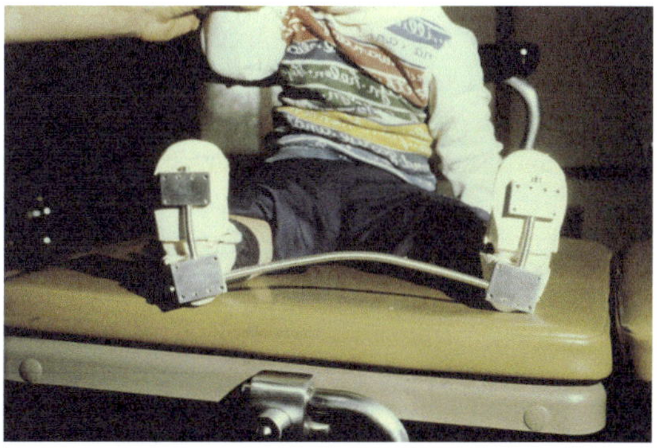

Fig. 6.17 Ganley splint attached and worn by child

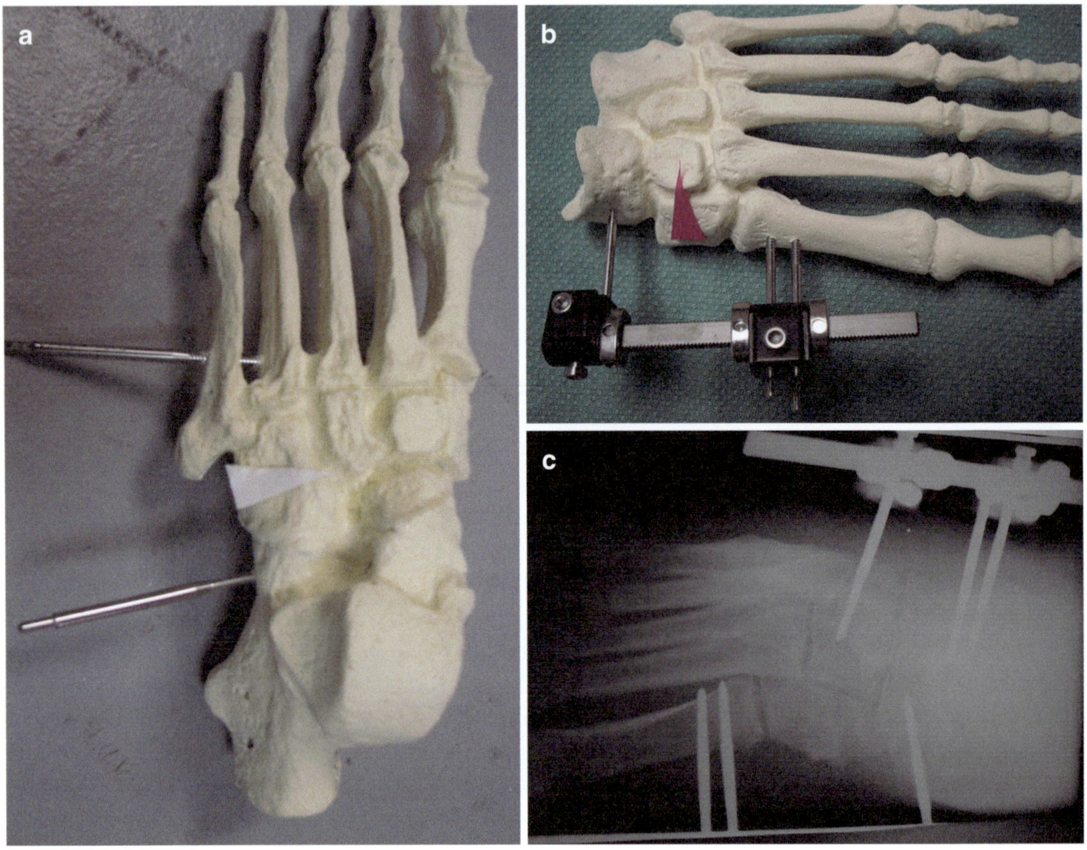

Fig. 6.18 (**a**–**c**) positioning bayonets and frames with osteotomies in planning

These are as follows: surgery at the site of deformity, less osteotomies, and better healing bones than distally. Operating at the site of deformity, instead of creating a second deformity to improve the appearance of the organ, is better. The greater the number of surgical procedures, the greater the cumulative potential for complications. There is more cancellous bone in the tarsal bones than the metatarsals, so faster bone healing may be anticipated (Fig. 6.18a–c).

Rear foot osteotomies are rarely employed as standalone procedures for midfoot adduction. Rear foot surgery may be necessary and beneficial to resolve coincidental deformities and compensatory derangement caused by uncorrected midfoot adduction. Examples may include medial calcaneal displacement osteotomies to reduce overpronation in compensated midfoot adduction, or laterally to correct cavus deformity in uncompensated midfoot adduction. Shortening lateral column osteotomies/calcaneal cuboid arthrodesis may improve the appearance of midfoot adduction and correct cavus deformity simultaneously. Lengthening osteotomies of the lateral column may correct overpronation seen in compensated midfoot adduction, but may also exacerbate the outward appearance of the midfoot adduction more than other surgical approaches to correct overpronation. Subtalar arthroereisis may correct overpronation with less exacerbation of midfoot adduction.

Summary

Principles of management of midfoot adduction include the following:

1. Early recognition
2. Cautiously identifying potential contributing factors such as neurologic, muscular, and connective tissue diseases
3. Realistic and completely honest prognostication
4. Early gentle effective intervention
5. Age-appropriate intervention when a suboptimal age of presentation occurs

References

1. Kite HJ. The clubfoot. New York: Grune & Stratton; 1964.
2. Wegner DR, Rang M. The art and practice of children's orthopedics. New York: Raven Press; 1993.
3. McDonough MW. Fetal positions a cause of right and left-sided foot and leg disorders. J Am Podiatry Assoc. 1981;7:65–8.
4. Ponseti IV, Becker JR. Congenital metatarsus adductus: the results of treatment. J Bone Joint Surg Am. 1996;48:702.
5. Agnew PS. Evaluation of the child with ligamentous laxity. Clin Podiatr Med Surg. 1997;14:117–30.
6. Wynne-Davies R. Family studies and the cause of congenital clubfoot, talipes equino-varus, talipes calcaneovalgus and metatarsus varus. J Bone Joint Surg Br. 1964;445(9):46.
7. Hunziker UA, Largo RH, Due G. Growth and development neonatal metatarsus adductus, joint mobility, access and rotation in preterm and term children 0-5 years of age. Eur J Pediatr. 1988;148:19–23.
8. Morcuende JA, Ponseti IV. Congenital metatarsus adductus in early human fetal development: a histological study. Clin Orthop. 1996;46:376.
9. Sgarlato TE. A discussion of metatarsus adductus. Arch Podiatr Med Foot Surg. 1973;1:35.
10. Ganley JV, Ganley TJ. Metatarsus adductus deformity. In: Mcglamry ED, Banks AS, Downey MS, editors. Comprehensive textbook of foot surgery. 2nd ed. Baltimore: Williams & Wilkins; 1992. p. 829–52.
11. Halvac HF. Differences in x-ray findings with varied positioning of the foot. J Am Podiatry Assoc. 1987;57:465–71.
12. Root ML, Orien WP, Weed JH, et al. Biomechanical examination of the foot. Los Angeles: Clinical Biomechanics; 1971. p. 33.
13. Yu GV, DiNapoli DR. Surgical management of hallux abductovalgus with concomitant metatarsus adductus. In: Mcglamry ED, editor. Reconstructive surgery of the foot and leg: update '89. Tucker: Podiatry Institute; 1989. p. 262–8.
14. Weissman SD. Biomechanically acquired foot types. In: Weissman SF, editor. Radiology of the foot. Baltimore: Williams & Wilkins; 1982. p. 50–76.
15. Heatherington VJ, Lehtinen J, Grill F. The pediatric patient. In: Levy LA, Heatherington VJ, editors. Principles and practice of podiatric medicine. New York: Churchill Livingstone; 1990. p. 571–612.
16. McCormick D, Blount WP. Metatarsus adducto varus. JAMA. 1949;449(5):141.
17. Berg EE. A reappraisal of metatarsus adductus and skewfoot. J Bone Joint Surg Am. 1986;68:1185.
18. Paulos L, Coleman SS, Samuelson KM. Pes cavo varus. J Bone Joint Surg Am. 1980;62:942–53.
19. Valmassy RL. Torsional and frontal plane conditions of the lower extremity. In: Thompson P, editor. Introduction to podopaediatrics. London: WB Saunders; 1993.
20. Banks AS, Hsu YS, Marish S, et al. Juvenile hallux abducto valgus association with metatarsus adductus. J Am Podiatr Med Assoc. 1994;84:219–24.
21. Hardy RH, Chlapham JCR. Observations on hallux valgus. J Bone Joint Surg Br. 1951;33:376–91.
22. LaReaux RL, Lee BR. Metatarsus adductus and hallux abducto valgus: their correlation. J Foot Surg. 1987;26:304–8.
23. Ganley JV. Lower extremity examination of the infant. J Am Podiatry Assoc. 1981;71:92–8.
24. Kight HJ. Congenital metatarsus varus. J Bone Joint Surg Am. 1967;49:388–97.
25. Yoho RM, Vardaxis V, Dikis J. A retrospective review of the effect of metatarsus adductus on healing time in the fifth metatarsal jones fracture. Foot. 2015;25:215–9.
26. Yoho RM, Carrington S, Dix B, Vardaxis V. The association of metatarsus adductus to the proximal fifth metatarsal Jones fracture. J Foot Ankle Surg. 2012;51(6):739–42.
27. Crawford AH, Gabriel KR. Foot and ankle problems. Orthop Clin North Am. 1987;18:649–66.
28. Scheimer OM. Chiropodical management of infantile metatarsus varus. J Mat Assoc Chirop. 1957;47:435.
29. Ganley JV. Corrective casting in infants. Clin Podiatry. 1984;1:501–16.
30. Lynch FR. The Ganley splint: indications and usage. Clin Podiatry. 1984;1(15):517–34.
31. Thompson GH, Simons GW. Congenital talipes equino varus (clubfeet) and metatarsus adductus.

In: Drennan JC, editor. The child's foot and ankle. New York: Raven Press; 1992.
32. Lichtblu S. Section of the abductor hallucis tendon for correction of metatarsus adductus varus deformity. Clin Orthop. 1975;110:227–32.
33. Heyman CH, Herndon CH, Strong JM. Mobilization of the tarsometatarsal and intermetatarsal joints for correction of resistant adduction of the forepart of the foot in congenital clubfoot or congenital metatarsus varus. J Bone Joint Surg Am. 1958;40:299–310.
34. Stark JG, Johanson JE, Winter RB. The Heyman-Herndon tarsometatarsal capsulotomy for metatarsus adductus: results in 48 feet. J Pediatr Orthop. 1987;7:305–10.
35. Yu GV, Wallace GF. Metatarsus adductus. In: McGlamry ED, editor. Comprehensive textbook of foot surgery, vol. 1. Baltimore: Williams and Wilkins; 1987. p. 324–53.
36. Fowler SB, Brools AL, Parrish TF. The cavovarus foot. J Bone Joint Surg Am. 1959;41:75.
37. Harley BD, Fritzhand AJ, Little JM, et al. Abductory midfoot osteotomy procedure for metatarsus adductus. J Foot Ankle Surg. 1995;34:153–62.

Juvenile Hallux Abductovalgus

7

Michelle L. Butterworth and John T. Marcoux

There is a lack of consensus regarding the precise definition of hallux abductovalgus; however, most clinicians describe the condition as the presence of a varus deviation of the first metatarsal in combination with a valgus deviation of the hallux occurring in a skeletally immature child [1, 2]. Goldner and Gaines, however, classified the entity as occurring in an individual less than 20 years of age [3]. Zollinger found the presence of hallux abductovalgus in adolescence to be only 3.5%, making it a relatively uncommon finding [4]. Other studies, however, have shown that for 50% of adults with hallux valgus, the deformity began in adolescence [1, 4, 5]. Coughlin and Mann found that 40% of juvenile patients with hallux abductovalgus develop the deformity early in childhood, before the age of 10 [2]. Chell and Dhar also confirm that approximately half of the children with hallux abductovalgus note the presence of the deformity before the age of 10 [6]. These studies have also shown that over 80% of the children who presented with juvenile hallux valgus were female [2, 6]. It has also been shown that race plays a role in the development of juvenile hallux valgus with black children being affected five times as often as white children [7]. Helal also reported that 75% of the cases occurred bilaterally [8].

M. L. Butterworth (✉)
Williamsburg Regional Hospital, Kingstree, SC, USA
e-mail: mbutter@ftc.net

J. T. Marcoux
Steward – St. Elizabeth's Medical Center,
Brighton, MA, USA

Etiology

Intrinsic and extrinsic factors have both been investigated as an etiology in the development of the hallux abductovalgus deformity. Footwear, particularly narrow-toed shoes, has been identified as an extrinsic factor exacerbating the progression of a hallux valgus deformity [9–11]. Studies have shown that the incidence of hallux valgus is more common in those that wear shoes over those that walk barefoot [12, 13]. In juvenile hallux valgus, however, constricting footwear was noted to contribute to the development of the deformity in only 24% of the patients [2].

Several authors have noted a positive family history for hallux valgus ranging from 58% to 80% [14–16]. Johnson believed that hallux valgus was inherited through an autosomal dominant trait with incomplete penetrance [17]. In 2007, Pique-Vidal et al. also agreed with Johnson when evaluating inheritance as an intrinsic factor for the development for hallux valgus and found an autosomal dominant trait with 56% incomplete penetrance. They examined the pedigree charts of 350 patients and found a family history present in 90% of probands, affecting some family members across three generations [18].

M. L. Butterworth, J. T. Marcoux (eds.), *The Pediatric Foot and Ankle*,
https://doi.org/10.1007/978-3-030-29788-6_7

The biomechanical basis for the development of this pathologic deformity has been debated over the years. Many structural abnormalities have been implicated in the development of hallux valgus including pes planus, equinus, medial column insufficiency, metatarsus adductus, ligamentous laxity, the shape and/or deviation of the articular cartilage on the first metatarsal head, and structural obliquity of the first metatarsal cuneiform joint [8, 19, 20]. Juvenile hallux valgus can also be seen as a manifestation of other conditions such as cerebral palsy due to muscular imbalance and spasticity as well as ligamentous laxity and decreased muscle tone seen in Down syndrome. It is important to get a family history to see if other siblings, parents, or relatives have hallux valgus or other foot deformities.

Recent literature has brought a new theory to our understanding of the hallux abductovalgus deformity as a whole. Research has determined that the hallux abductovalgus deformity is often a combination of frontal and transverse plane deformities with the apex of the deformity proximally. The first metatarsal is rotated into a valgus (pronated, eversion, external rotation) position with the sesamoids still aligned in the crista on sesamoid axial radiographs. The authors coined the term hallux abductovalgus with metatarsus primus adducto valgus to better define the pathology [21]. Failure to address the frontal plane component during surgical reconstruction is a major factor in the development of recurrent deformity [21]. Mortier and his colleagues performed a prospective single-center radiologic and anatomic study on 100 feet operated on for hallux valgus. Baseline radiographs determined the preoperative position of the first metatarsal head in the coronal plane. The study confirmed the existence of pathological pronation of the metatarsophalangeal apparatus in hallux valgus [22].

Clinical Presentation

Often times, the parents of children with juvenile hallux valgus are more concerned about the deformity than the child. In the young child, the condition is not typically painful nor does it limit activity. The child may present for other orthopedic complaints such as pes valgus and arch strain or heel pain, and the hallux abductovalgus deformity is an incidental finding and of no complaint to the child. If the deformity is painful, it is usually related to irritation with shoe gear or abutment of the hallux with the second toe. The teenage years is the most common age group for complaints with the deformity. The hallux valgus deformity often becomes problematic in shoes, especially for those athletic children, and often can be a significant cosmetic concern for developing young adults.

Clinically, juveniles with hallux abductovalgus typically have a smaller medial eminence and less valgus rotation of the hallux than adults with the deformity (Fig. 7.1). They also usually have less pain involved with the deformity than adults, and their first metatarsophalangeal joint is free of degenerative changes in most cases. Although hypermobility may be present, the juvenile hallux valgus deformity is typically a much more stable deformity than that seen in the adult. Also, juvenile hallux valgus is commonly associated with other structural abnormalities, most notably metatarsus adductus and pes planus. The incidence of metatarsus adductus in patients presenting with juvenile hallux abductovalgus is much higher than what is seen in the normal population. It has ranged from 22% to 75% in various studies [2, 23, 24] (Fig. 7.2). The incidence of pes planus deformity contributing to the development of juvenile hallux valgus deformity has varied considerably in the literature from no increase to a 41% increased incidence [2, 25–27] (Fig. 7.3).

Radiographic Evaluation

Radiographic assessment of a juvenile hallux valgus deformity should include weightbearing dorsoplantar, medial oblique, lateral, and sesamoid axial views to appreciate the deformity in all planes. The problem with standard radiographs is that they provide two-dimensional

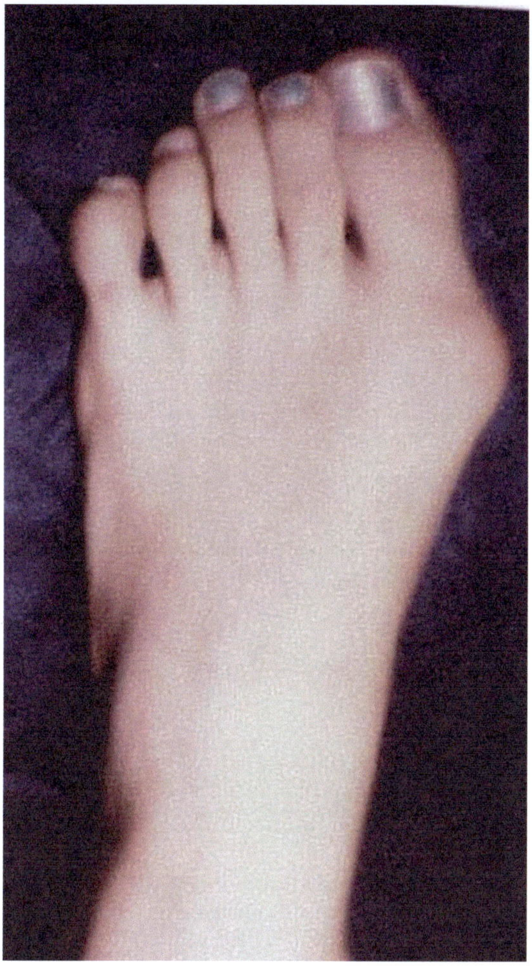

Fig. 7.1 Typical clinical presentation of a pediatric bunion deformity. Notice there is not a lot of valgus rotation of the hallux

findings for a three-dimensional deformity. The hallux abductus angle, intermetatarsal angle, and sesamoid position via the sesamoid axial projection provide the most reliable and reproducible assessment of the deformity [28, 29]. The proximal articular set angle (PASA) is also important to be evaluated in the juvenile hallux valgus deformity. PASA is defined as the relationship between a line connecting the medial and lateral articular margins of the first metatarsal head and the longitudinal axis of the first metatarsal. Measurements between 0° and 8° are considered normal; however, Vittetoe et al. also recommended evaluating PASA intraoperatively since there is only a 95% chance of estimating this angle within 5° of the true angle [30]. An increased PASA indicates functional adaptation of the first metatarsal due to chronic malpositioning of and abnormal forces of the hallux. An increased PASA is a common finding in the radiographic evaluation of the pediatric hallux valgus deformity. This lateral deviation of the articular surface results in a congruent valgus deformity of the first metatarsophalangeal joint (Fig. 7.4). This congruent valgus deformity renders the first metatarsophalangeal joint stable and less prone to degenerative changes. This is in contrast to the adult deformity, where PASA is not commonly increased and there is an incongruent valgus positioning of the first metatarsophalangeal joint. This incongruency renders the first metatarsophalangeal joint unstable; therefore, subluxation is common and the joint is prone to degeneration.

It is also important to look at the length of the first metatarsal when evaluating this pediatric deformity. According to McLuney et al. and Munuera et al., a long first metatarsal is a significant component and predictor of juvenile hallux abductovalgus development and has been shown to be 94.3% accurate [31, 32]. Other factors to assess radiographically include the physis, the articulation of the first metatarsal and medial cuneiform, and other concomitant deformities. The physis is located at the base of the first metatarsal and is typically closed by the age of 17. It should also be noted that the growth plate usually closes at an earlier age in females than in their male counterparts. It is also very important to evaluate the metatarsus adductus angle in pediatric patients. The existence of an increased metatarsus adductus angle has been shown to be a common finding in patients with juvenile hallux abductovalgus [23, 24]. Although the intermetatarsal angle (IMA) may be low when assessing the juvenile bunion deformity, one has to take into account the underlying increased metatarsus adductus angle (MAA) when present in order to calculate a more accurate angle. The true or effective IMA was defined by Yu et al. by the following formula: IMA + (MAA − 15) = true IMA

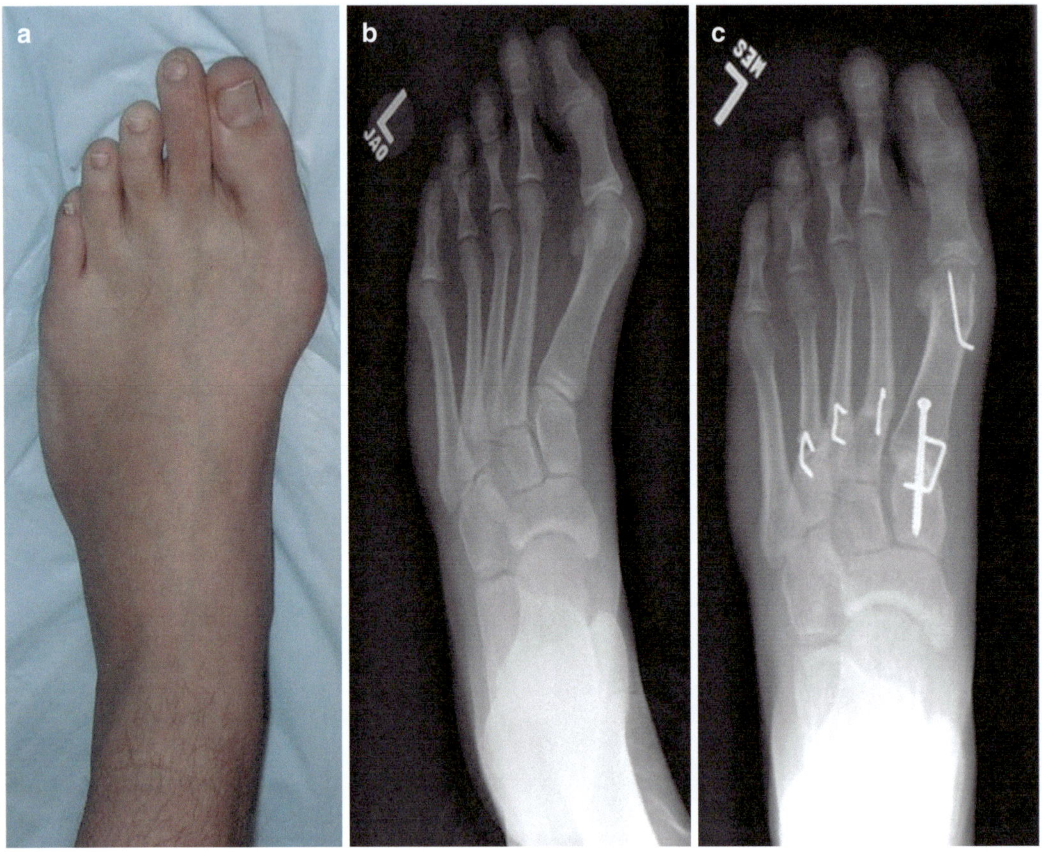

Fig. 7.2 (**a**, **b**) Clinical and radiographic appearance of a 15-year-old male with juvenile hallux valgus and underlying metatarsus adductus deformity. (**c**) Surgical correction of the hallux abductovalgus deformity with a Lapidus arthrodesis and a Reverdin osteotomy. The metatarsus adductus deformity was also corrected

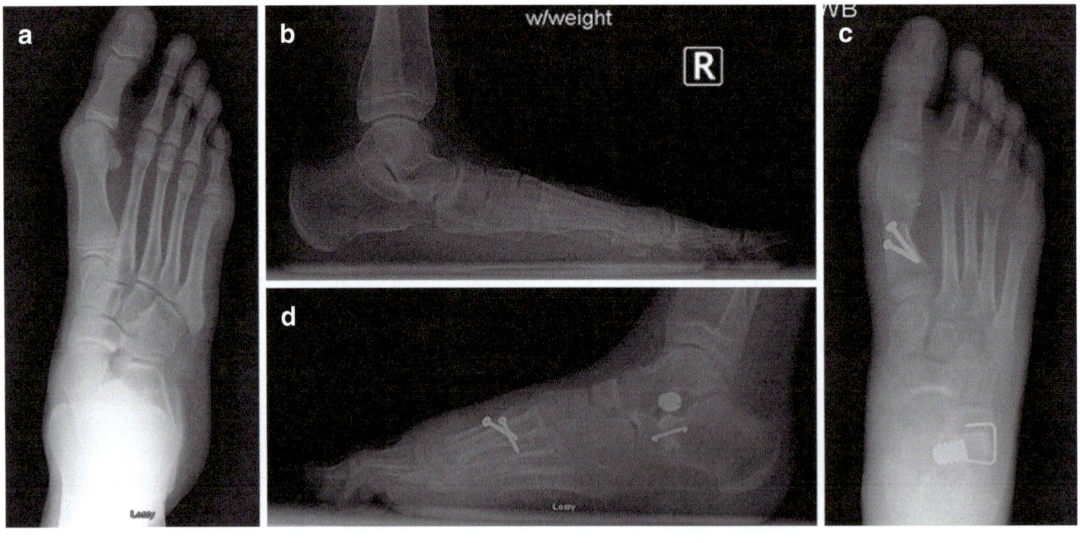

Fig. 7.3 (**a**, **b**) Radiographs of a 13-year-old female with a painful hallux abductovalgus deformity and underlying pes planovalgus. (**c**, **d**) Postoperative radiographs showing surgical correction of all deformities with a closing base wedge osteotomy, Evans calcaneal osteotomy with allogeneic bone graft, and a subtalar joint arthroereisis

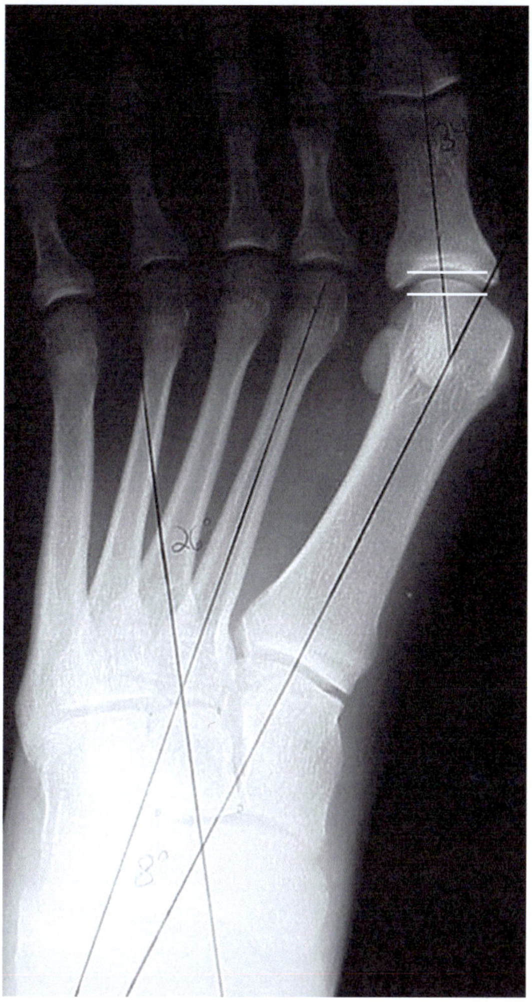

Fig. 7.4 This is the radiograph of the clinical bunion deformity in Fig. 7.1. Notice the small medial eminence and long first metatarsal. There is also a very large hallux abductus angle (HAA), low intermetatarsal angle (IMA), increased metatarsus adductus angle, and increased proximal articular set angle (PASA). This lateral deviation of the articular cartilage results in a congruent valgus deformity and renders the first metatarsophalangeal joint stable. This is in contrast to the adult deformity where PASA is typically not increased, resulting in an incongruent valgus positioning of the first metatarsophalangeal joint and rendering it unstable and prone to subluxation

[33]. So, when taking the MAA into account, the true IMA is larger than one expects. This is very important when deciding on surgical procedures. The presence of a pes planovalgus deformity should also be assessed as it may also coexist with a hallux abductovalgus deformity.

Griffiths and Palladino found that in the pediatric bunion deformity, there was a statistically significant direct relationship between an increased metatarsus adductus angle, an increased hallux abductus angle, and an increased proximal articular set angle, but a trend of a decreased intermetatarsal angle [24, 34, 35]. This is quite different than the adult that tends to have a higher intermetatarsal angle, a moderate hallux abductus angle, but a low metatarsus adductus angle, and a low proximal articular set angle (Fig. 7.5).

Treatment Considerations

Treatment options are based upon many factors and should not be performed for solely cosmetic reasons. Considerations that the surgeon needs to take into account prior to developing a treatment plan include the age of the patient, skeletal maturity, open physis, flexibility of deformity, onset and progression of deformity, underlying etiologic factors, concomitant deformities, severity of symptoms and the patients and parents expectations. Nonoperative treatments for the pediatric bunion deformity focus on managing the symptoms and trying to address any underlying structural problems that are present. Symptomatic relief of painful bunions can be achieved with wider toebox shoes, accommodative padding, activity modification, and anti-inflammatory measures. Structural issues are often addressed with the use of functional foot orthoses and the use of bunion splints. It is important to continue to monitor for progression of the bunion deformity and reassess the treatment plan as the child matures.

Surgical intervention should only be entertained after conservative measures have failed and if there is pain and interference with activities. It is extremely important to obtain a complete history and physical examination of the patient. It is essential to obtain from parents or caretakers any familial or hereditary disease processes that may result in joint laxity. The patient must be evaluated for any concomitant deformities such as metatarsus adductus, pes planovalgus, equinus, internal tibial torsion, and femoral anteversion which may have led to the development of the hallux abductovalgus deformity. Failure to identify

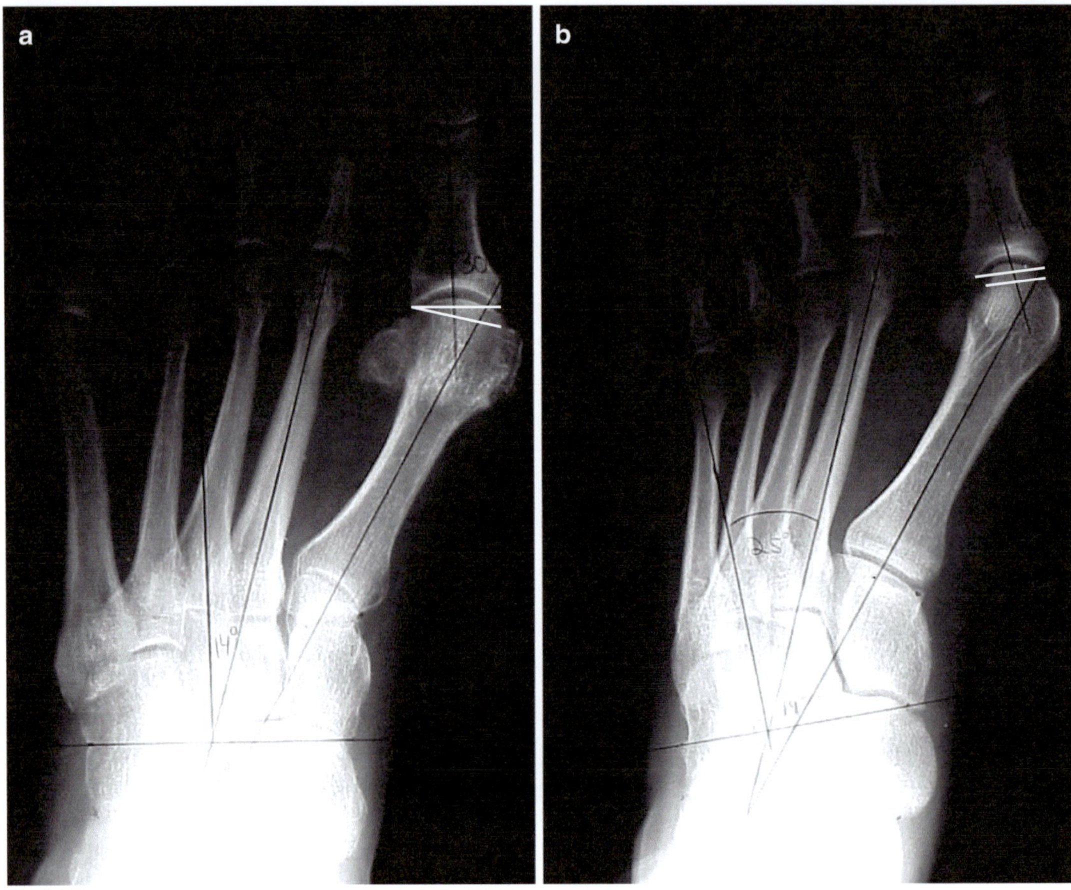

Fig. 7.5 (**a**) Common radiographic presentation of an adult bunion deformity including a low MAA, moderate HAA, low PASA, and incongruent valgus deformity and subluxation of the 1st MTPJ. (**b**) Common radiographic presentation of a pediatric bunion deformity including a high MAA, high HAA, high PASA, and a congruent valgus deformity and stable 1st MTPJ. Also note the long first metatarsal

and address concomitant pathology may lead to insufficient correction or recurrence of the bunion deformity.

Although the age of the patient is important to consider when evaluating surgical options with a child, the patient's skeletal maturity is key to the timing of surgical intervention. There is limited effectiveness with bunion surgery in a child under the age of six, and it should be avoided. The first metatarsal is very small and immature and has only achieved 40 to 50% of its normal growth. The first metatarsal has obtained 60–80% of its length between the age of 6 to 10 years old, and the growth plate is still open. Although the metatarsal is becoming similar in size and shape to the adult version, surgical intervention should still be avoided in these patients if possible. Surgery in this age group should be reserved for very severe, painful, and rapidly progressive deformities.

Girls tend to reach skeletal maturity at an earlier age than boys. By the age of 12, 95% of the normal metatarsal length is obtained in females and 90% has been obtained in males. The epiphyseal plate generally closes between the ages of 13 and 15 in girls and between 15 and 17 years of age in boys. The presence of an open physis at the base of the first metatarsal may lead to either a delay in surgical correction or placement of an osteotomy in a more distal location to avoid injury to the growth plate. Currently, the authors prefer to wait until the patient reaches skeletal maturity, meaning the growth plate is closed and the first metatarsal has reached normal length, before proceeding with elective bunion surgery in the pediatric population. Therefore, surgical intervention is most favorable when the child is typically over 16 years old.

Surgical Intervention

As with any type of deformity correction, the basis for surgical intervention for hallux abductovalgus involves realigning the bone and rebalancing the soft tissue structures around the joint back into proper position. Historically, surgical treatment options for juvenile bunion correction have focused on distal metatarsal osteotomies and basilar procedures. Since the juvenile hallux abductovalgus deformity usually warrants greater and more aggressive surgical intervention than the adult, a distal metatarsal osteotomy alone is typically not enough to gain and maintain full correction of the deformity (Fig. 7.6). When performed,

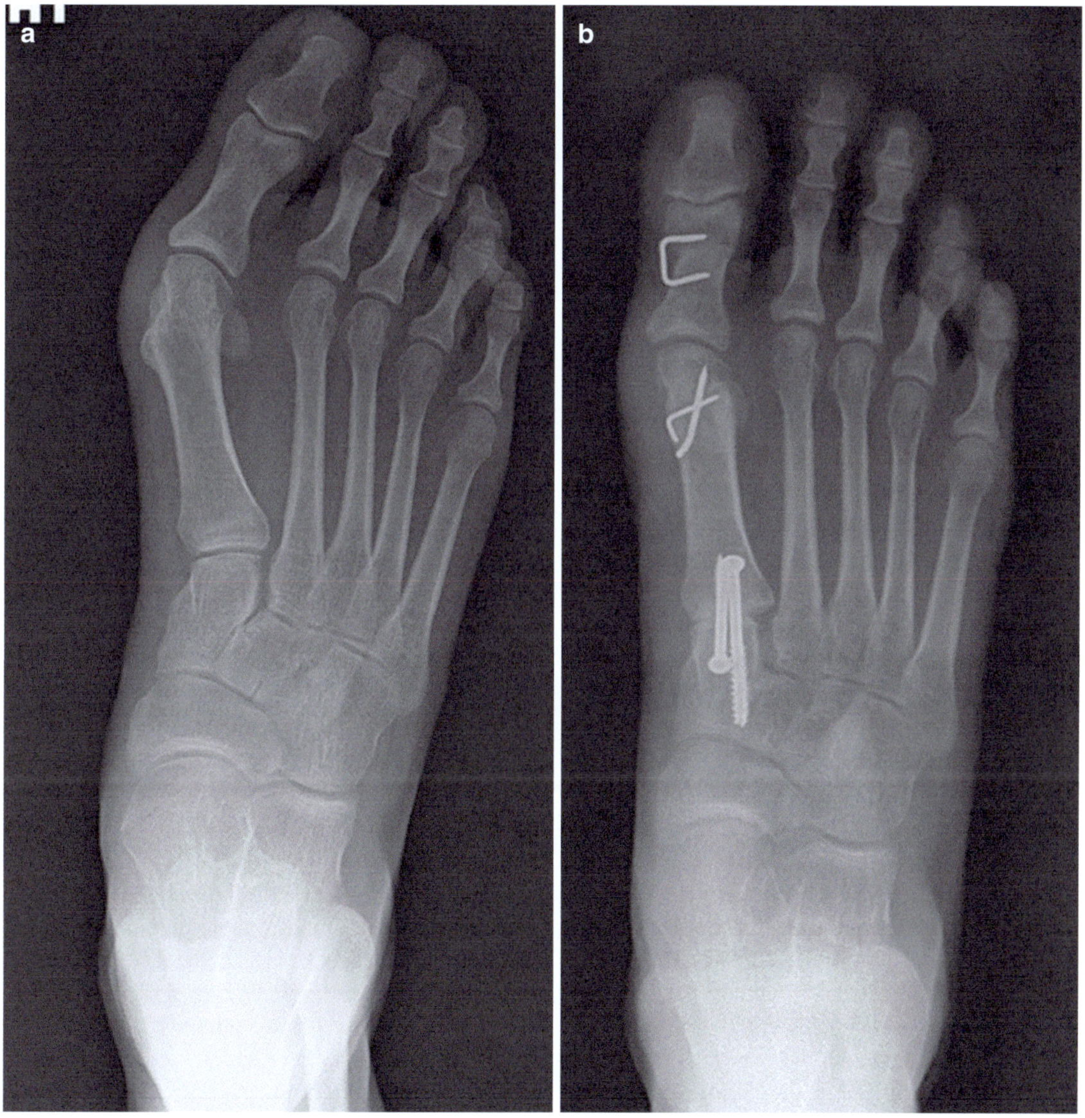

Fig. 7.6 (**a**) A 16-year-old female with cerebral palsy underwent a Silver bunionectomy 1 year prior. This procedure was inadequate to correct the deformity, and additional surgery was warranted. (**b**) Revisional surgery including a Lapidus bunionectomy, Reverdin osteotomy, and distal Akin was performed, and full correction was obtained

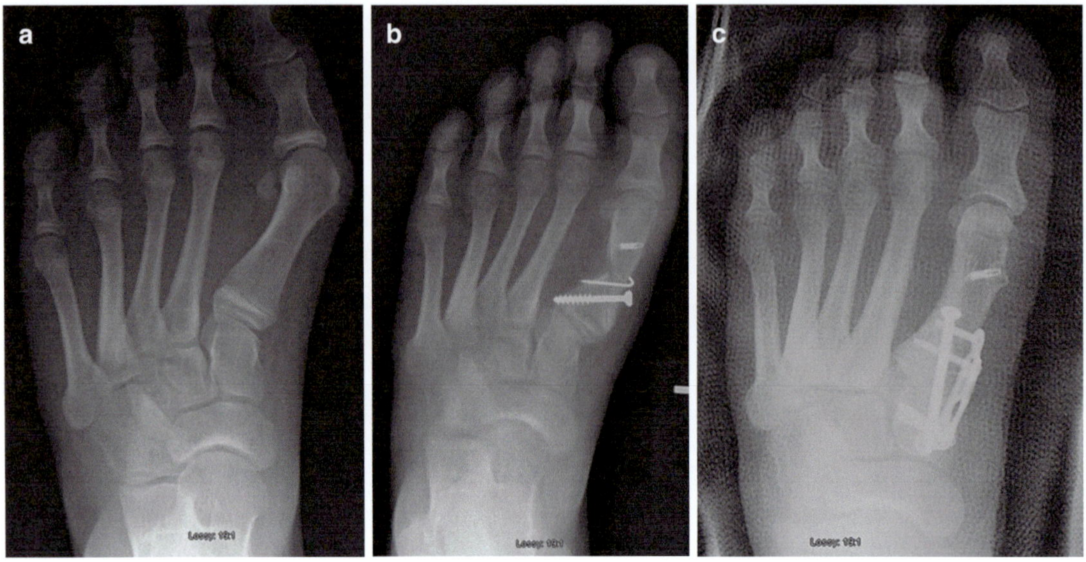

Fig. 7.7 (**a**) Preoperative radiograph of a 12-year-old female with severe juvenile bunion deformity. (**b**) First surgical intervention was a closing base wedge osteotomy with an adductor hallucis tendon transfer. (**c**) She returned 6 years later with recurrence of the bunion deformity and lesser metatarsalgia due to medial column insufficiency necessitating a Lapidus procedure

distal metatarsal osteotomies are usually used in combination with basilar procedures to correct for adaptation of the first metatarsal articulation. The most common basilar procedures performed are the closing base wedge osteotomy and the first metatarsal cuneiform arthrodesis. They are both effective procedures in correcting the bunion deformity, and it is usually surgeon preference which procedure is performed. If the growth plate is still open, the closing base wedge osteotomy is favorable because it allows for the execution of the osteotomy and placement of fixation without interfering with the growth plate. If hypermobility is present or frontal plane correction of the deformity is warranted, the first metatarsal cuneiform arthrodesis is typically the procedure of choice (Fig. 7.7). Other procedures that have also been performed for the correction of juvenile hallux abductovalgus deformity include the opening base wedge osteotomy, crescentic osteotomy, and epiphysiodesis.

Distal Metatarsal Osteotomies

Distal osteotomies have the advantage of avoiding the physis at the base of the first metatarsal, but the amount of intermetatarsal angle correction obtained can be limited. The Reverdin osteotomy, and its modification, is a popular procedure to realign the articular surface of the first metatarsal by removing a medially based wedge from the dorsal arm. The osteotomy can also be modified to include a plantar arm to avoid damage to the sesamoids. The capital portion of the osteotomy can also be shifted laterally for intermetatarsal angle correction. A Chevron-type osteotomy and its modifications are another type of distal osteotomy that can be utilized to decrease the intermetatarsal angle and in some instances be swiveled to address articular adaptation that is noted intraoperatively. Fixation for distal osteotomies is often achieved with a Kirschner wire or small screw(s) (Fig. 7.8).

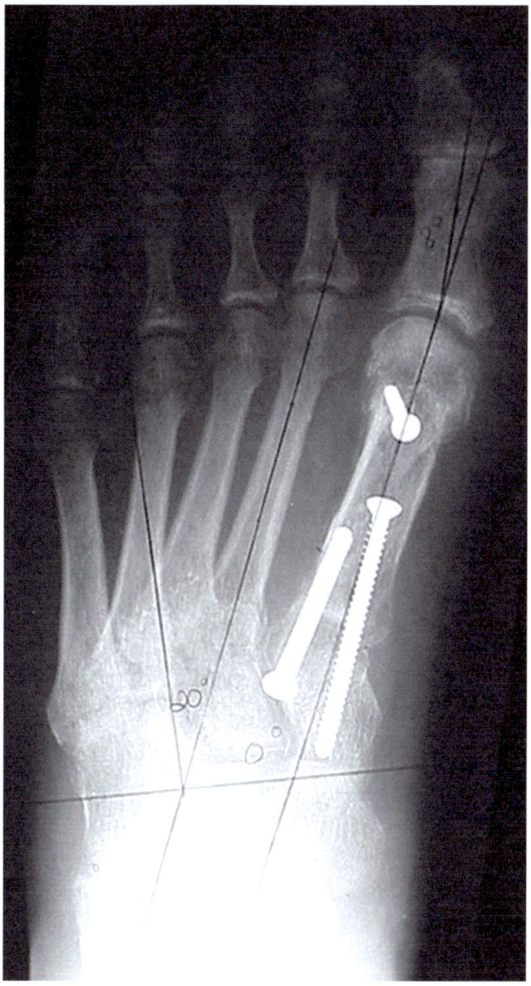

Fig. 7.8 In addition to a Lapidus arthrodesis, a Reverdin osteotomy was performed with screw fixation to realign the articular cartilage on the first metatarsal and gain full correction of the deformity

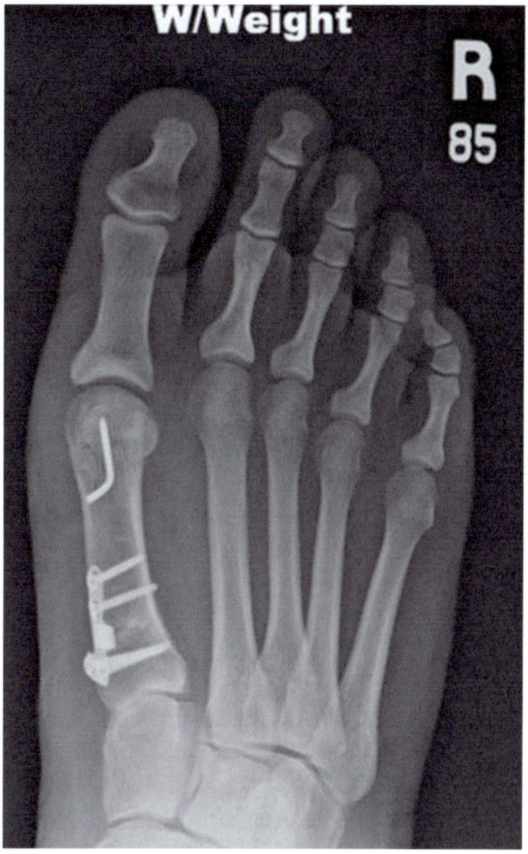

Fig. 7.9 An opening wedge osteotomy with plate fixation was performed on this patient with a short first metatarsal. A Reverdin osteotomy was also performed to correct for PASA

Proximal Metatarsal Osteotomies

The crescentic osteotomy has been shown to provide correction of the juvenile bunion deformity in several planes, including the frontal plane, and it also avoids shortening of the metatarsal. Fixation of the osteotomy has proven to be difficult however, and it is not commonly used in this patient population. The opening base wedge osteotomy has also been mentioned, but rarely utilized, in the correction of juvenile bunion deformities. This osteotomy actually lengthens the first ray and may cause jamming and stiffness in the first metatarsophalangeal joint. Since most juveniles have a long first metatarsal, this procedure is not ideal. Also, the opening wedge osteotomy requires bone grafting and/or special spacers and fixation (Fig. 7.9).

The more common proximal metatarsal osteotomy is the closing base wedge. The closing base wedge osteotomy has been performed

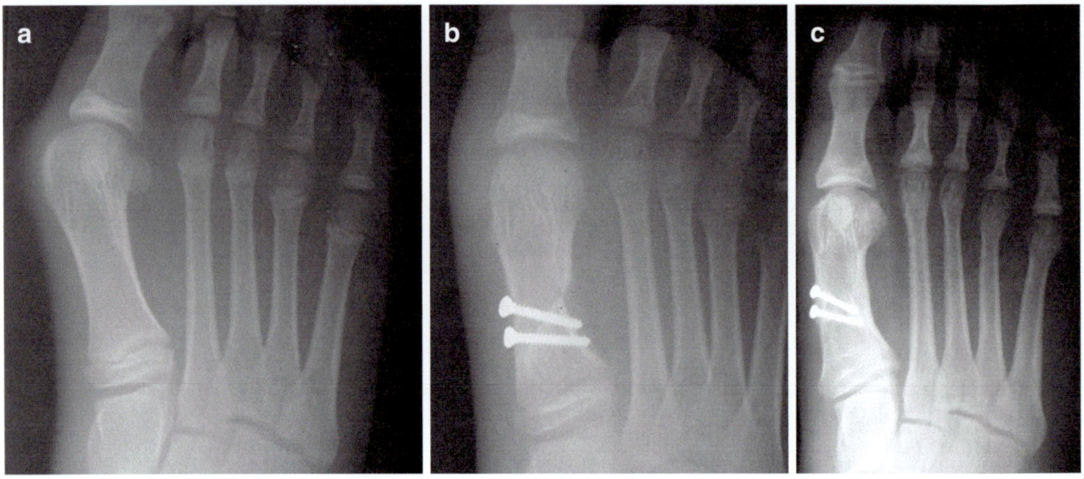

Fig. 7.10 (**a**) Preoperative radiograph of an 11-year-old male with a very painful hallux valgus deformity interfering with his daily activities and warranting surgical intervention. Notice the open growth plate in the base of the first metatarsal. (**b**) A closing base wedge osteotomy was performed distal to the open growth plate. (**c**) Radiograph of the same patient 10 years after the closing base wedge osteotomy was performed. Notice how distal the screws appear in the metatarsal once full growth has been obtained

for years in the pediatric patient with a large bunion deformity. This procedure can be carefully performed with an open growth plate with the apex of the osteotomy distal to the physis. Unfortunately, the more distal the osteotomy is made, the less the intermetatarsal correction can be obtained, and there is a greater likelihood of exacerbating any cartilage malposition of the first metatarsal head (Fig. 7.10). When performing the osteotomy, care is taken to try and maintain the hinge on the proximal medial aspect at the apex. Fixation is typically obtained with two-screw fixation with an anchor screw perpendicular to the long axis of the metatarsal and a compression screw perpendicular to the osteotomy (Fig. 7.11). If greater deviation of the proximal articular set angle of the first metatarsal is noted intraoperatively, then a distal osteotomy such as a Reverdin can be performed in conjunction with the closing base wedge osteotomy. Base wedge osteotomies in conjunction with the distal Reverdin procedure have been shown to produce excellent results in the correction of juvenile hallux abductovalgus deformities, particularly those associated with metatarsus adductus and an increased PASA [23].

One of the main disadvantages to a patient having a proximal metatarsal osteotomy is that postoperatively, they must remain nonweightbearing on that foot until osseous union is achieved. This is typically 6–8 weeks in a short leg cast prior to beginning progressive protected weightbearing in a removable walking boot. Devastating results, including elevation of the osteotomy, nonunion, malunion, and hardware failure, can happen with a non-compliant patient.

First Metatarsal Cuneiform Arthrodesis

Lapidus first described the first metatarsal cuneiform arthrodesis for the correction of juvenile hallux abductovalgus in 1934 [36]. If the physis is closed, a Lapidus first metatarsal cuneiform joint fusion with capsule tendon balancing about the first metatarsal phalangeal joint is a viable option in correcting the pediatric bunion deformity. The Lapidus procedure allows for correction in all three cardinal planes and can help provide stability along the medial column. This procedure,

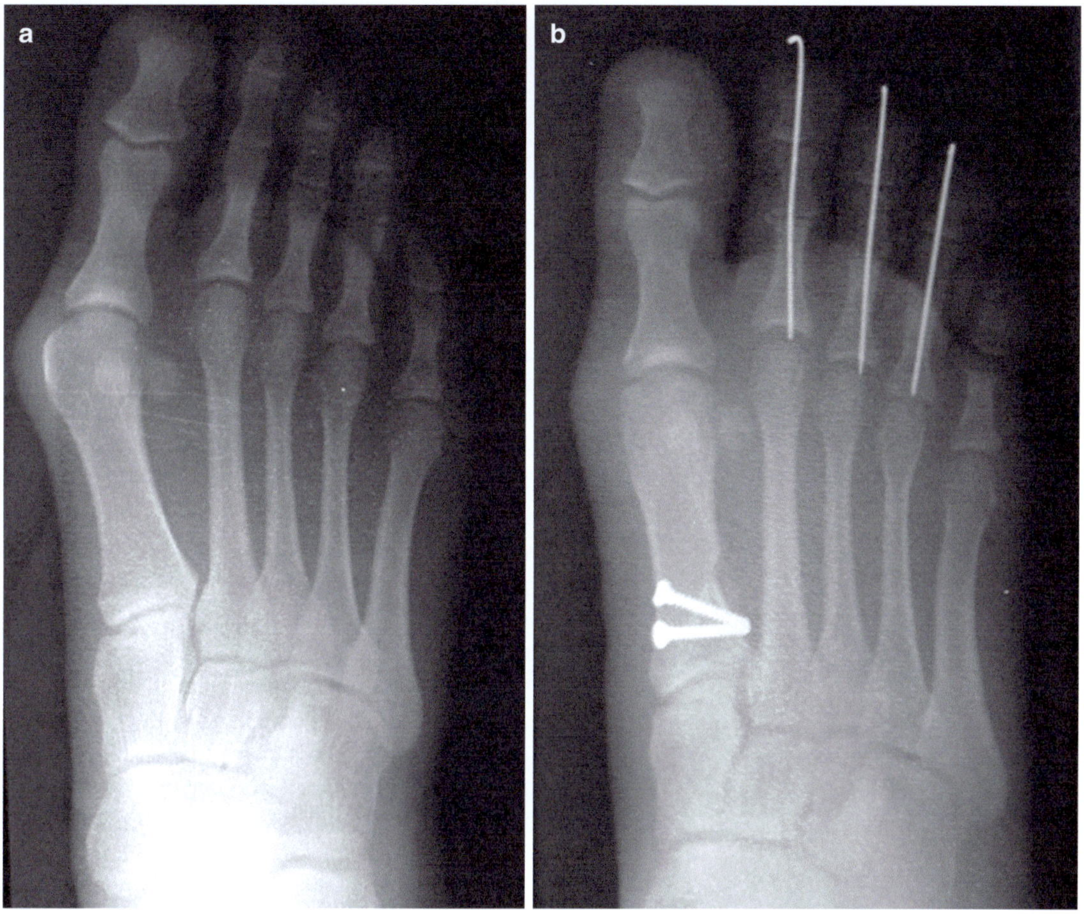

Fig. 7.11 (**a**) Preoperative radiograph of a 15-year-old female. The growth plate is closed, and the first metatarsal is not elongated, so the procedure of choice was a closing base wedge osteotomy. (**b**) Closing base wedge osteotomy with two screw fixation. The anchor screw is perpendicular to the long axis of the first metatarsal, and the compression screw is perpendicular to the osteotomy

therefore, is very beneficial in patients with frontal plane deformity and/or hypermobility.

Adequate joint preparation of the first metatarsal cuneiform joint using either hand or power instrumentation is performed. Historically, a laterally based wedge was removed at the joint to afford adequate intermetatarsal correction; however, this resulted in shortening of the first metatarsal which was often problematic. To account for the shortening, the metatarsal was often transposed plantarly. More recently, contoured or planar joint preparation has been utilized which leads to much less shortening and does not require plantar translocation of the first metatarsal. Since most pediatric bunion deformities have a long first metatarsal, this procedure can effectively reduce the first metatarsal length as needed.

Following joint resection, the first metatarsal can be corrected in all three planes to improve the intermetatarsal angle, frontal plane rotation, and sagittal plane positioning of the first metatarsal as needed. Various forms of fixation constructs have been utilized to stabilize the Lapidus procedure including screws, staples, plates, intramedullary nails, and external fixation (Fig. 7.12). Since the fixation utilized for this procedure crosses the joint and would interfere with an open phy-

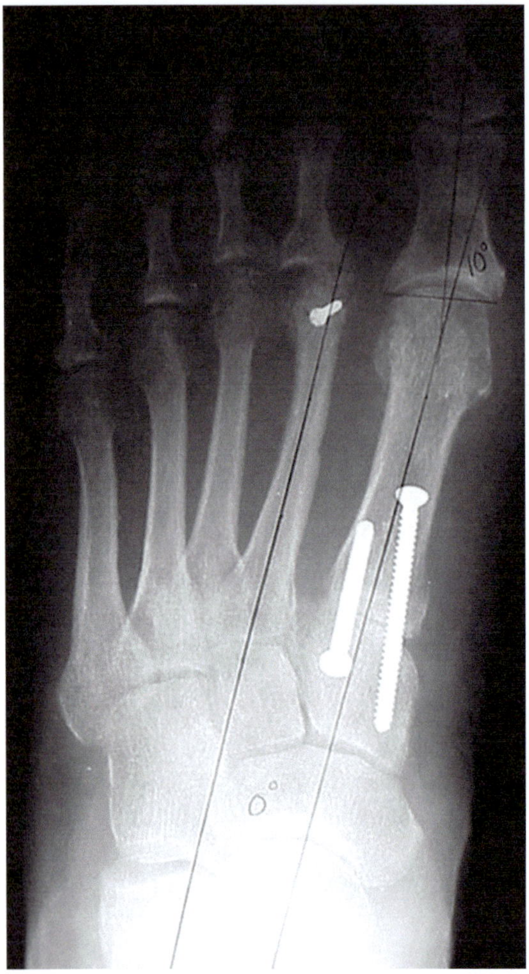

Fig. 7.12 A Lapidus arthrodesis with two-screw fixation was performed on this 17-year-old female with hypermobility

sis, this procedure is not recommended for those patients undergoing surgical correction with an open growth plate. Although smooth Kirschner wires could be utilized for fixation if an open physis is present, it is not ideal.

One of the drawbacks of performing the Lapidus arthrodesis procedure for bunion correction is the need for non-weightbearing postoperatively. However, with enhanced fixation techniques, the need for non-weightbearing has been dramatically reduced. Some surgeons begin weightbearing as early as 2 weeks without showing detrimental effects such as nonunion or disruption of the arthrodesis site.

Epiphysiodesis

Less commonly, a lateral hemiepiphysiodesis, can be performed for a skeletally immature patient with a juvenile hallux abductovalgus deformity. This epiphysiodesis technique was first described in the 1930s to correct angular deformities in children [37]. The procedure offers a surgical alternative to a first metatarsal osteotomy in patients with a significant bunion deformity and remaining growth of the metatarsal. Ablation of the physis on the lateral side results in asymmetric growth of the metatarsal on the medial aspect, which can lead to reduction of the intermetatarsal angle and correction of the deformity over time. According to Green et al., the pattern of growth of first metatarsal follows a logarithmic regression curve. This allows for clinical prediction of first metatarsal growth based on age and sex and, in turn, guides the timing of the lateral hemiepiphysiodesis procedure. Unfortunately, at the current time, the clinical results of hemiepiphysiodesis have not been able to be correlated with the anatomic predictions that the authors provided [38].

Summary

Successful management of juvenile hallux abductovalgus necessitates thorough knowledge of the deformity itself and treatment options. The surgeon has to be able to recognize all causative factors, concomitant deformities, and biomechanical influences that have contributed to the development of the hallux abductovalgus deformity. If contributory conditions are not addressed, maintenance of long- term correction is unlikely. The physician must also recognize that the pediatric deformity differs from the adult deformity and should direct treatments accordingly. Skeletal maturity is key for successful surgical intervention. Surgery performed prior to complete skeletal maturity runs a higher risk for complications including damage to the growth plate. Typically, a combination of distal and proximal surgical procedures is warranted for complete correction of the hallux abductovalgus deformity. The surgeon has to individualize the treatment plan according to clinical and radiographic findings and select the surgical procedures that are best for each patient. Successful correction of juvenile hallux abductovalgus can be consistently obtained if the physician recognizes and address all contributing factors of the deformity, skeletal maturity is reached prior to surgical intervention, and the treatment plan is individualized.

References

1. Piggot H. The natural history of hallux valgus in adolescence and early adult life. J Bone Joint Surg Br. 1960;42B:749–60.
2. Coughlin MJ. Juvenile hallux valgus: etiology and treatment. Foot Ankle Int. 1995;16(11):682–97.
3. Goldner JL, Gaines RW. Adult and juvenile hallux valgus: analysis and treatment. Orthop Clin North Am. 1976;7:863.
4. Zollinger H, Fellman J, Brumm C. Juvenile hallux valgus. Orthopade. 1996;25:349–53.
5. Hardy R, Clapham J. Observations on hallux valgus based on a controlled series. J Bone Joint Surg Br. 1951;33:376–91.
6. Chell J, Dhar S. Pediatric hallux valgus. Foot Ankle Clin N Am. 2014;19:235–43.
7. Gould N, Schneider W, Ashikagu T. Epidemiological survey of foot problems in the United States. Foot Ankle Int. 1980;1:8.
8. Helal B. Surgery for adolescent hallux valgus. Clin Orthop Relat Res. 1981;(157):50-63.
9. Coughlin MJ, Thompson FM. The high price of high-fashion footwear. Instr Course Lect. 1955;44: 371–7.
10. Coste F, Desoille H, Illouz G, Chavy AL. Locomotor apparatus and classical dancing. Rev Rheum Mal Osteoartic. 1960;27:259–67.
11. Coughlin MJ, Thompson FM. Women's shoe wear and foot disorders. West J Med. 1995;163:569–70.
12. Shine IB. Incidence of hallux valgus in a partially shoe-wearing community. Br Med J. 1965;1:1648–50.
13. Sim-Fook L, Hodgson AR. A comparison of foot forms among the non-shoe and shoe-wearing Chinese population. J Bone Joint Surg Am. 1958;40-A:1058–62.
14. Geissele AE, Stanton RP. Surgical treatment of adolescent hallux valgus. J Pediatr Orthop. 1990;10:642.
15. Meier PJ, Kenzora JE. The risks and benefits of distal first metatarsal osteotomies. Foot Ankle Int. 1985;6:7.
16. Glynn MK, Dunlop JB, Fitzpatrick D. The Mitchell distal metatarsal osteotomy for hallux valgus. J Bone Joint Surg Br. 1980;62:188.
17. Johnson O. Further studies of the inheritance of hand and foot anomalies. Clin Orthop. 1954;8:146.
18. Pique-Vidal C, Sole MT, Antich J. Hallux valgus inheritance: pedigree research in 350 patients with bunion deformity. J Foot Ankle Surg. 2007;46: 149–54.
19. Craigmile DA. Incidence, origin, and prevention of certain foot defects. Br Med J. 1953;2:1953.
20. Cole S. Foot inspection of the school child. J Am Podiatry Assoc. 1959;49:446.
21. Dayton P, Kauwe M, Feilmeier M. Clarification of the anatomic definition of the bunion deformity. J Foot Ankle Surg. 2014;53(2):160–3.
22. Mortier JP, Bernard JL, Maestro M. Orthop Trauma Surg Res. 2012;98:677–83.
23. Pontious J, Mahan KT, Carter S. Characteristics of adolescent hallux abducto valgus; a retrospective review. J Am Podiatr Med Assoc. 1994;84:208–18.
24. Ferrari J, Malone-Lee J. A radiographic study of the relationship between metatarsus adductus and hallux valgus. J Foot Ankle Surg. 2003;42(1):9–14.
25. Trott A. Hallux valgus in the adolescent. Am Acad of Orthopaedic Surgeons Instructional Course Lectures, XXI. St. Louis: CV Mosby; 1972. p. 262–8.
26. Scranton P. Adolescent bunions: diagnosis and management. Pediatr Ann. 1982;11:518–20. Kalen V, Brecher A. Relationship between adolescent bunions and flatfeet. Foot Ankle Int. 1988;8:331–6.
27. Kilmartin TE, Barrington RI, Wallace WA. Metatarsus primus varus. A statistical study. J Bone Joint Surg Br. 1991;73:937–40.
28. Dayton P, Kaume M, Feilmeier M. Is our current paradigm for evaluation and management of the bunion deformity flawed? A discussion of procedure philosophy relative to anatomy. J Foot Ankle Surg. 2015;54(1):102.
29. Dayton P, Feilmeier M, Kaume M, Hirschi J. Relationship of frontal plane rotation of first metatarsal to proximal articular set angle and hallux alignment in patients undergoing tarsometatarsal arthrodesis for hallux abducto valgus: a case series and critical review of the literature. J Foot Ankle Surg. 2013;52(3):348.
30. Vittetoe D, Saltzman C, Krieg J, et al. Validity and reliability of the first distal metatarsal articular angle. Foot Ankle Int. 1994;15(10):541–7.
31. McCluney JG, Tinley P. Radiographic measurements of patients with juvenile hallux valgus compared with age-matched controls: a cohort investigation. J Foot Ankle Surg. 2006;4(1):63–74.
32. Munuera PV, Polo J, Rebollo J. Length of the first metatarsal and hallux in hallux valgus in the initial stage. Int Orthod. 2008;32(4):489–95.

33. Yu GV, Landers P, Lo K, et al. Juvenile and adolescent hallux abducto valgus deformity. In: DeValentine SJ, editor. Foot and ankle disorders in children. New York: Churchill Livingstone; 1992.
34. Griffiths TA, Palladino SJ. Metatarsus adductus and selected radiographic measurements of the first ray in normal feet. J Am Podiatr Med Assoc. 1992;82:616.
35. Banks AS, Hsu YS, Mariash S, and Zirm R. Juvenile Hallux Abductovalgus Association with Metatarsus Adductus. J Am Podiatr Med Assoc. 1994;84:219.
36. Lapidus PW. The operative correction of the metatarsus primus varus in hallux valgus. Surg Gynecol Obstet. 1934;58:183.
37. Phemister DB. Operative arrest of longitudinal bones in the treatment of deformities. J Bone Joint Surg Am. 1993;15:1.
38. Green JD, Nicholson AD, Sander JO, Cooperman DR, Liu RW. Analysis of serial radiographs of the foot to determine normative values for the growth of the first metatarsal to guide hemiepiphysiodesis for immature hallux valgus. Pediatr Orthop. 2017;37(5):338–43.

Pediatric Equinus Deformity

8

Patrick A. DeHeer

Introduction

Equinus has been called "the worst foot in the world," "the most profound causal agent in foot pathomechanics," and "the primary causal agent in a significant proportion of foot pathology" [1–3]. Up to 95.5% of all biomechanically related lower extremity pathologies are associated with equinus leading to equinus being described as "extremely prevalent" [3]. The role of equinus in the pediatric patient is similar to that of the adult patient, with noted specific pathologies related to equinus that are unique to the pediatric patient. Historically, equinus in the pediatric patient has predominately been discussed in the neurological patient. Much has been written on this topic especially in the cerebral palsy patient. On the other hand, little has been written on functional equinus in the non-neurological pediatric patient. Documentation of the pathologic effect of equinus on the lower extremity in the literature dates back for well over 100 years [4].

In 1913 John Joseph Nutt, MD, described the relationship of equinus and its effect on the arch, essentially describing gastrocnemius equinus [4]. The literature continues to shed light on this topic as evident by the Foot and Ankle Clinics of North America, December 2014 edition, dedicated solely to the gastrocnemius. Despite the abundance of literature on equinus, it continues to be under-evaluated and treated. Pierre Barouk, MD, discussed this in his Introduction as guest editor for the Gastrocnemius Edition of Foot and Ankle Clinics of North America [5]:

> Looking for a retraction of the gastrocnemius should be an essential part of the foot and ankle examination for practitioners, not just surgeons. Even though the equinus has been recognized for 50 years as having an influence on the foot, only a few practitioners routinely search for it. The proportion of gastrocnemius tightness is high in the normal population, but it is significantly higher in populations that have foot and ankle problems.
>
> Attaching some symptoms (calf cramps, lower limb instability, difficulty in walking without a heel, lumbar pain) to gastrocnemius tightness is essential to treating patients in a global manner. I hope you will be convinced of the importance of this, and no longer do without!

Anatomy

Grasping the anatomy of the gastrocnemius-soleus complex (GSC) is essential to understanding equinus. The GSC is in the superficial posterior compartment of the leg and is made up of the gastrocnemius, soleus, and plantaris [6].

P. A. DeHeer (✉)
St. Vincent Hospital, Indianapolis, IN, USA

Private Practice Hoosier Foot & Ankle, Franklin, IN, USA

M. L. Butterworth, J. T. Marcoux (eds.), *The Pediatric Foot and Ankle*,
https://doi.org/10.1007/978-3-030-29788-6_8

Achilles Tendon

The Achilles tendon is the strongest, thickest, largest tendon in the body approximately 15 cm long (11–26 cm) with a mean width at its origin of 6.8 cm (4.5–8.6 cm) narrowing distally to mean width of 1.8 cm (1.2–2.6 cm) and then widening at the insertion to a mean width of 3.4 cm (2.0–4.8 cm) [7]. The Achilles is made up of contributions from the gastrocnemius and soleus muscles. The exact contribution of each component was documented by Cummins et al., who discovered in 52 of 100 cadavers that the Achilles tendon consisted of 52% by the soleus and 48% by the gastrocnemius, 35% had equal contributions from both muscles, and in 13% the gastrocnemius contributed more than 60% [8]. The tendon inserts into the middle third of the posterior aspect of the calcaneus with a retrocalcaneal bursae between the two. The Achilles tendon fibers spiral approximately 90° with the gastrocnemius muscle fibers inserting laterally and the soleus muscle fibers inserting primarily medially. The Achilles does not have a true tendon sheath but rather a paratenon that covers the tendon allowing for gliding. The paratenon provides protection and nourishment. The tendon's vascular supply is from the myotendinous junction, paratenon, and calcaneal periosteum [6]. The "watershed" area of the tendon is approximately 4 centimeters from the insertion and is often the site of rupture due to inadequate blood flow [6]. See Figs. 8.1, 8.2, and 8.3.

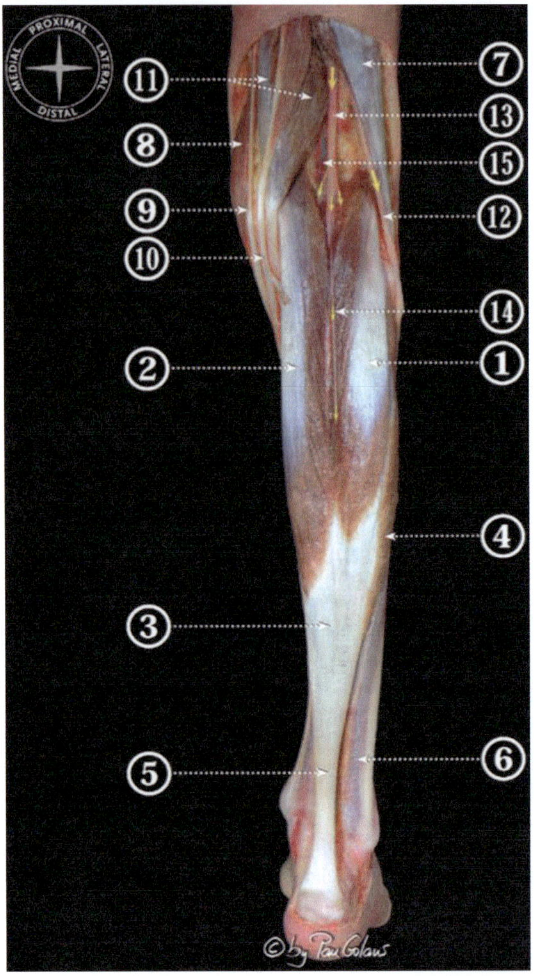

Fig. 8.1 Superficial dissection of the leg and popliteal area showing a posterior view of the triceps surae and its components and surrounding structures. (1) Lateral head of the gastrocnemius muscle; (2) medial head of the gastrocnemius muscle; (3) gastrocnemius aponeurosis; (4) soleus muscle; (5) calcaneal tendon; (6) posterior deep fascia of the leg; (7) biceps femoris muscle; (8) sartorius muscle; (9) gracilis tendon; (10) semitendinosus tendon; (11) semimembranosus muscle; (12) common peroneal nerve; (13) tibial nerve and branches; (14) sural nerve; (15) popliteal artery and vein (Copyright © Pau Golano′ 2014.) (Reprinted with permission from *Foot and Ankle Clinics* 19.4 (2014): 603–635. Copyright 2014, Elsevier)

Gastrocnemius, Soleus, and Plantaris Muscles

The anatomical specifications of the muscles that make up the GSC complex are described in Table 8.1 [6–8].

The pathologic influence caused by a contracture of the GSC is the result of the gastrocnemius muscle crossing the knee, ankle, and subtalar joints. The extension of the knee while the foot is dorsiflexed in late midstance puts the gastrocnemius under maximal tension. When the GSC is pathologically tight, abnormal biomechanical consequences ensue.

Clinical Diagnosis

A significant amount in the literature on the clinical examination of equinus exists, most of it showing the unreliability of clinical examination of ankle joint dorsiflexion [10]. Specifically,

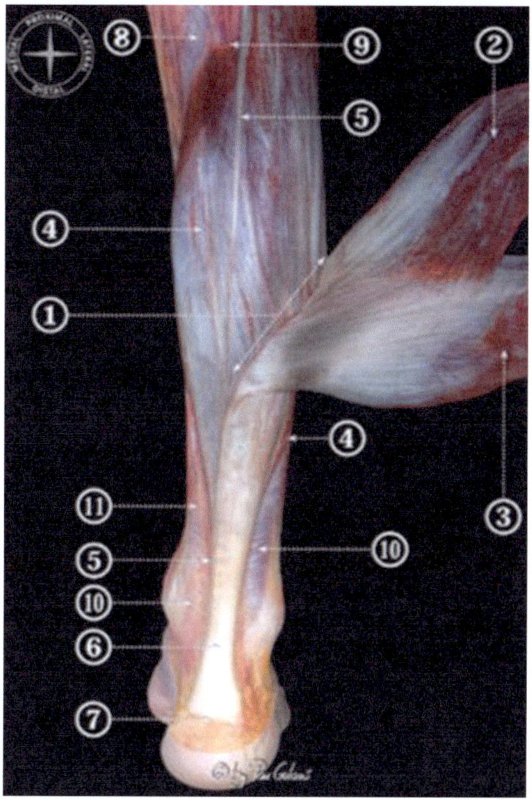

Fig. 8.2 Muscular dissection of the leg to show the components of the triceps surae (gastrocnemius muscle is reflected to reveal soleus posterior aponeurosis). (1) Area of insertion of the gastrocnemius aponeurosis into the soleus posterior aponeurosis (conjoint junction); (2) lateral head of the gastrocnemius muscle; (3) medial head of the gastrocnemius muscle; (4) soleus posterior aponeurosis; (5) plantaris tendon; (6) calcaneal tendon; (7) insertional area of the calcaneal tendon; (8) popliteus muscle; (9) tendinous arch of the soleus muscle; (10) posterior deep fascia of the leg; (11) medial intermuscular septum (Copyright © Pau Golano' 2014.) (Reprinted with permission from *Foot and Ankle Clinics* 19.4 (2014): 603–635. Copyright 2014, Elsevier)

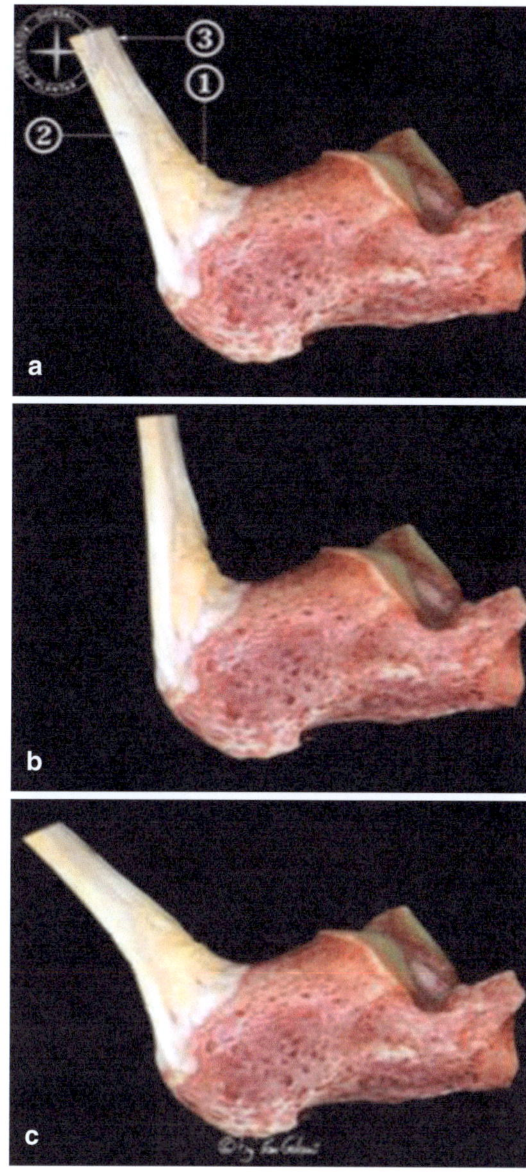

Fig. 8.3 Dissection of the calcaneal tendon and its insertion on the calcaneus showing the retrocalcaneal bursa through ankle's range of motion (calcaneus has been disarticulated from the foot skeleton). (**a**) Ankle in neutral position. (**b**) Ankle in dorsiflexion. (**c**) Ankle in plantarflexion. (1) Retrocalcaneal bursa; (2) calcaneal tendon; (3) plantaris tendon (Copyright © Pau Golano' 2014.) (Reprinted with permission from *Foot and Ankle Clinics* 19.4 (2014): 603–635. Copyright 2014, Elsevier)

the use of a goniometer to measure ankle joint dorsiflexion has been questioned [10–13]. Although the utilization of a goniometer may have poor intra- and inter-rater reliability, it is still the most practical method. The key is using proper technique when measuring. Barouk and Barouk described the correct method to evaluate equinus by correcting any hindfoot valgus to neutral or varus (to prevent dorsiflexion occurring at the STJ or midtarsal joint), avoiding contracture of the extensors (especially the tibialis anterior tendon), applying the proper amount of force (10 nm/2 kg) [9, 14]. With over 23 methods described in the literature on how to evaluate ankle joint dorsiflexion, it is easy to

Table 8.1 Anatomy of the gastrocsoleus complex

	Gastrocnemius muscle	Soleus muscle	Plantaris muscle
Origin	Posterior aspect femoral condyles and knee capsule	Head and proximal 1/3 of the posterior fibula, middle 1/3 of the medial border of the tibia, soleal line, and interosseous membrane	Medial and above the lateral head of gastrocnemius at lateral condyle of femur coursing lateral to medial
Aponeurosis	Anterior to muscle	Posterior to muscle	None – insertion is either conjoined with Achilles tendon or medial to Achilles tendon insertion
Innervation	Tibial nerve (S1 and S2)	Tibial nerve (S1 and S2)	Tibial nerve (S1 and S2)
Vascular supply	Sural branches of the popliteal artery	Sural branches of the popliteal artery, posterior tibial artery, peroneal artery	Sural branches of the popliteal artery, posterior tibial artery, peroneal artery
Joints crossed	Knee, ankle, subtalar joints	Ankle, subtalar joints	Knee, ankle, subtalar joints
Action	Plantarflexion of the ankle joint, flexion of the knee	Plantarflexion of the ankle joint, stabilizing the leg in standing	Assists with plantarflexion of the ankle joint and flexion of the knee

understand much of the confusion associated with equinus [78]. Ankle dorsiflexion can vary by as much as 8.5° to 10° based on a supinated or pronated foot position [78]. When the entire foot is supinated and then the foot is dorsiflexed, this limits midtarsal joint motion to 2.5°, a clinically insignificant amount resulting in improved evaluation consistency [78]. Consistency among research findings by different authors is reassuring. Dayton et al. compared radiographic evaluation of ankle joint dorsiflexion radiographically and clinically with the foot supinated, pronated, and in neutral position [79]. The authors found significant difference with clinical examination depending on foot position (approximately 14° between a pronated foot position and a supinated foot position and approximately 9° between supinated and neutral), while radiographically the tibiotalar angle did not change significantly [79]. The article concluded: "Motion of the foot between the neutral and supinated positions introduced an additional source of potential error from the measurement technique when using the neutral position as the standard, which has been recommended in the past. We recommend a supinated foot position as a more reliable foot position for measuring the clinical ankle joint range of motion and propose it as a potential standard" (see Fig. 8.4) [79].

Definition of Equinus

DiGiovanni et al., in the *Journal of Bone and Joint Surgery (JBJS) 2002*, established an evidenced-based definition [9]. The study consisted of 34 symptomatic patients and 34 control patients examining two central points; the amount of ankle joint dorsiflexion in each group and how often the diagnosis was correct using a goniometer [9]. The patient group averaged 4.5° ± 4.5° dorsiflexion with the knee extended and 17.9° ± 9.0° dorsiflexion with the knee flexed [9]. The control group averaged 13.1° ± 8.2° and 22.3° ± 10.9° dorsiflexion, respectively [9]. The difference between the two groups with the knee extended was statistically significant, while the difference between the two groups with the knee flexed was not statistically significant [9]. The percent of the symptomatic patients with less than 5° dorsiflexion was 65%, and the control group was 24%, and for less than 10° dorsiflexion, the totals were 88% and 44%, respectively [9]. The diagnosis was found to be correct with a goniometer, confirmed with an equinometer, for less than 5°of dorsiflexion in 76% of the patient group and 94% of the control group and for less than 10° dorsiflexion in 88% and 79%, respectively [9]. The authors stated, "We have selected <5° of maximal ankle dorsiflexion with the knee in

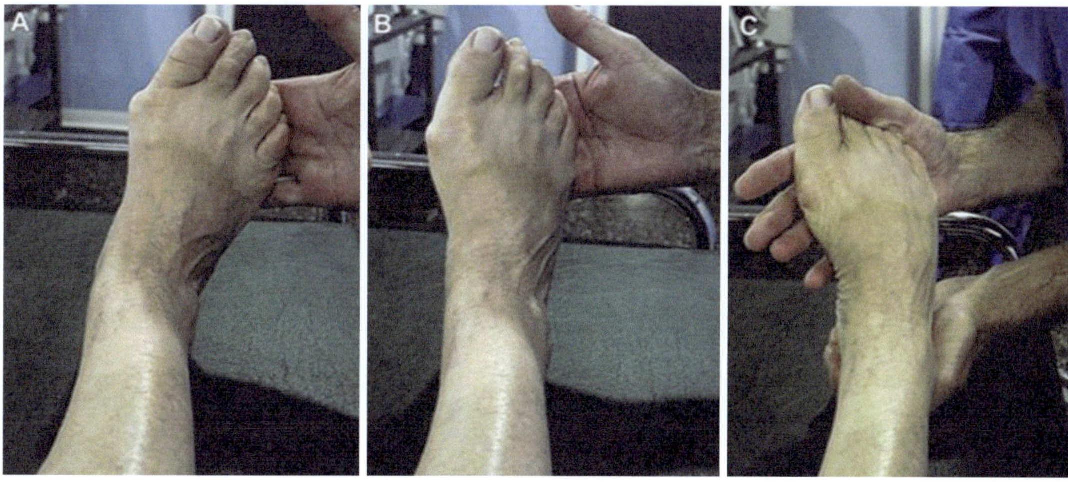

Fig. 8.4 Examination of ankle joint dorsiflexion with the hindfoot in valgus (**a**), neutral position (**b**), and varus position (**c**) (Reprinted with permission from *Foot and Ankle Clinics* 19.4 (2014): 659–667. Copyright 2014, Elsevier)

full extension as our definition because it allowed us to diagnose the problem in those who were at risk (symptomatic patients) with fairly good reproducibility (76%) and, more importantly, we were able to reliably avoid (in 94% of the cases) unnecessary treatment of those who were not at risk (asymptomatic people)" [9].

Gatt el al. went one step farther, correlating the static measurement with dynamic function occurring in late midstance prior to heel off [78]. It is well established in late midstance prior to heel off, and 10° to 15° of ankle joint dorsiflexion is required to move the body from behind the foot over the top of the planted foot [78]. Gatt et al.'s study consisted of two groups: group A measured $<-5°$ ankle joint dorsiflexion with the foot maximally supinated, and group B measured $\leq -5°$ to 0° [78]. In late midstance, ankle joint dorsiflexion measured 4.4° in group A and 13.9° in group B [78]. Clearly, 4.4° is inadequate ankle joint dorsiflexion in late midstance and will require proximal and/or distal compensation. The authors concluded: "There is no relationship between a static diagnosis of ankle dorsiflexion at 0° with dorsiflexion during gait. On the other hand, those subjects with less than −5° of dorsiflexion during static examination did exhibit reduced ankle range of motion during gait" [78].

Silverskoild in 1924 described the technique for examining ankle joint dorsiflexion with the knee extended and flexed to differentiate gastrocnemius equinus from gastrocsoleus equinus [15]. Using the parameters established by Gatt et al., when ankle joint dorsiflexion with the foot maximally supinated is $\leq -5°$ with the knee extended and $\geq 10°$ with the knee flexed, the deformity is a gastrocnemius equinus. If ankle joint dorsiflexion with the foot maximally supinated is $\leq -5°$ with the knee extended and $\leq 10°$ with the knee flexed, the deformity is considered a gastrocsoleus or osseous equinus. An abrupt end range of motion necessitates a lateral charger view (maximal dorsiflexion) x-ray to rule out an anterior ankle boney block (see Fig. 8.6). If ankle joint dorsiflexion with the foot maximally supinated is $\geq -5°$ with the knee extended and $\geq 10°$ with the knee flexed, there is no equinus deformity.

Classification of Equinus

Classification of equinus consists of muscular or osseous equinus deformities and then is further subdivided based on clinical examination; see Diagram 8.1 or Diagram 8.2.

Psuedoequinus occurs when the forefoot is plantarflexed relative to the rearfoot and the ankle dorsiflexes to get the forefoot parallel to the rearfoot, resulting in limited available ankle joint dorsiflexion. This is not a true equinus, and care must

Diagram 8.1 Muscular equinus diagram

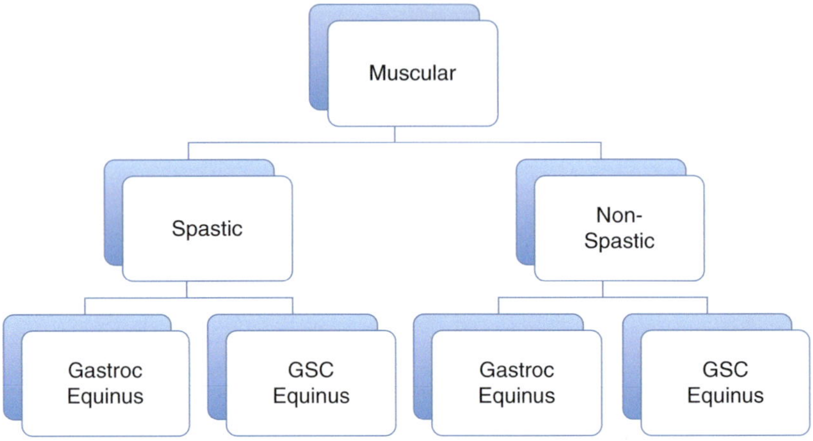

Diagram 8.2 Osseous equinus diagram

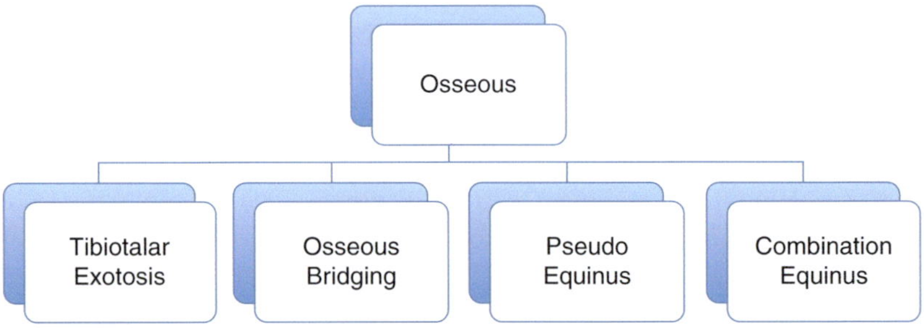

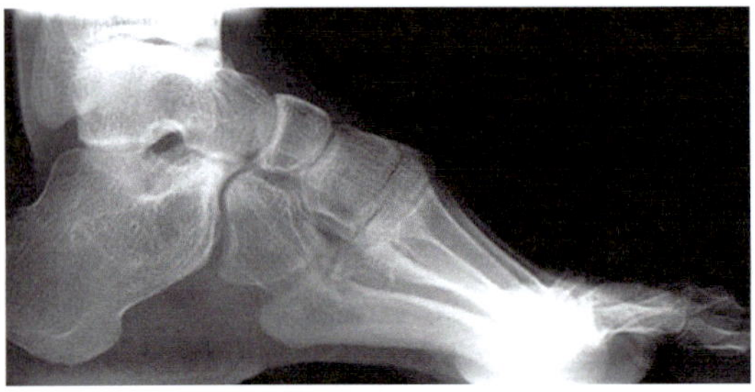

Fig. 8.5 Lateral weight-bearing foot x-ray demonstrating a cavus deformity with a pseudoequinus

be taken when evaluating ankle joint dorsiflexion in the cavus foot (see Fig. 8.5). With plantarflexion of the forefoot to the rearfoot, the horizontal arm of the goniometer is aligned to the 5th metatarsal base and not the metatarsal head. Osseous equinus is best evaluated with a lateral x-ray in maximal ankle joint dorsiflexion (charger view) and examining for anterior impingement (see Fig. 8.6).

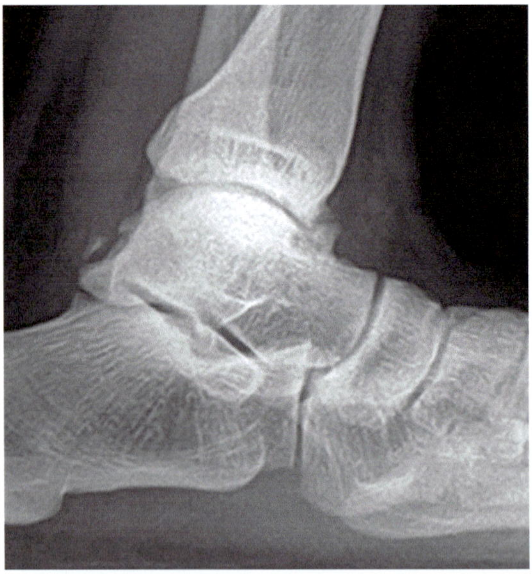

Fig. 8.6 Lateral weight-bearing foot x-ray with maximal dorsiflexion showing anterior impingement of the tibiotalar joint

Frequency of Equinus

Hill studied the frequency of equinus in 206 new patients over a 6-week period, excluding 26 of the patients that did not meet the study inclusion criteria [3]. Six patients were found to have normal ankle joint dorsiflexion using a definition of ≤3° dorsiflexion with the knee extended, resulting in 168 patients with equinus (3 with gastrocnemius equinus and 165 with gastrocsoleus equinus) [3]. The study findings showed a 96.5% rate of equinus in patients with foot and ankle pathologies [3]. Other authors echo the high frequency of equinus described by Hill [5, 16].

Associated Pediatric-Related Pathologies

Becerro de Bengoa Vallejo et al. and Szames et al. both described the relationship between Sever's disease and equinus [17, 18]. Pediatric flatfoot is another common pediatric lower extremity condition associated with an underlying equinus deformity [19, 20]. Several authors have described the relationship between hallux abducto valgus and equinus [3, 9, 21–27]. Achilles tendonitis is another commonly associated condition with equinus [3, 16, 26, 34, 39–46]. Other conditions that are less commonly associated with equinus include ankle sprains, ankle fractures, patellofemoral syndrome, iliotibial band syndrome, hammer toes/claw toes, shin splints/medial tibial stress syndrome, chronic ankle instability, genu recurvatum, and stress fractures [22, 26, 28–38].

Biomechanics of Equinus

In addition to understanding the anatomy of the GSC, understanding the biomechanics of the GSC is equally important to grasp fully the influence of equinus deformity on the lower extremity. Root described the functions of the gastrocnemius and soleus muscles as they relate to lower extremity biomechanics [1]. See Table 8.2.

Table 8.2 Functions of the gastrocnemius and soleus muscles according to Root et al. [1]

Gastrocnemius functions	Soleus functions
Maintains flexion tension knee – late contact to late midstance	Stabilize lateral forefoot – late contact and throughout midstance
Stabilize knee – prevents hyperextension	Decelerate pronation – end of contact
Decelerates STJ pronation – end of contact	Decelerates knee flexion – midstance
Accelerates STJ supination – midstance and propulsion	Decelerates tibialforward momentum – midstance
Locking MTJ – supination STJ and MTJ	Heel lift – stopping AJ DF during propulsion
Lifting heel and knee flexion – initiates propulsion	
Toe clearance – continued knee flexion during first ½ of propulsion	

STJ subtalar joint, *MTJ* midtarsal joint

Two landmark articles that discuss the role of the GSC on the medial arch and first ray provide the basis for understanding the biomechanics of equinus. Thordarson et al. conducted a study on the "dynamic support of the human longitudinal arch by the leg muscles active in the stance phase of gait and by the plantar aponeurosis" [47]. Progressive loading of various leg muscles and the angular displacement of the medial arch in the sagittal plane (talus to 1st metatarsal) and transverse plane (navicular to talus) were measured [47]. The study showed the GSC produced the greatest amount of arch deformation in both the transverse and sagittal planes with increasing loading, while the plantar fascia and tibialis posterior tendon increased the arch the greatest in the sagittal and transverse planes, respectively [47].

Johnson and Christensen studied the effect of the GSC on the first ray using cadavers with sensors placed on the talus, navicular, first cuneiform, and first metatarsal [2]. With progressive loading of the GSC, there was a dampening effect on the peroneus longus leading to unlocking of the midtarsal joints (hypermobility) and plantarflexion of the naviculocuneiform joint (dorsiflexion of the first metatarsal and first cuneiform, plantarflexion of the talus and navicular) [2]. This finding corresponds to the distal compensation that occurs when the GSC limits normal advancement of the tibia relative to the foot during the late midstance phase of gait. The plantarflexion of the naviculocuneiform joint via unlocking of the midtarsal joint (parallel alignment of the oblique and longitudinal midtarsal joint axes) occurs due to the increased pronation moment caused by the anterior and lateral movement of the center of pressure relative to the subtalar joint axis exceeding the supinatory moment created by the GSC. The net effect is a pronatory moment on the foot. This increased net pronatory moment is the ultimate cause of the pathological conditions with an underlying equinus component.

Nonsurgical Management of Equinus

The nonsurgical management of equinus presents several questions answered by the literature. The initial question is as follows: What is stretching? Is it the muscle or tendon? Konrad and Tilp examined the effect of a short-term static stretching program on the structural components of various muscles [48]. Participants utilized the runner's stretch for four 30-second stretches per day per leg for a total of 6 weeks [48]. The stretching group showed a statistically increased ankle joint range of motion at the completion of the study compared to the control group. The structural components of the muscle or the tendon showed no significant change [48]. The conclusion was the increased range of motion was possibly the result of adaptations of nociceptive nerve endings [48].

The next question for consideration is how long daily stretching should be done? The literature ranges from 30 seconds daily to all night via a night splint [49–57]. In a meta-analysis conducted by Radford et al. to determine if static calf stretching increased ankle joint range of motion, stretching time was also evaluated [58]. Stretching times consisted of ≤15 minutes, 15–30 minutes, and ≥30 minutes of stretching resulting in increased ankle joint dorsiflexion of 2.07°, 3.03°, and 2.49°, respectively [58]. The general trend was the longer the stretch, the greater the increase in ankle dorsiflexion, except the ≥30 minute group [58]. The authors attributed this to an underpowered sample for this group [58].

Does subtalar joint position matter with stretching of the GSC? Johanson et al. examined the effect of subtalar joint position with ankle joint dorsiflexion [30]. The study consisted of 27 patients that stretched for 30-seconds five times a day with the foot supinated and pronated [30]. The initial measurements for ankle joint dorsiflexion with the knee extended were right (4.6° ± 4.1°) and left (4.6° ± 2.9°) [30]. The findings revealed an increase in midfoot/forefoot dorsiflexion when stretching with the subtalar joint pronated compared to supinated, significantly more knee extension with supination (supination externally rotates the tibia allowing for full knee extension via the "screw-home mechanism") compared to pronation, and vertical ground reactive forces normalized with supination [30]. There was no significant change in ankle/rearfoot dorsiflexion between the two positions [30].

What is the effect on range of motion with stretching? This is the ultimate question when considering nonsurgical treatment of equinus. If there is no significant increase in ankle joint range of motion with stretching, then this method of treatment for equinus becomes invalid. Macklin et al. examined range of motion, peak plantar pressures, heel contact time, and stance phase time with calf stretching [59]. The study examined 13 runners without a foot or ankle pathology and ≤ 6° ankle joint dorsiflexion with the knee extended [59]. Extremes in foot structure (pes planus or pes cavus) were excluded from the study using the foot posture index criteria (inclusion included foot posture index ≤ +8 to ≥ −8) [59]. The GSC complex was stretched with an adjustable ramp for

4 minutes twice a day with measurements taken after 4 and 8 weeks using a goniometer (average of three measurements) [59]. Initial ankle joint dorsiflexion with the knee extended measured 5° on both right and left legs [59]. Ankle joint range of motion increased by approximately 200% following 8 weeks of stretching with a total increase in range of motion for the left of 11° and right of 10° [59]. Peak plantar pressures were hypothesized to decrease with normalization of ankle range of motion, but the results showed an increase in peak plantar pressures beneath the first and second metatarsal heads bilateral and fifth metatarsal head right. Heel contact time was also expected to be higher with improved ankle joint dorsiflexion, but it decreased [59]. The authors attributed these results to improved foot mechanics resulting in higher peak plantar pressures being distributed more evenly for shorter durations of time [59]. They theorized this was less harmful to the foot [59]. They concluded: "These results also strongly indicate that this specific non-invasive stretching regime could be considered before resorting to more invasive options."

When considering different nonsurgical treatment of equinus, manual stretching has been described most often in the literature. There are significant obstacles this method of treatment presents. As stated previously, the time required to stretch daily has never been established in the literature. If a time of 30 minutes per day per leg were a reasonable time frame, then manual stretching would require a patient to perform the runner's stretch for a total of one per day. Additionally, it is accepted that 6 weeks of stretching is required to reach normality (I believe it is more like 8 to 12 weeks based on my clinical experience). These factors lead to low rates of compliance with any manual stretching program and ultimate failure. Finally, the runner's stretch is technically demanding to do correctly; back heel must be completely on the ground, back knee straight and front knee bent, avoiding bending at the hips too much, and supination of the subtalar joint is mandatory (pronation results in dorsiflexion through the midfoot and ineffective stretching of the GSC). The reality of manual stretching is that it is a technically demanding maneuver to perform correctly. In the pediatric patient, all of these factors become more pronounced resulting in a very low compliance rate.

If manual stretching is not the solution, are night splints the answer? Night splints do not go above the knee and are incapable of maintaining the knee in full extension resulting in suboptimal stretching. This is particularly true if the patient tries to sleep with them on because the sleeping position with a night splint on is almost always on the side with knees bent. This does not stretch the gastrocnemius at all and therefore inadequately treats the deformity. Indeed, a patient could wear a night splint and extend the leg, but fully extending the knee while dorsiflexing the foot is uncomfortable, and the natural position of the knee is slight flexion. If the knee is not locked into full extension and held externally, the tendency will be to flex it slightly to reduce the discomfort and assume a natural state of slight knee flexion. Also, if the subtalar joint is not supinated, the tibia will not externally rotate allowing for full knee extension. Finally, night splints do not allow for precisely controlled dorsiflexion of the ankle joint resulting in either over- or under stretching. The ideal bracing solution would include an above-the-knee extension; an adjustable, controlled ankle hinge; and a method to supinate the subtalar joint. This is only available in the The Equinus Brace® (IQ Med, Carmel, Indiana). This brace is recommended to be used daily for 1 hour per day. If bracing is utilized to treat equinus, the patient should be evaluated monthly, and dorsiflexion increased until the patient reaches 5° ankle joint dorsiflexion with the knee extended. This typically takes between 8 and 12 weeks. In high-demand patients, such as runners or other athletes that participate in running-related sports, a maintenance therapy program is recommended to prevent recurrence. During the running gait cycle, the knee is never fully extended while the ankle is dorsiflexed. According to the law of Davis (over time soft tissue contracts to the shortest length possible), this shortened functioning of the GSC during the running gait cycle puts the runner or athlete that participates in running-related sports to recurrence of deformity [4]. This scenario is also a problem in diabetic patients as they are prone to a tightness of the GSC due to glycosylation of the tendon requiring a maintenance program [62]. In the pediatric patient, bone has been shown to grow faster than muscle (GSC) during growth spurts leading to an equinus deformity [17, 18]. A child experiencing a growth spurt may require maintenance therapy. Customized maintenance therapy based on the patient's response to the treatment provides a logical treatment algorithm. For example, have the patient stretch 1 day a week, with their ankle joint dorsiflexion being examined monthly to determine any required treatment modification. If the ankle joint dorsiflexion is falling below the 5° mark, then the patient should stretch twice weekly and be reevaluated in another month. The exact number of days per week required of stretching should be based on the patient's results and customized accordingly.

Conservative treatment of several pediatric foot and ankle conditions is considered the standard of care. If an equinus deformity is related to the pathology, it must be treated either prior or simultaneously with the pathology. For example, when treating a pediatric flatfoot with orthotics, it is recommended to correct the equinus component before implementing orthotic therapy. Orthotic tolerance by the patient improves when the plantarflexion of the naviculocuneiform joint resolves with treatment of the equinus deformity. Conversely in Sever's disease, treatment is most optimal treating the equinus and the Sever's disease simultaneously.

One final consideration regarding the nonsurgical management of equinus is bilateral vs. unilateral therapy. In cases where the pathology is unilateral, should the asymptomatic leg be treated? The answer is evident in both the structural evaluation of the muscle-tendon unit and from research on stretching therapy for equinus. Manal et al. examined the pennation angle of lower leg muscles and found no significant difference between right and left sides for any of the studied muscles [61]. Additionally, studies like Johanson et al. and Macklin et al. both showed similar findings on right and left sides with initial measurements of 4.6° and 5° of ankle joint dorsiflexion with the knee extended for both right and left sides, respectively [30, 59]. These findings and others indicate that both legs under normal circumstances have equivalent ankle joint dorsiflexion, and when it is abnormally limited, the equinus deformity is present bilaterally. In cases when a patient has a unilateral pathology, it is recommended to treat the equinus bilaterally as deformity is most likely symmetrical and treating only the symptomatic side can result in a functional limb length inequality.

Surgical Treatment of Equinus Deformity

The surgical management of equinus consists of five operative zones within the GSC [60] (see Figs. 8.7 and 8.8). Historically, the surgical approach to equinus deformity has centered on lengthening of the Achilles tendon (TAL). Recently there has been a transition to gastrocnemius recession via the Baumann or Strayer procedures. Review of the literature on this topic provides a clear picture why gastrocnemius recession has become preferable, particularly the Baumann procedure. The most concerning complication associated with TAL is over-lengthening resulting in a calcaneal deformity. This can become a limb-threating deformity. Holstein et al. used TAL to treat diabetic forefoot ulcers with an 80% success rate, but there was an 11% heel ulcer transfer rate [63]. Similar over-lengthening results can be seen in other studies (13%, 2% to 10%, 22%) [64–66]. Conversely, the complications

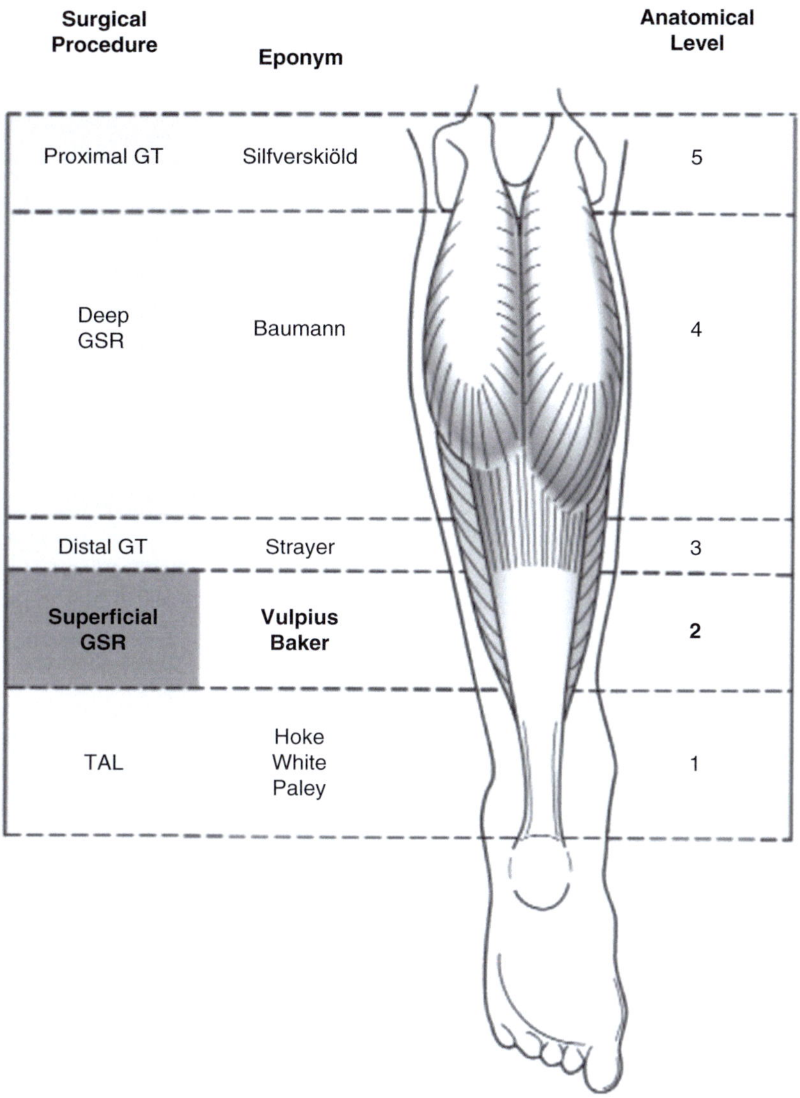

Fig. 8.7 The posterior leg can be divided into five anatomical levels. Based on anatomical level and clinical assessment, specific surgical procedures are indicated. The location for superficial gastrocnemius soleus recession is highlighted. GT gastrocnemius tenotomy, GSR gastrocnemius soleus recession, TAL tendo-Achilles lengthening (Reprinted with permission from the Journal of the American Podiatric Medical Association; 95(1):18–25. Copyright 2005, The American Podiatric Medical Association)

associated with gastrocnemius recession are relatively minor ranging from nerve injury to delayed wound healing [67]. Furthermore, TAL has been demonstrated to have higher recurrence rates in neurologically based equinus deformities compared to gastrocnemius recession [68].

Baumann and Koch described an intramuscular gastrocnemius fascial lengthening consisting of multiple recessions of the gastrocnemius to increase ankle joint dorsiflexion [69, 70]. The Baumann procedure differs from the Strayer gastrocnemius recession, which lengthens the gastrocnemius aponeurosis and possibly results in more weakness [71]. Herzenberg et al. examined the Baumann procedure looking at the ankle joint dorsiflexion with successive recessions of the gastrocnemius and soleus and Achilles tenotomy [72]. A summary of the data from the study is shown in Table 8.3.

The interesting finding from this study is that the amount of dorsiflexion increase from one

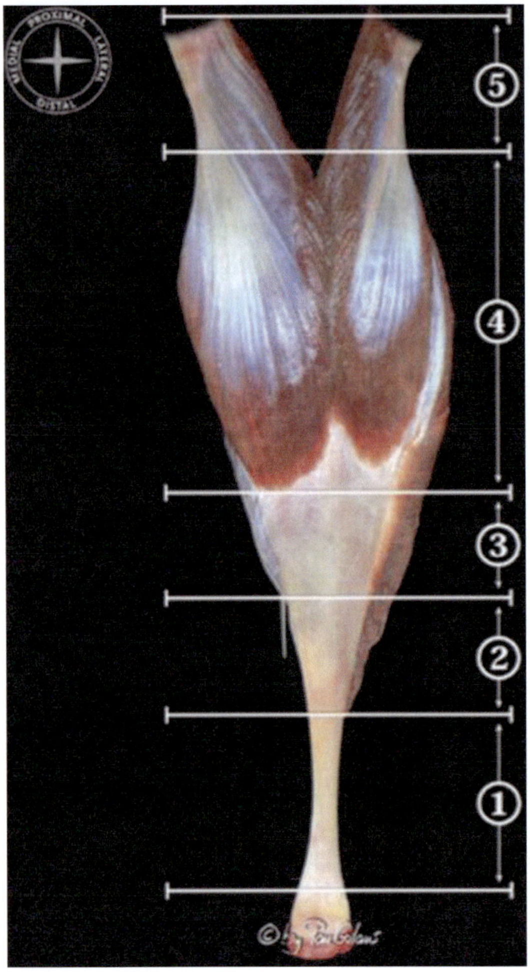

Fig. 8.8 Surgical anatomy of the triceps surae. The triceps surae is divided into 5 levels for a better understanding of the structures resected during surgery at each level, following the division proposed by Lamm and colleagues. (1) Level 1, calcaneal tendon; (2) Level 2, starts in the common aponeurotic tendon of the soleus and gastrocnemius and finishes at the distal end of the soleus muscle; (3) Level 3, starts where the muscle bellies of the gastrocnemius merge to form the calcaneal tendon and finishes where the aponeuroses of the soleus and gastrocnemius merge; (4) Level 4, comprises the medial and lateral bellies of the gastrocnemius; (5) Level 5, comprises the proximal insertion and tendons of the medial and lateral heads of the gastrocnemius (Copyright © Pau Golano' 2014.) (Reprinted with permission from *Foot and Ankle Clinics* 19.4 (2014): 603–635. Copyright 2014, Elsevier)

gastrocnemius recession to a second gastrocnemius recession was 6°, whereas adding a soleus recession increased dorsiflexion by only 1° [72]. The amount of dorsiflexion achieved after one recession was 8°, which is well above the definition of equinus described by DiGiovanni et al. of ≥5° [9, 72]. An important intraoperative recommendation in addition to using multiple recessions within the gastrocnemius fascial layer is to cut the plantaris tendon as well. This provides a noticeable increase in ankle range of motion.

Rong et al. demonstrated that a Baumann procedure with two recessions provides an equal amount of increased ankle dorsiflexion compared to a Strayer gastrocnemius recession without the weakness associated with the Strayer [80].

Saraph et al.'s retrospective study examined the Baumann procedure as part of the multilevel single-stage surgical correction of 22 cerebral palsy patients with 28 limbs [73]. The findings showed significantly increased ankle joint dorsiflexion without weakness of the GSC [73]. Additionally, improvement of the popliteal angle postoperatively (an important component of treatment in the cerebral palsy patient) and reversal of abnormal energy generation during midstance to a typical pattern of energy absorption were noted [73]. Similarly, El-Adwar et al. showed 80% satisfactory results for the use of the Baumann procedure in cerebral palsy pediatric patients [74]. Rong et al. examined the use of the Baumann procedure as part of the comprehensive treatment of both adult and pediatric flatfoot reconstructions [75]. The post-procedure mean increase in ankle joint dorsiflexion was 13.6° with the knee extended and 9.7° with the knee flexed [75]. The average American Orthopaedic Foot & Ankle Society ankle-hindfoot (AOFAS-AH) scores improved from 56.8 to 72.1 [75].

The recurrence of contracture post-GSC lengthening of any type has been documented to

Table 8.3 Summary of ankle joint dorsiflexion preoperative, post single gastrocnemius recession, post double gastrocnemius recession, post soleus recession, and post Achilles tenotomy

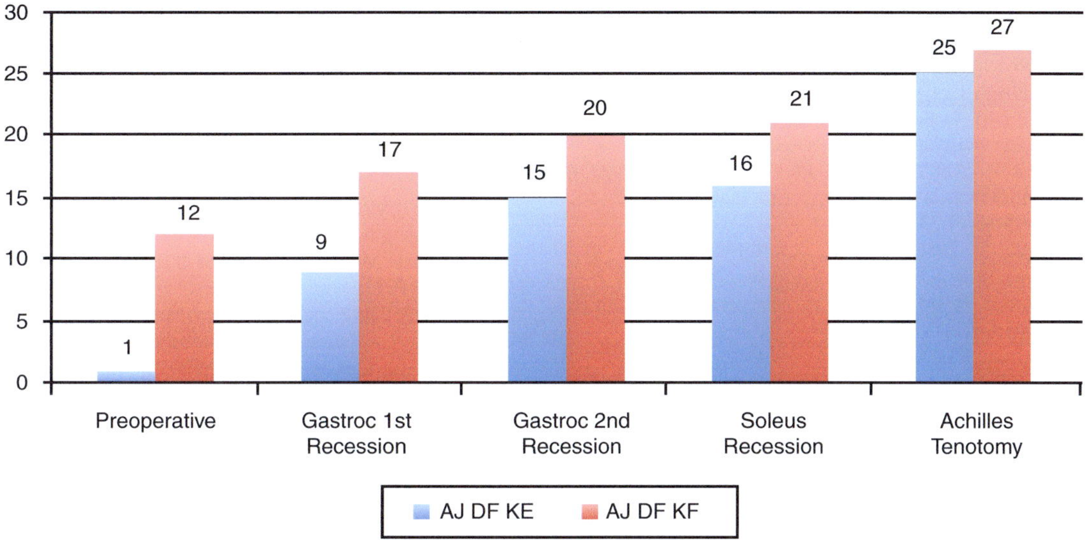

Blue = ankle joint dorsiflexion with knee extended, Red = ankle joint dorsiflexion with knee flexed

range from 9.1% to 35% [68, 74–77]. With this high recurrence percentage of equinus deformity, consideration for post-surgical bracing may be beneficial and should be considered.

Conclusion

Equinus deformity is prevalent and especially so in the biomechanically related pathologic patient. In fact, often the equinus is the "root" or "primary causal agent" of the deformity. James Amis, MD, in his article from *Foot and Ankle Clinics of North America 2014* stated it best [16]:

> It has been postulated that epidemiologic factors, such as obesity, sedentary lifestyle, medical comorbidities, shoe wear, concrete floors, advanced age, female gender, and overuse issues, to name a few, are responsible for a variety of foot and ankle pathology. Although these factors might consistently coexist with a variety of foot and ankle problems and seem to have a causal relationship, it is my assertion that they have little if any direct relationship.
>
> The singular and real association of each of these epidemiologic factors is a contracture of the gastrocnemius muscle, which is camouflaged in this list. Most every other cause of these foot and ankle problems is likely mediated by contributing to the degree and/or rate of an already contracting gastrocnemius. These problems promote gastrocnemius tightness, which in time causes incremental damage to the foot and/or ankle.

I concur with Dr. Amis in his assertion that equinus is the "singular and real association" etiologic factor of most biomechanically related lower extremity pathologies. With the ever-emerging evidence on the significance of equinus deformity in the adult or pediatric patient, a thorough understanding of equinus and treating it accordingly is essential to optimal patient outcomes.

Disclosure Patrick A. DeHeer is the inventor of The Equinus Brace® and an owner of IQ Med.

References

1. Root M, Orien W, Weed J. Normal and abnormal function of the foot. Clinical Biomechanics Corp.: Los Angeles; 1977.
2. Johnson C, Christensen J. Biomechanics of the first ray part V: the effect of equinus deformity. J Foot Ankle Surg. 2005;44(2):114–20.
3. Hill R. Ankle equinus. Prevalence and linkage to common foot pathology. J Am Podiatr Med Assoc. 1995;85(6):295–300.
4. Nutt J. Diseases and deformities of the foot. New York: E.B. Treat & Company; 1913.
5. Barouk P. Introduction to gastrocnemius tightness. Foot Ankle Clin. 2014;19(4):xv.
6. Dalmau-Pastor M, Fargues-Polo B, Casanova-Martínez D, Vega J, Golanó P. Anatomy of the triceps surae. Foot Ankle Clin. 2014;19(4):603–35.
7. Doral M, Alam M, Bozkurt M, Turhan E, Atay O, Dönmez G, et al. Functional anatomy of the Achilles tendon. Knee Surg Sports Traumatol Arthrosc. 2010;18(5):638–43.
8. Cummins E, Anson B, Carr B, Wright R, Hauser E. The structure of the calcaneal tendon (of Achilles) in relation to orthopedic surgery, with additional observations on the plantaris muscle. Surg Gynaecol Obst. 1946;83:107–16.
9. Digiovanni C, Kuo R, Tejwani N, Price R, Hansen S, Cziernecki J, et al. Isolated gastrocnemius tightness. J Bone Joint Surg. 2002;84-A(6):962–70.
10. Van Gheluwe B, Kirby K, Roosen P, Phillips R. Reliability and accuracy of biomechanical measurements of the lower extremities. J Am Podiatr Med Assoc. 2002;92(6):317–26.
11. Lundgren P, Nester C, Liu A, Arndt A, Jones R, Stacoff A, et al. Invasive in vivo measurement of rear-, mid- and forefoot motion during walking. Gait Posture. 2008;28(1):93–100.
12. Martin R, McPoil T. Reliability of ankle goniometric measurements. J Am Podiatr Med Assoc. 2005;95(6):564–72.
13. Evans A, Scutter S. Sagittal plane range of motion of the pediatric ankle joint. J Am Podiatr Med Assoc. 2006;96(5):418–22.
14. Barouk P, Barouk L. Clinical diagnosis of gastrocnemius tightness. Foot Ankle Clin. 2014;19(4):659–67.
15. Silfverskiold N. Reduction of the uncrossed two joint muscles of the leg to one joint muscle in spastic conditions. Acta Chir Scand. 1924;56:315–30.
16. Amis J. The gastrocnemius. Foot Ankle Clin. 2014;19(4):637–47.
17. Becerro de Bengoa Vallejo R, Losa Iglesias M, Rodríguez Sanz D, Prados Frutos J, Salvadores Fuentes P, Chicharro J. Plantar pressures in children with and without Sever's disease. J Am Podiatr Med Assoc. 2011;101(1):17–24.
18. Szames S, Forman W, Oster J, Eleff J. Sever's disease and its relationship to equinus: a statistical analysis. Clin Podiatr Med Surg. 1990;7(2):377–84.
19. Reimers J, Pedersen B, Brodersen A. Foot deformity and the length of the triceps surae in Danish children between 3 and 17 years old. J Pediatr Orthop B. 1995;4(1):71–3.
20. DiGiovanni C, Langer P. The role of isolated gastrocnemius and combined Achilles contractures in the flatfoot. Foot Ankle Clin. 2007;12(2):363–79.
21. Downey M, Banks A. Gastrocnemius recession in the treatment of nonspastic ankle equinus. A retrospective study. J Am Podiatr Med Assoc. 1989;79(4):159–74.
22. Sgarlato T, Morgan J, Shane H, Frenkenberg A. Tendo achillis lengthening and its effect on foot disorders. J Am Podiatr Med Assoc. 1975;65(9):849–71.
23. Hansen S Jr. Hallux valgus surgery. Morton and Lapidus were right! Clin Podiatr Med Surg. 1996;13(3):347–54.
24. Holstein A. Hallux Valgus – an acquired deformity of the foot in cerebral palsy. Foot Ankle Int. 1980;1(1):33–8.
25. Barouk L. The effect of gastrocnemius tightness on the pathogenesis of juvenile hallux valgus. Foot Ankle Clin. 2014;19(4):807–22.
26. Phisitkul P, Rungprai C, Femino J, Arunakul M, Amendola A. Endoscopic gastrocnemius recession for the treatment of isolated gastrocnemius contracture: a prospective study on 320 consecutive patients. Foot Ankle Int. 2014;35(8):747–56.
27. Pinney S, Hansen S Jr, Sangeorzan B. The effect on ankle dorsiflexion of gastrocnemius recession. Foot Ankle Int. 2002;23(1):26–9.
28. Tabrizi P, McIntyre W, Quesnel M, Howard A. Limited dorsiflexion predisposes to injuries of the ankle in children. J Bone Joint Surg. 2000;82(8):1103–6.
29. Lun V. Relation between running injury and static lower limb alignment in recreational runners. Br J Sports Med. 2004;38(5):576–80.
30. Johanson M, DeArment A, Hines K, Riley E, Martin M, Thomas J, et al. The effect of subtalar joint position on dorsiflexion of the ankle/rearfoot versus midfoot/forefoot during gastrocnemius stretching. Foot Ankle Int. 2013;35(1):63–70.
31. Neely F. Biomechanical risk factors for exercise-related lower limb injuries∗. Sports Med. 1998;26(6):395–413.
32. Messier S, Pittala K. Etiologic factors associated with selected running injuries. Med Sci Sports Exerc. 1988;20(5):501–5.
33. Green D, Ruch J, McGlamry E. Correction of equinus-related forefoot deformities: a case report. J Am Podiatr Med Assoc. 1976;66(10):768–80.
34. Wilder R, Sethi S. Overuse injuries: tendinopathies, stress fractures, compartment syndrome, and shin splints. Clin Sports Med. 2004;23(1):55–81.
35. Lilletvedt J, Kreighbaum E, Phillips R. Analysis of selected alignment of the lower extremity related to the shin splint syndrome. J Am Podiatr Med Assoc. 1979;69(3):211–7.
36. Pope R, Herbert R, Kirwan J. Effects of ankle dorsiflexion range and pre-exercise calf muscle stretching on injury risk in Army recruits. Austr J Physiother. 1998;44(3):165–72.

37. McGlamry E, Banks A. McGlamry's comprehensive textbook of foot and ankle surgery. Philadelphia: Lippincott Williams & Wilkins; 2001.
38. Fredericson M. Common injuries in runners. Sports Med. 1996;21(1):49–72.
39. Verrall G, Schofield S, Brustad T. Chronic Achilles tendinopathy treated with eccentric stretching program. Foot Ankle Int. 2011;32(09):843–9.
40. Gurdezi S, Kohls-Gatzoulis J, Solan M. Results of proximal medial gastrocnemius release for Achilles tendinopathy. Foot Ankle Int. 2013;34(10):1364–9.
41. Lamm B, Paley D, Herzenberg J. Gastrocnemius soleus recession. J Am Podiatr Med Assoc. 2005;95(1):18–25.
42. Kiewiet N, Holthusen S, Bohay D, Anderson J. Gastrocnemius recession for chronic noninsertional Achilles tendinopathy. Foot Ankle Int. 2013;34(4):481–5.
43. Duthon V, Lübbeke A, Duc S, Stern R, Assal M. Noninsertional Achilles tendinopathy treated with gastrocnemius lengthening. Foot Ankle Int. 2011;32(04):375–9.
44. Gentchos C, Bohay D, Anderson J. Gastrocnemius recession as treatment for refractory Achilles tendinopathy: a case report. Foot Ankle Int. 2008;29(6):620–3.
45. Laborde J, Weiler L. Achilles tendon pain treated with gastrocnemius-soleus recession. Orthopedics. 2011;34(4):289–91.
46. Cychosz C, Phisitkul P, Belatti D, Glazebrook M, DiGiovanni C. Gastrocnemius recession for foot and ankle conditions in adults: evidence-based recommendations. Foot Ankle Surg. 2015;21(2):77–85.
47. Thordarson D, Schmotzer H, Chon J, Peters J. Dynamic support of the human longitudinal arch. Clin Orthop Relat Res. 1995;(316):165–72.
48. Konrad A, Tilp M. Increased range of motion after static stretching is not due to changes in muscle and tendon structures. Clin Biomech. 2014;29(6):636–42.
49. Grady J, Saxena A. Effects of stretching the gastrocnemius muscle. J Foot Surg. 1990;30(5):465–9.
50. Youdas J, Krause D, Egan K, Therneau T, Laskowski E. The effect of static stretching of the calf muscle-tendon unit on active ankle dorsiflexion range of motion. J Orthop Sports Phys Ther. 2003;33(7):408–17.
51. Zito M, Driver D, Parker C, Bohannon R. Lasting effects of one bout of two 15-second passive stretches on ankle dorsiflexion range of motion. J Orthop Sports Phys Ther. 1997;26(4):214–21.
52. Barry L, Barry A, Chen Y. A retrospective study of standing gastrocnemius-soleus stretching versus night splinting in the treatment of plantar fasciitis. J Foot Ankle Surg. 2002;41(4):221–7.
53. Batt M, Tanji J, Skattum N. Plantar Fasciitis. Clin J Sport Med. 1996;6(3):158–62.
54. Porter D, Barrill E, Oneacre K, May B. The effects of duration and frequency of Achilles tendon stretching on dorsiflexion and outcome in painful heel syndrome: a randomized, blinded, control study. Foot Ankle Int. 2002;23(7):619–24.
55. Evans A. Podiatric medical applications of posterior night stretch splinting. J Am Podiatr Med Assoc. 2001;91(7):356–60.
56. Roos E, Engström M, Söderberg B. Foot orthoses for the treatment of plantar fasciitis. Foot Ankle Int. 2005;27(8):606–11.
57. Berlet G, Anderson R. A prospective trial of night splinting in the treatment of recalcitrant plantar fasciitis: the Ankle Dorsiflexion Dynasplint. Orthopedics. 2002;25(11):1273–5.
58. Radford J, Burns J, Buchbinder R, Landorf K, Cook C, Rome K. Does stretching increase ankle dorsiflexion range of motion? A systematic review * Commentary. Br J Sports Med. 2006;40(10):870–5.
59. Macklin K, Healy A, Chockalingam N. The effect of calf muscle stretching exercises on ankle joint dorsiflexion and dynamic foot pressures, force and related temporal parameters. Foot. 2012;22(1):10–7.
60. Lamm B, Paley D, Herzenberg J. Gastrocnemius soleus recession. J Am Podiatr Med Assoc. 2005;95(1):18–25.
61. Manal K, Roberts D, Buchanan T. Optimal pennation angle of the primary ankle plantar and dorsiflexors: variations with sex, contraction intensity, and limb. J Appl Biomech. 2006;22(4):255–63.
62. Grant W, Sullivan R, Sonenshine D, Adam M, Slusser J, Carson K, et al. Electron microscopic investigation of the effects of diabetes mellitus on the Achilles tendon. J Foot Ankle Surg. 1997;36(4):272–8.
63. Holstein P, Lohmann M, Bitsch M, Jørgensen B. Achilles tendon lengthening, the panacea for plantar forefoot ulceration? Diabetes Metab Res Rev. 2004;20(S1):S37–40.
64. Mueller M, Sinacore D, Hastings M, Strube M, Johnson J. Effect of Achilles tendon lengthening on neuropathic plantar ulcers. J Bone Joint Surg. 2003;85-A(8):1436–45.
65. Nishimoto G, Attinger C, Cooper P. Lengthening the Achilles tendon for the treatment of diabetic plantar forefoot ulceration. Surg Clin N Am. 2003;83(3):707–26.
66. Chilvers M, Malicky E, Anderson J, Bohay D, Manoli A. Heel overload associated with heel cord insufficiency. Foot Ankle Int. 2007;28(6):687–9.
67. Rush S, Ford L, Hamilton G. Morbidity associated with high gastrocnemius recession: retrospective review of 126 cases. J Foot Ankle Surg. 2006;45(3):156–60.
68. Sharrard W, Bernstein S. Equinus deformity in cerebral palsy. J Bone Joint Surg Br. 1971;54-B(2):272–6.
69. Baumann J, Koch H. Ventrale aponeurotische Verlängerung des Musculus gastrocnemius. Oper Orthop Traumatol. 1989;1(4):254–8.
70. Baumann J, Koch H. Lengthening of the anterior aponeurosis of musculus gastrocnemius through multiple incisions. Orthop Traumatol. 1992;1(4):278–82.
71. Strayer L. Recession of the gastrocnemius. J Bone Joint Surg. 1950;32(3):671–6.
72. Herzenberg J, Lamm B, Corwin C, Sekel J. Isolated recession of the gastrocnemius muscle: the Baumann procedure. Foot Ankle Int. 2007;28(11):1154–9.

73. Saraph V, Zwick E, Uitz C, Linhart W, Steinwender G. The Baumann procedure for fixed contracture of the gastrosoleus in cerebral palsy. J Bone Joint Surg. 2000;82(4):535–40.
74. El-Adwar K, El-Rashidi A, Al-Magrabri E. The treatment of fixed contracture of the gastrosoleus in cerebral palsy using the Baumann procedure: preliminary results of a prospective study. Curr Orthop Pract. 2009;20(4):448–53.
75. Rong K, Ge W, Li X, Xu X. Mid-term Results of Intramuscular Lengthening of Gastrocnemius and/or Soleus to Correct Equinus Deformity in Flatfoot. Foot & Ankle International. 2015;36(10):1223–8.
76. Chung C, Sung K, Lee K, Lee S, Choi I, Cho T, et al. Recurrence of equinus foot deformity after Tendo-Achilles lengthening in patients with cerebral palsy. J Pediatr Orthop. 2015;35(4):419–25.
77. Firth G, Passmore E, Sangeux M, Thomason P, Rodda J, Donath S, et al. Multilevel surgery for equinus gait in children with spastic Diplegic cerebral palsy. J Bone Joint Surg Am. 2013;95(10):931.
78. Gatt A, et al. A pilot investigation into the relationship between static diagnosis of ankle equinus and dynamic ankle and foot dorsiflexion during stance phase of gait: time to revisit theory? Foot. 2017;30: 47–52.
79. Dayton P, et al. Experimental comparison of the clinical measurement of ankle joint dorsiflexion and radiographic Tibiotalar position. J Foot Ankle Surg. 2017;56(5):1036–40.
80. Rong K, et al. Comparison of the efficacy of three isolated gastrocnemius recession procedures in a cadaveric model of gastrocnemius tightness. Int Orthop. 2016;40(2):417–23.

9 Calcaneovalgus and Congenital Vertical Talus

Marissa S. David and Glenn M. Weinraub

Congenital pes planovalgus describes a spectrum of flatfoot deformity present at birth with varying degrees of severity. Calcaneovalgus is a flexible dorsiflexion and eversion deformity of the foot and is reducible with manipulation (Fig. 9.1). Congenital vertical talus is a more severe convex deformity defined by irreducibility of the navicular on the vertically oriented talus, combined with dorsolateral and Achilles tendon contractures. This distinction of flexibility versus rigidity determines diagnosis and treatment.

Calcaneovalgus

Introduction

Calcaneovalgus is a flexible dorsiflexion and eversion deformity of the entire foot. It is the most common neonatal foot and ankle deformity [1]. Estimations of incidence vary widely from 1:1000 to as much as 30%, as mild cases may go unnoticed and undiagnosed and are self-correcting [2]. Incidence is greater in females than males and greater in first-born children. This postural deformity is most likely caused by intrauterine malposition and compression within the small uterine space, a theory consistent with the greater incidence in first-born children [3]. Importantly, there are no osseous changes, hypoplasia, subluxations, or dislocations limiting correction. Treatment aims to identify those cases which may benefit from gentle manipulation or serial casting. Surgery is not indicated.

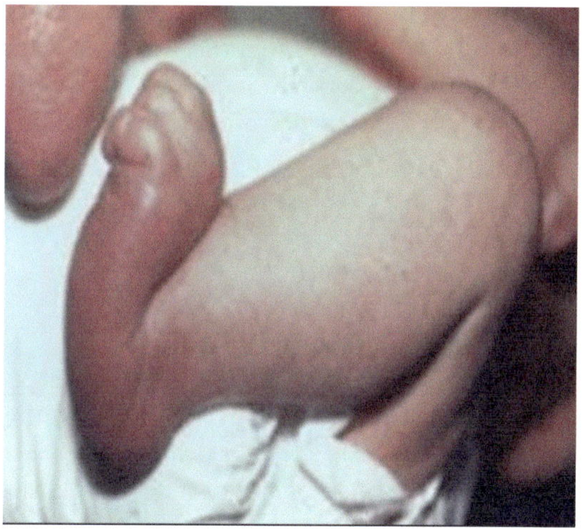

Fig. 9.1 Calcaneovalgus is a flexible dorsiflexion and eversion deformity of the entire foot

M. S. David
Podiatric Surgery Resident (PGY-III), Kaiser Permanente Santa Clara and GSAA, Santa Clara, CA, USA

G. M. Weinraub (✉)
Department of Orthopaedic Surgery, TPMG- GSAA, San Leandro, CA, USA

Midwestern University, Glendale, AZ, USA

Western University, Pomona, CA, USA

M. L. Butterworth, J. T. Marcoux (eds.), *The Pediatric Foot and Ankle*,
https://doi.org/10.1007/978-3-030-29788-6_9

Diagnosis

In mild cases the foot may appear mildly dorsiflexed, everted, and abducted, but in severe presentations the foot may touch the anterior aspect of the leg. With gentle plantarflexion, inversion, and adduction, the foot is brought into rectus alignment. A variable degree of tightness of the dorsal-lateral structures may be appreciated. The reducibility of the deformity is crucial in distinguishing calcaneovalgus from complex congenital pes planovalgus or congenital vertical talus, which is a rigid talonavicular dislocation that produces a characteristic "rocker-bottom" appearance of the plantar surface and is discussed in greater detail below. If the foot is fully reducible, radiographs are not indicated. In severe cases with excessive dorsal-lateral soft tissue contracture, plains films should rule out osseous adaptations.

Treatment

Though all cases of calcaneovalgus are flexible, the severity of the deformity is defined by reducibility: mild cases can be plantarflexed and inverted beyond neutral, moderate cases can be brought to neutral alignment with some difficulty, and severe cases display flexibility but cannot be fully plantarflexed and inverted to neutral position. Severity also dictates treatment. Mild cases are self-correcting within 3–6 months. Moderate cases are treated with frequent stretching of the foot by the child's parents with the goal of gently manipulating the foot to neutral position and stretching the contracted dorsal-lateral soft tissues. The stretch is comfortably held for 10–20 seconds and performed up to dozens of times daily. Stretches are well tolerated by the infant and can be incorporated into repetitive child care routines to ensure compliance. Severe cases require serial casting weekly for 4–6 weeks. The deformity can be fully corrected without surgical intervention.

Prognosis is excellent regardless of severity. Comparison between calcaneovalgus treated with manipulation and elastic bandaging versus observation alone suggests even stretching may not be necessary to yield excellent outcomes, as one early series of 125 patients demonstrated no significant difference between treatment groups at a follow-up of 3–11 years [4]. The majority of feet display normal architecture and function at long-term follow-up. Parents and clinicians can remain vigilant for symptomatic flexible flatfoot as the affected child grows, as a high correlation between pathologies has historically been suggested [5]. More recent evidence in a 16-year follow-up of 13 children treated for calcaneovalgus suggests no tendency toward the development of pes planus [6].

Congenital Vertical Talus

Introduction

In contrast to calcaneovalgus, congenital vertical talus (CVT) presents at birth with a rigid convex flatfoot. The navicular is irreducibly dislocated upon the talar head. The Achilles tendon and dorsal-lateral soft tissues are contracted. The calcaneocuboid articulation may be subluxed or dislocated. As suggested in nomenclature, the talus is vertically oriented, parallel to the tibial axis viewed radiographically. The condition is rare but disabling if left untreated. Advances in minimally invasive surgical techniques combined with serial casting have improved markedly upon historically performed extensive soft tissue releases, and outcomes are now promising.

Diagnosis

Pediatric flatfoot may be the presenting feature of multiple deformities including flexible calcaneovalgus, tibial bowing, oblique talus, idiopathic pes planus, and CVT. The neonatal foot with CVT displays a convex plantar surface with fixed forefoot abduction and hindfoot valgus. The talar head is palpable plantar medially. In cases presenting later in childhood, the child may already be walking, as CVT does not delay progression to ambulation. A "peg-leg" gait without normal shock absorption or toe-off is characteristic. The forward progression of gait is without normal ground contact of the heel, lateral column, or digits. The medial longitudinal arch is fully collapsed and convex and is the primary weight-bearing surface of the foot. The foot is maximally pronated throughout the entire gait cycle [7].

The defining feature of CVT is irreducibility and may be appreciated immediately upon initial examination, prompting further radiographic confirmation. Examination should include anterior-posterior, lateral, and dynamic films. Incomplete ossification of the pediatric foot can limit full visual delineation of the deformity, but characteristic findings are visible nonetheless and can confirm the diagnosis. The anterior-posterior view will show an abnormally increased talocalcaneal angle beyond 30°. On lateral plain radiographs, the talotibial, talocalcaneal, tibiocalcaneal, and talo-first metatarsal angles are abnormal. The talo-first metatarsal angle exceeds 35°. The talus will be oriented vertically, paralleling the tibial axis, with a talotibial angle approaching 180 degrees (Fig. 9.2). Midfoot dorsiflexion will not reduce under dynamic visualization. Though the non-ossified navicular will not be visualized, the talo-first metatarsal angle will not reduce to normal. The combination of a clinically convex, rigid pes planovalgus with non-reducible midfoot dislocation on dynamic stress radiographs confirms the CVT diagnosis [8].

CVT produces or is the result of anatomical changes across the mid- and hindfoot that together combine in a convex plantar surface and dorsal-lateral contractures. The breadth of anatomical changes is correlated with the severity of the deformity. Dorsal dislocation of the navicular leads to hypoplasia of its plantar aspect. The extent of articular cartilage on the adjacent dorsal talar head expands to accommodate the abnormal articulation. The talar dome articulates within the talocrural joint only in its posterior one-third. The articular surfaces of the calcaneus are malformed to accommodate the vertically aligned talus: the sustentaculum tali no longer supports the talus, and the now nonarticular middle and anterior facets of the subtalar joint are reduced in size or fibrotic. The calcaneocuboid articulation may be intact, subluxed, or dislocated.

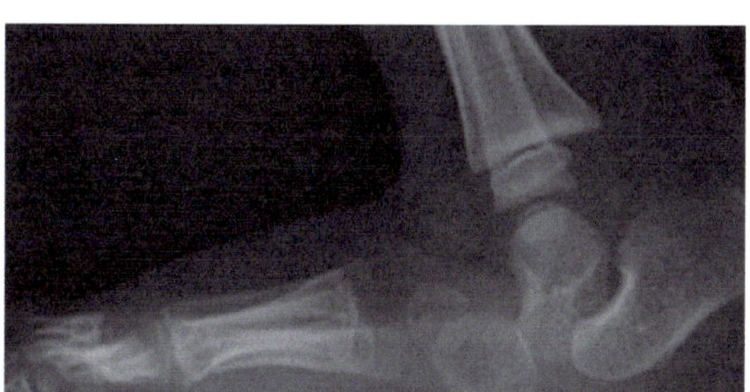

Fig. 9.2 Lateral radiograph of congenital vertical talus. Note the increased talo-first metatarsal angle as well as the vertical orientation of the talus yielding a tibial-talo angle of almost 180 degrees

Plantar-medial ligamentous structures are elongated or attenuated to accommodate the plantar-medial bulge of the talar head. Conversely, the dorsal-lateral and posterior structures including the dorsal talonavicular and calcaneofibular ligaments and the posterior ankle and subtalar joint capsules are contracted. The extensor retinaculum is thickened and accentuates the dorsiflexory power of the extensor musculature. Both the triceps surae and anterior group are shortened, consistent with both equinus and midfoot dorsal contracture.

Etiology

CVT is a rare defect, affecting approximately 1 in 10,000 births [2]. CVT may present as an "isolated" deformity defined by the absence of any associated medical comorbidities, but approximately 50% of cases are "non-isolated" and associated with genetic or neuromuscular conditions. Non-isolated cases of CVT are generally more severe, with even greater rigidity of the deformity. Muscular and neurological conditions most frequently associated with CVT include arthrogryposis and myelomeningocele. Diastematomyelia, cauda equina lipoma, sacral agenesis, and neurofibromatosis have also been associated with CVT, as have a plethora of rare genetic syndromes [9]. An inheritance pattern evident in approximately 20% of cases suggests autosomal dominant transmission with incomplete penetrance. Though specific mutations of HOXD10 and GDF5 have been noted in specific familial lineages with isolated CVT, genetic factors and heritability of the condition remain poorly understood [10–13]. CVT is idiopathic in the majority of cases and correlational in much of the remainder. Treatment is not dictated by etiology, but the greater contracture and rigidity of non-isolated CVT has historically required more prolonged or invasive treatment. More recent evidence suggests that isolated and non-isolated CVT can be treated identically with similar outcomes [9].

Treatment

The goal of treatment is to reduce the rigid dorsiflexion deformity to a relatively mobile, plantigrade, pain-free, and functional foot. Treatment has evolved since the first complete anatomical description of CVT in 1914. Conservative cast treatment alone proved minimally successful and was succeeded first by early attempts at excision of the talus or navicular and later by two-staged tendon lengthening and posterior capsulotomies described between 1956 and 1970 [14–16]. A single-stage medial approach with soft tissue release was then described in 1979 [17]. A more popular dorsal approach was popularized by Seimon in 1987 with a promising case series describing extensor hallucis longus and peroneus tertius tenotomies, talonavicular capsulotomy, percutaneous tendo-Achilles lengthening, and Kirschner wire fixation of a reduced talonavicular joint [18]. A comparison between the dorsal single-stage release and a multiple incision posterior approach by Mazzocca et al. in 2001 confirmed successful reduction and maintenance of the talonavicular joint with better clinical outcomes, fewer complications, and less surgical time with a single dorsal approach [19]. Despite a decades-long trend toward progressively less invasive surgical correction, single and double incisional soft tissue releases continued to be frustratingly complicated by peri-incisional soft tissue necrosis, rearfoot and ankle stiffness or arthrofibrosis, incomplete reduction, and avascular necrosis of the talus.

The preferred treatment of CVT underwent a dramatic change in 2006 with the publication by Dobbs et al. of a method combining serial casting, percutaneous Kirschner fixation of the talonavicular joint, and percutaneous tendo-Achilles lengthening (TAL) [20]. The dramatic success of the Ponseti method of clubfoot treatment – in which the cavovarus deformity is gradually manipulated around the talar head – prompted a similar application of principles to the correction of the dorsal-laterally dislocated foot in CVT, albeit in reverse. The foot is manipulated into plantarflexion and inversion with pressure applied to the plantar-medial talar head and progressively corrected with serial casts weekly for 5 weeks. The talo-navicular joint is then pinned in a corrected position with a single Kirschner wire. A percutaneous TAL is performed. In cases with incomplete talonavicular reduction with casting alone, a minimal incision is made dorsal-laterally to allow the insertion of an elevator to facilitate reduction; no extensive capsulotomy is performed. Eleven patients (19 feet) were followed for a minimum of 2 years. Three patients experienced re-subluxation of the navicular. At final follow-up, all patients displayed significant improvement in all measured radiographic variables, which were now within normal limits. Importantly – and in contrast with more extensive soft tissue releases – rearfoot motion was preserved, with 33° of ankle plantarflexion and 25° of dorsiflexion. Subsequent studies have shown similarly promising outcomes in both isolated and non-isolated CVT over the short term [21–24].

These promising early results were followed in 2015 by long-term follow-up confirming superior ankle range of motion and pain scores with the combined Dobbs or reverse-Ponseti approach compared to extensive soft tissue release [9]. Yang and Dobbs followed 27 patients (42 feet) for mean of 7 years (range, 5–11.3 years). Sixteen patients (24 feet) were treated with the combined minimally invasive approach at an average age of 6.6 months, while 11 patients (18 feet) underwent extensive soft tissue release including posterior capsulotomy of the ankle and subtalar joints, calcaneofibular ligament transectioning, and midtarsal capsulotomy at an average of 15.2 months. Patients were assessed radiographically, clinically, and subjectively with the PODCI questionnaire. Angle dorsiflexion, plantarflexion, and total range of motion were significantly better with the minimally invasive approach, yielding mean dorsiflexion of 18.5°, plantarflexion of 23.9°, and total range of motion of 42.4°, compared to 5°,7.7°, and 12.7°, respectively, in the more extensively release group. The mean normative pain score was significantly less (51.0 versus 34.1), and normative global function was greater (48.3 versus 34.3) in the minimally invasive group. Radiographic correction was identical. The extensive release group required more repeat soft tissue releases, and one patient suffered soft tissue necrosis.

Summary and Recommendations

CVT is a rare, potentially disabling deformity characterized by a convex weight-bearing surface of the affected foot, with dorsal dislocation of the navicular and contracture of the Achilles and dorsal-lateral soft tissue pedal structures. Calcaneovalgus may appear similar but can easily be distinguished by reducibility of the deformity to neutral alignment. This distinction dictates treatment.

Mild calcaneovalgus requires no intervention and is self-correcting. Moderate calcaneovalgus benefits from simple stretching. Severe calcaneovalgus rapidly improves with serial casting. Children and parents can anticipate normal development, and recent literature suggests no proclivity to develop symptomatic pes planus in adolescence.

The optimal treatment of CVT now combines serial casting and minimally invasive surgery to reduce the deformity and maintain correction, regardless of etiology. Serial casting for 4–6 weeks stretches contracted dorsal-lateral soft tissues and partially or completely reduces the dorsally dislocated navicular. The improved alignment of the foot is then maintained with percutaneous pinning of the talonavicular joint. A small stab incision may be required to facilitate complete talonavicular reduction. A percutaneous TAL is performed. The combined approach has been shown to maintain normal ankle joint ROM, minimize pain, reduce complications, and maintain reduction. No follow-up of the combined method has been carried into adulthood to date, but long-term follow-up at an average of 7 years is excellent.

References

1. Tachdjian MO. The child's foot. Philadelphia: WB Saunders Company; 1985.
2. Sullivan JA. Pediatric flatfoot: evaluation and management. J Am Acad Orthop Surg. 1999;7:44–53.
3. Graham JM, Sanchez-Lara PA. Calcaneovalgus (pes planus) in *Smith Recognizable Patterns of Human Deformation*. 4th ed. Philadelphia: Elsevier; 2016.
4. Larsen B, et al. Congenital calcaneovalgus. Acta Orthop Scand. 1974;45:145.
5. Giannestras NJ. Recognition and treatment of flatfeet in infancy. Clin Orthop Relat Res. 1970;70:10–29.
6. Widhe T. Foot deformities at birth: a longitudinal prospective study over a 16-year period. J Pediatr Orthop. 1997;17:20–4.
7. Jacobsen ST, Craford AH. Congenital vertical talus. J Pediatr Orthop. 1983;3(3):306–10.
8. Mickie J, Radomisli T. Congenital vertical talus: a review. Clin Podiatr Med Surg. 2010;27:145–56.
9. Yang JS, Dobbs MB. Treatment of congenital vertical talus: comparison of minimally invasive and extensive soft tissue release procedures at minimum five-year follow-up. J Bone Joint Surg. 2015;97:1354–65.
10. Levinsohn EM, et al. Congenital vertical talus and its familial occurrence: an analysis of 36 patients. Skelet Radiol. 2004;33:649–54.
11. Shrimpton AE, et al. A HOX gene mutation in a family with isolated congenital vertical talus and Charcot-Marie-tooth disease. Am J Hum Genet. 2004;75:92–6.
12. Gurnett, et al. Absence of HOXD10 mutations in idiopathic clubfeet and sporadic vertical talus. Clin Orthop Rel Res. 2007;462:27–31.
13. Merrill, et al. Skeletal muscle abnormalities and genetic factors related to vertical talus. Clin Orthop Relat Res. 2011;469(4):1167–74.
14. Osmond-Clarke H. Congenital vertical talus. J Bone Joint Surg Br. 1956;38(1):334–41.
15. Herndon CH, Heyman CH. Problems in the recognition and treatment of congenital pes valgus. J Bone Surg Am. 1963;45:413–29.
16. Coleman SS, et al. Pathomechanics and treatment of congenital vertical talus. Clin Orthop Relat Res. 1970;70:62–72.
17. Ogata K, et al. Congenital vertical talus and its familial occurrence: an analysis of 36 patients. Clin Orthop Relat Res. 1979;139:128–32.

18. Seimon LP. Surgical correction of congenital vertical talus under the age of 2 years. J Pediatr Orthop. 1987;7(4):405–11.
19. Mazzocca AD, et al. Comparison of the posterior approach versus the dorsal approach in the treatment of congenital vertical talus. J Pediatr Orthop. 2001;21(2):212–7.
20. Dobbs, et al. Early results of a new treatment for idiopathic congenital vertical talus. J Bone Joint Surg. 2006;88(6):1192–200.
21. Chalayon O, et al. Minimally invasive approach for the treatment of non-isolated congenital vertical talus. J Bone Joint Surg Am. 2012;94(11):73.
22. Eberhardt O, et al. The talar-axis-first metatarsal-base angle in CVT treatment: a comparison of idiopathic and non-idiopathic cases treated with the Dobbs methods. J Child Orthop. 2012;6(6):491–6.
23. Aslani, et al. Primary outcomes of the congenital vertical talus correction using the Dobbs method of serial casting and limited surgery. J Child Orthop. 2012;6(4):307–11.
24. Wright et al. Reverse Ponseti-type treatment for children with congenital vertical talus: comparison between idiopathic and teratological patients. Bone Joint J. 2014;96(2):274–8.

Pediatric Flexible Pes Valgus Deformity

10

Kieran T. Mahan and Caitlin Mahan Madden

Terminology

The terminology used to describe this deformity has led to confusion about the nature of the condition. The terms "flatfoot" and "pes planus" are particularly problematic. Both terms describe a low arch foot, but not necessarily an unstable low arch foot. As such, these terms end up being viewed as descriptors of one range of normal anatomy and function. Because some of these patients have a stable but low arch, they have no need for intervention and they can be confused with those patients who have a truly pathological foot.

Sigvard Hansen used the term "peritalar subluxation" in the adult flatfoot, while McGlamry used the term collapsing pes valgo planus [1]. In either event, it is important to use terminology that captures the fact that we are dealing with a pathological condition. Pes valgus deformity is the term that the authors most frequently use.

K. T. Mahan (✉)
Department of Podiatric Surgery, Temple University School of Podiatric Medicine, Philadelphia, PA, USA

Department of Podiatric Medicine and Surgery, Temple University Hospital, Philadelphia, PA, USA

Faculty, The Podiatry Institute, Decatur, GA, USA

College of Physicians of Philadelphia, Philadelphia, PA, USA
e-mail: kmahan@temple.edu

C. M. Madden
Private Practice, Podiatry Care Specialists, West Chester, PA, USA

Functional Anatomy

Support of the foot depends on a number of factors, including osseous architecture, ligamentous stability, and muscular activity. Basmajian and Stecko [2] demonstrated that extrinsic muscle stability does not significantly contribute to arch stability during stance. Rather, osseous and ligamentous structures provide the majority of the stability in static stance. The stability that these muscles provide is significantly dependent on their location compared to the axes of motion of the joints of the foot. For example, those muscles on the supinatory side of the subtalar joint axis can contribute significantly to decelerating pronation. The tibialis posterior is the most powerful of those muscles because of its size, long lever arm, and the deep integration of its many insertional fibers with ligamentous structures. Pes valgus deformity patients demonstrate increased activity of tibialis anterior and posterior, soleus, and peroneus longus in comparison to the rectus foot. The effect of the tendoachillis serves to greatly accentuate pronation in a valgus foot when the tendon falls on the pronating side of the joint.

The truss and beam concept has been used to describe the stability of the arch. In this model,

M. L. Butterworth, J. T. Marcoux (eds.), *The Pediatric Foot and Ankle*,
https://doi.org/10.1007/978-3-030-29788-6_10

the metatarsals and lesser tarsals are the anterior strut, while the talus and calcaneus are the posterior strut, and the plantar fascia acts as the tie rod connecting them. As the posterior strut is loaded and the struts attempt to separate, the tie rod (fascia) becomes loaded under tension. The central band of the plantar fascia, or plantar aponeurosis, provides the majority of this stability.

Intrinsic muscle activity supports ligamentous function particularly during gait [3]. Mann and Inman showed that individuals with flatfeet require greater intrinsic muscle activity during walking to stabilize the foot [4]. Ligamentous integrity provides tremendous stability in both stance and gait. The foot can also be thought of as an articulated beam with load creating compression on the dorsal convex side and tension on the plantar concave side.

The complexity of arch stability is exemplified by the variety of tissue failures that can create collapse. The spring ligament is one of those tissues whose compromise is known to produce a collapsed foot in the adult. The spring ligament is a broad thick ligament with the superomedial calcaneal ligament providing medial to lateral articular stability to the head of the talus. In the severely deformed pediatric foot, it is logical to expect that a valgus foot will present with a deformed spring ligament and that correction of the deformity may leave the ligament in a stretched position that may require repair. Tibialis posterior rupture is well known to cause arch collapse in the adult flatfoot, particularly with an intact peroneus brevis that now has nothing to counteract it. Rupture of the spring ligament has also been identified as an isolated cause of collapse of the medial arch in adults [5], [6]. Peroneus longus rupture disrupts the stability of the first ray, which can result in a cascade of events causing collapse of the medial longitudinal arch. Rupture of the plantar fascia can also result in long-term arch collapse. The spring, deltoid, and interosseous talocalcaneal ligaments are most important in stabilizing the arch [7].

Epidemiology

Given the lack of a standard definition and diagnostic tools, a discussion of epidemiology based upon past studies is difficult. Staheli's [8] longitudinal study of asymptomatic children and adult footprints is often cited as proof that flatfeet are within the normal range in children and adults. Although the study contributed to the understanding that children's feet, under most circumstances, develop from flat to rectus, the study was severely limited by the use of footprint technology which could not assess function [9]. Nonetheless, even with this limitation, and with the possibility that changing fat pad development alters the findings, it is clear that stability of the child's foot increases with age as part of normal development [10].

The need for objective studies was highlighted by the study by Cowan et al. (1994) who measured consistency of visual assessment of arch height among clinicians [11]. The probability of a clinician identifying a foot as clearly flat, given that another clinician had identified it as clearly flat, had a median probability of 0.57, indicating that inter-reporter reliability is poor. Hillstrom and Song described the Center of Pressure Excursion Index (CPEI) to capture dynamic instability and successfully were able to differentiate between rectus and pronated feet [12]. This technique objectively quantifies the degree of pronation during gait. The Malleolar Valgus Index (MVI) is a technique described by Song et al. who utilized readily available scanning technology to quantify static stability [13, 14].

Menz et al. (2013) examined the association of foot posture and pronated foot function with foot pain in the Framingham Foot Study [15]. Pronation foot function was associated with an increased likelihood of generalized foot pain in men. Planus foot posture was also significantly associated with an increased likelihood of arch pain in men. They concluded that planus foot posture and pronated foot function are associated with foot symptoms and that interventions that modify foot posture and function may have a role in the prevention and treatment of foot pain.

Pathogenesis

A number of factors may contribute to the development of a pathological pes valgus. Harris and Beath examined adult patients and identified that 23% have flatfeet. They subdivided them into rigid (peroneal spastic), flexible, and flexible with a short tendoachillis [16]. In evaluating children with flexible pes valgus, those born with a short tendoachillis seemed to be the most problematic due to the location of the short tendon on the pronating side of the subtalar joint. Equinus is one of the most powerful etiologies for the pathological pes valgus.

Compensation for forefoot varus, internal tibial torsion, metatarsus adductus, knee valgus, and other deformities can result in rearfoot valgus. Assessing the impact of metatarsus adductus can be done preoperatively with neutral position x-rays. The talonavicular joint is relocated and the subtalar joint placed in neutral position. A dorsal plantar x-ray is taken, and the metatarsus adductus angle is assessed. This is particularly important if an Evans calcaneal osteotomy were planned which would add adduction to the foot and unmask a compensated metatarsus adductus.

Ligamentous laxity clearly can be a powerful etiology for a pathological pes valgus. Although more extreme conditions such as Ehlers-Danlos or Marfan's syndrome with generalized ligamentous laxity can demonstrate the most significant instability, there are ranges of ligamentous laxity short of this that can also create significant instability. This is important to identify preoperatively because these patients require special consideration and do not generally respond as well to typical sets of procedures. Chen et al. reported that joint laxity, W-sitting position, obesity, males, and younger age were associated with a higher risk of flatfoot in preschool children aged 3–6 years [17].

The increasing prevalence of obesity is another significant issue. Pourghasem et al. (2016) in a study of 1158 school children found that body mass index (BMI) correlated significantly with flexible flatfoot as measured by contact footprints [18]. Stolzman et al. published a systematic review that identified a significant correlation between pes planus and obesity across 13 cross-sectional studies [19]. However, due to different definitions of pes planus and the different methodologies in the studies, a direct correlation among foot pain, pes planus, and obesity could not be determined. Children who are both obese and have a painful flatfoot deserve to have good communication between the foot and ankle surgeon and the pediatrician.

Biomechanics

The concept of planal dominance, as illustrated by Green and Carol, is a simple concept that helps to explain some aspects of the valgus foot deformity. It is particularly useful for surgical planning. Compensation for deforming forces occurs perpendicular to the axis of motion. When the subtalar axis is vertical, compensation occurs in the transverse plane with an increased calcaneal cuboid angle and talonavicular dislocation, whereas a horizontal subtalar axis would compensate in the sagittal plane with a lowered calcaneal angle inclination angle, an increased talar declination angle, and a navicular cuneiform sag. This is an oversimplification of what occurs in practice, but can be a useful way of organizing an approach to the foot.

Evaluation

The interview of the pediatric patient with pes valgus deformity is usually much more challenging than that with the adult patient. Having experienced pain for most of their lives, they may not be able to adequately articulate the type, nature, or duration of symptoms. The painful accessory navicular will usually be an exception. Children may avoid more vigorous activities because of symptoms, and this may be a clue in the history. It is important to listen carefully to the child, particularly for adolescents, and not only to the parents.

Careful attention is paid to identify rigid flat feet, ligamentous laxity, and medical conditions that may affect the connective tissues such as Ehlers-Danlos syndrome, Marfan's syndrome, and Down syndrome. Down syndrome can be associated with severe pes valgus [20]. Examining patients for general ligamentous laxity should be a standard part of the examination, as specific considerations are necessary for addressing this foot type. The ability of the patient to hyperextend their wrist or elbow or generalized "double jointedness" can indicate a variation of a ligamentous laxity syndrome. Benign hypermobility syndrome which is associated with elevated relaxin levels demonstrates a statistically significant association with pes planus [21].

Physical examination should include hip alignment and range of motion, knee alignment, tibial torsion, malleolar alignment, weightbearing and non-weightbearing foot postures, and examination of range of motion of the ankle, rearfoot, and forefoot joints. The relaxed calcaneal stance position should be noted along with the degree of abduction of the forefoot on the rearfoot and the navicular drop with weightbearing. The flexibility of the deformity should be evaluated. A rigid deformity may be associated with a coalition or a peroneal spastic flatfoot. The Hubscher maneuver or toe test of Jack is useful in this regard [22]. The ability of the patient to balance on one foot was noted to correlate with the width of footprint measures [23]. In a flexible flatfoot, tiptoe standing will generally cause recreation of the medial arch and inversion of the heels. The diagnosis and evaluation of coalitions is beyond the scope of this chapter, but clinical examination and radiographs are usually sufficient to make the diagnosis, and the differentiation from the flexible flatfoot is critical. The calcaneal axial or Harris Beath views will identify the middle facet coalition. The medial oblique view demonstrates the calcaneonavicular bar.

The gait examination is critical and should be documented in the record. This is an opportunity to look for planes of compensation, the absence of resupination, and adduction and plantarflexion of the talar head. From posterior to the heel, there may be a "too many toes sign," as in the adult flatfoot. Early heel off, with midtarsal breech, should be documented if present. Angular or rotational deformities will often be visibly worse during gait.

Examination for equinus is an important part of the exam and documentation. The Silfverskiold test can help to determine whether or not equinus is present. The subtalar joint is held in the neutral position and the foot dorsiflexed on the leg with the knee extended and then flexed (to eliminate the effect of the gastrocnemius muscle that crossed the knee joint) [24]. The patients who may go on to surgical intervention for adolescent pes valgus deformity may very well have a short tendoachillis or gastrocnemius equinus. In addition, intraoperative examination should be performed after the Evans calcaneal osteotomy is performed because of the increase in apparent equinus from plantarflexion of the forefoot on the rearfoot.

Metatarsus adductus can be observed clinically by holding the foot from the plantar heel and looking for forefoot adduction. Should surgical intervention with the Evans calcaneal osteotomy be considered, a subtalar neutral position dorsal plantar x-ray can be performed. Because of the adductory effects of the Evans, its use should be limited or modified in the presence of metatarsus adductus. Routine radiographic imaging is not necessary in every patient with pes valgus, particularly in younger children. However, if there is a question about the rigidity of the foot, then x-rays are necessary. Symptomatic feet may also benefit from radiographic examination. On the dorsal plantar x-ray, particular attention should be paid to the uncovering of the talar head and the talocalcaneal angle. These, along with the cuboid abduction angle, indicate transverse plane compensation. The metatarsus adductus angle should be noted. On the lateral view, the talar declination angle and the calcaneal inclination angle are indicative of sagittal plane compensation. Meary's angle (talo-first metatarsal angle) can be helpful in identifying the apex of deformity. Noting any radiographic navicular cuneiform fault is helpful to correlate with the clinical examination and determine whether this joint needs to be stabilized. A calcaneal axial view can be useful in determining frontal plane deformity of the calcaneus. The long leg axial view can be used to determine the hind foot alignment. CT scans are reserved for the rigid flatfoot or when there are other diagnostic issues.

Conservative Care

Therapy for equinus can include home stretching, working with a physical therapist, and night splints. Initially, working with a physical therapist can help to ensure that the therapy gets off to a good start. Older children need education to understand the importance of the stretching and to be properly motivated. Children can keep their own calendar to motivate them to track their progress and compliance. Night splints are effective, but compliance can be difficult. Nonetheless, when the equinus is compensatory secondary to the valgus position of the rearfoot, these conservative therapies are particularly worthwhile [25].

It seems reasonable to state that over-the-counter insoles can be a first step for a mild pes valgus with symptoms although objective data is lacking. The more significantly collapsed foot can be treated with custom orthotics. These devices will not change the structure of the foot but may be very helpful in relieving symptoms. Although there are limitations to the study, the Cochrane Collaboration review of this topic is helpful. Their conclusion was that evidence from the current randomized controlled studies at that point was too limited to draw definitive conclusions about the use of nonsurgical interventions for "pediatric pes planus" [26].

Indications for Surgery

The most agreed-upon indication for surgery is pain that is not relieved by conservative care. This is often associated with a short tendoachillis. Many children and adolescents will have a pes valgus foot, but few will require surgery. The use of over-the-counter inserts or functional orthotics may bring sufficient pain relief such that surgery can be avoided.

General indications for surgery can include pain, deforming forces uncorrectable by conservative care, a painful accessory navicular, severe deformity, and postural symptoms or proximal mechanical effects (such as knee valgus) caused by the foot collapse. Each of these general indications has qualifiers. In most cases, the preference should be to give conservative care an attempt prior to surgical intervention.

Surgical Procedures

The selection of surgical procedures is based on the apex of the deformity, severity of deformity and symptoms, bone maturity, chronological and developmental age, weight, and plane of deformity and compensation, among other factors.

Evans Osteotomy

The Evans calcaneal osteotomy is a very powerful procedure [27]. In fact, its power can lead to complications. This osteotomy of the anterior beak of the calcaneus simultaneously lengthens the lateral column and puts tension on the plantar ligaments. Although it is primarily thought of as producing correction in the transverse plane, it also creates sagittal and frontal plane correction. The talonavicular joint becomes realigned, and there is dramatic correction of the calcaneocuboid joint and the talocalcaneal angle on the anterior posterior radiograph. Frontal plane correction occurs with a slight decrease in overall subtalar joint motion and a specific decrease in subtalar joint pronation. Sagittal plane correction is pronounced with an increase in the calcaneal inclination angle due to plantarflexion of the forefoot on the rearfoot as the plantar fascia and the long plantar ligament tighten [28]. The mechanism is adduction and plantarflexion of the midfoot relative to the hind foot. The cuboid and navicular move as a unit [29].

The incisional approach can be either oblique or longitudinal. The oblique incision is performed within the relaxed skin tension lines and results in a finer scar. The longitudinal incision parallels the sural and intermediate dorsal cutaneous nerves and is less likely to disrupt them. Either approach is acceptable. The authors' preference is for the oblique incision, but care must be taken to preserve the nerves. The extensor digitorum brevis is retracted dorsally, and the peroneal tendons are retracted inferiorly, along with the sural nerve. Although the calcaneocuboid joint is identified, it is not opened, which helps to preserve the stability of the joint. The osteotomy location is identified based upon the need to avoid the middle facet of the subtalar joint. Typically, the osteotomy is made 10–15 mm proximal to the calcaneocuboid joint. This usually allows for the cut to be made anterior to the middle facet. If there is any doubt about the location of the facet, an intraoperative C-arm view can be taken with an instrument such as a freer elevator marking the site of the osteotomy to confirm its location. The question of where to make the bone cut has received much attention, as the anatomy of the subtalar joint and the location of the osteotomy can imperil the middle facet [30]. The anterior and middle facets may be contiguous in many cases [31–34]. Canavese et al. performed postoperative CT scan 3D reconstructions of the calcaneus following the Evans osteotomy for flatfoot deformity in children. They identified the following as factors associated with risk of damage to the articular facets: [1] Bunning and Barnett's type B1 and B2 facets [2], osteotomy performed less than 10 mm or greater than 15 mm from the calcaneocuboid joint, and [3] incorrect direction of the osteotomy [35]. This is a good summary of the primary risk factors.

The osteotomy is made parallel to the calcaneocuboid joint and perpendicular to the weight-bearing surface. The Evans procedure has been described as a through and through cut to create a full lengthening osteotomy. However, it can be modified to preserve the medial hinge and make it a wedge osteotomy. The advantages to the hinge approach include less chance for dorsal displacement of the anterior beak and less chance for overcorrection. The primary disadvantage is that there is less correction per millimeter width of the graft. The authors' preferred technique is to leave the medial hinge intact allowing for increased stability of the graft and therefore more rapid healing. The various shapes of the graft will determine how much correction occurs. Rectangular grafts create the most correction, followed by a truncated wedge with a triangular graft creating the least correction by shape.

Material choices include allogeneic precut wedges, wedges that the surgeon cuts from allogeneic iliac crest, autogenous bone, and titanium foam wedges. The precut wedges come with a convenient instrumentation set of trial sizes and tamps. The wedges themselves are bi-cortical (lateral and dorsal surfaces) and may lack the strength of tri-cortical wedges. The trial sizers (for both Cotton and Evans osteotomies) can also be utilized with tri-cortical allogeneic iliac crest wedges. Because the performance of allogeneic bone is so good, the authors have not found a need to utilize autogenous bone [36]. Another alternative is the use of plates with metallic wedges in lieu of grafts [37]. The remaining space can be packed with chips or graft if so desired.

A current area of controversy is whether to fixate the osteotomy. It appears that elevation of the anterior beak, when it does occur, may decrease after the plantar soft tissues elongate with time [38, 39]. The authors' personal experience is that routine fixation is unnecessary. However, others have found that fixation prevents shifting of the anterior beak of the calcaneus and possibly less decrease in graft size with time. There does not appear to be any difference in union rates between fixated and non-fixated grafts [40]. The size of the graft plays into this decision. The primary author's own tendency is trending toward utilizing smaller grafts than what has been utilized through the years. For example, 30 years ago, the grafts used in adolescents might have been as large as 14–15 mm. Over the years it has become evident that these grafts are too large. They create excessive plantarflexion of the forefoot on the rearfoot, overly supinate the foot, and are more likely to create anterior beak shift because of the increased tension on the short and long plantar ligaments. Because the procedure can produce such dramatic radiographic effects, the temptation is to try and achieve full correction of all elements of the deformity. However, as the objective of the procedure is to produce a controllable foot, this may be unnecessary. More typically now, the senior author utilizes grafts for the Evans that are 8–9 mm truncated wedges or more triangular wedges, understanding that larger or smaller grafts may be necessary in individual circumstances.

Determining the ideal amount of correction for a patient is based upon realignment of the talonavicular joint. This can be checked with the sizers, with or without intraoperative x-ray. The block of iliac crest allogeneic graft can be shaped based upon the desired correction in terms of dimensions and shape.

Once the graft has been shaped, a distractor can be utilized to open up the area for insertion of the graft. Alternatively, a smooth lamina spreader can be utilized. The graft should be placed in its final position with a bone tamp in order to distribute the forces of compression more evenly across the graft. Otherwise, the graft wall can crack, which can cause collapse of the graft. The graft should be left slightly proud so that it does not collapse within the cancellous bone of the calcaneus.

Radiographic changes with the Evans calcaneal osteotomy are consistent and reproducible as has been demonstrated by many authors [28, 41–45]. These radiographic changes occur in multiple planes but are most noticeable in the transverse plane.

Complications can include an increase in forefoot pressures and calcaneocuboid pressures [30, 46–49]. Utilizing grafts just large enough for structural correction can reduce the frequency of these complications.

Z-Osteotomy

The Z-osteotomy can be useful for both shifting the valgus hind foot and lengthening the lateral column. The procedure as described by Weil involves more dissection than either the Evans or the medial calcaneal slide individually, but many authors have found it a reliable technique for reconstruction of the foot [50]. Xu et al. combined the Z-osteotomy with arthroereisis in adolescent pes valgus deformity [51]. Subtalar contact characteristics are affected in a manner similar to the Evans [52].

A 5 cm incision is made on the lateral side of the calcaneus with care taken to identify the sural nerve. This osteotomy usually requires mobilization of the peroneal tendons for visualization of the lateral calcaneus. The calcaneocuboid joint is identified, and the dorsal cut of the osteotomy is made approximately 1.5 cm proximal to the calcaneocuboid joint. The transverse arm of approximately 2.0 cm in length is directed posteriorly, and finally the inferior arm is cut. Trial sizers can be used to determine the amount of lengthening necessary [53].

Medial Calcaneal Slide/ Koutsogiannis

The "slide" osteotomy, described by Koutsogiannis, is a through and through osteotomy through the posterior calcaneus. It shifts the tendoachillis from the pronating side of the subtalar axis to the supination side of the axis. This procedure is based on that simple principle, but it is very effective (Figs. 10.1, 10.2, 10.3, 10.4, 10.5, 10.6, and 10.7). It is particularly suited to the compensatory metatarsus adductus foot where an Evans calcaneal osteotomy may adduct the foot too much. It also works well as a combination procedure with the Evans (Figs. 10.8, 10.9, 10.10, 10.11, 10.12, 10.13, and 10.14). It has gained particular popularity for the adult flatfoot.

The technical execution of the procedure begins with a lateral curvilinear incision posterior to the peroneal tendons. Care should be taken to avoid the sural nerve and to achieve hemostasis as the dissection is carried down through the superficial fascia. An incision to the bone through the periosteum is then performed. If fixation will be achieved through posterior to anterior screws, then the periosteal dissection will be minimal. Care should be taken regarding patients with an open apophysis. If one of the lateral plate systems will be used, then more dissection is performed with a key elevator. The peroneal

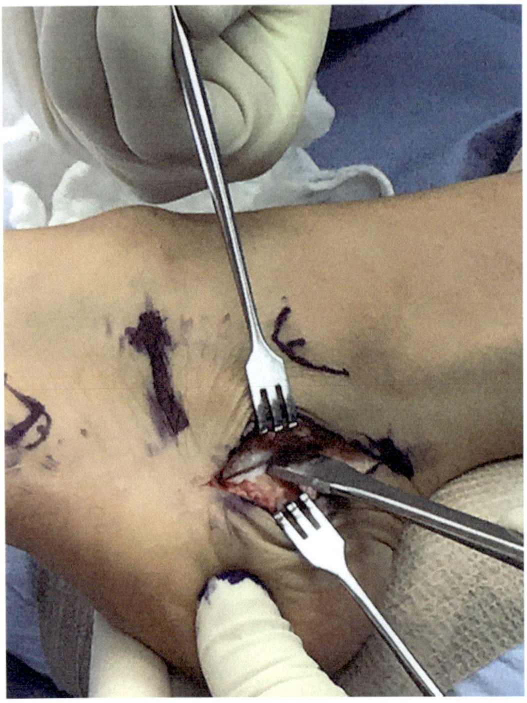

Fig. 10.1 Medial calcaneal slide osteotomy. Key elevator is used to shift the periosteum for plate application. Note outline for Evans osteotomy incision and tuberosity of the fifth metatarsal. Both incisions should be drawn prior to execution in order to ensure a skin bridge is maintained between the two osteotomies

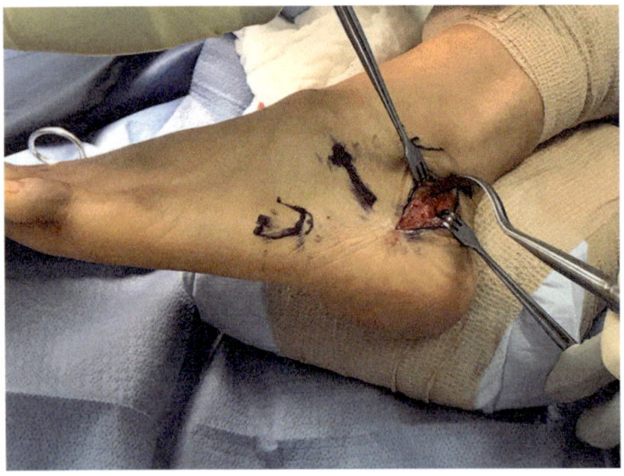

Fig. 10.2 Crego elevators can be used superiorly and inferiorly to protect the tarsal tunnel contents. These must be removed prior to the shift of the osteotomy

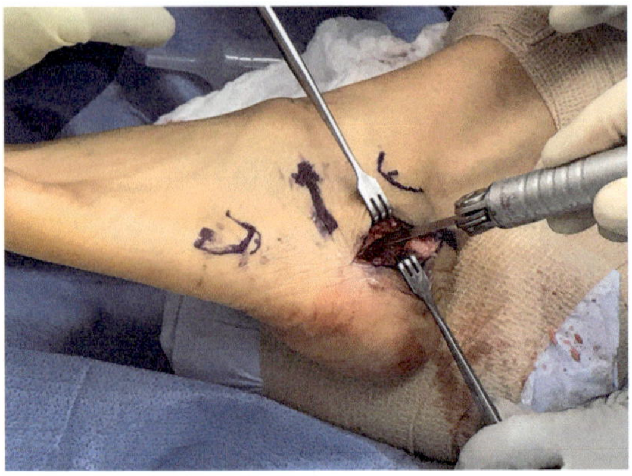

Fig. 10.3 The osteotomy is made perpendicular to the bone and parallel to the posterior facet

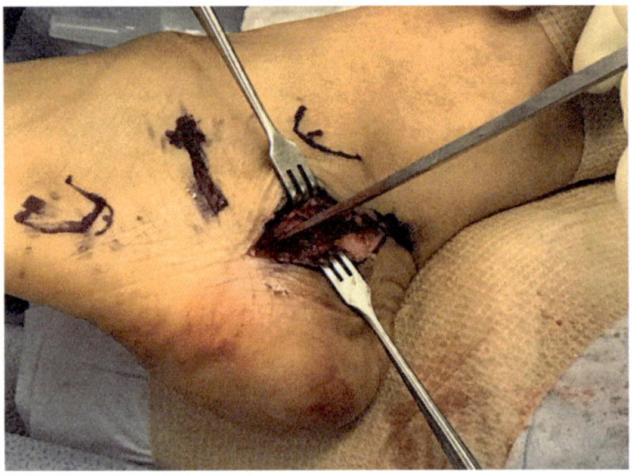

Fig. 10.4 An osteotome can be used to gently finish the osteotomy and to distract the soft tissues to make mobilization of the osteotomy easier

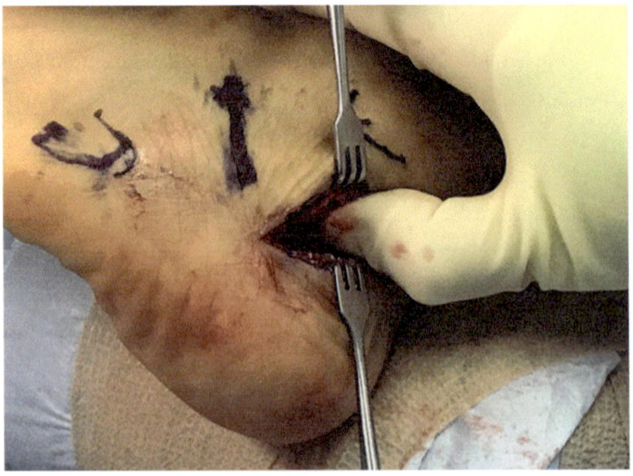

Fig. 10.5 The posterior calcaneus is shifted about 1 cm medially

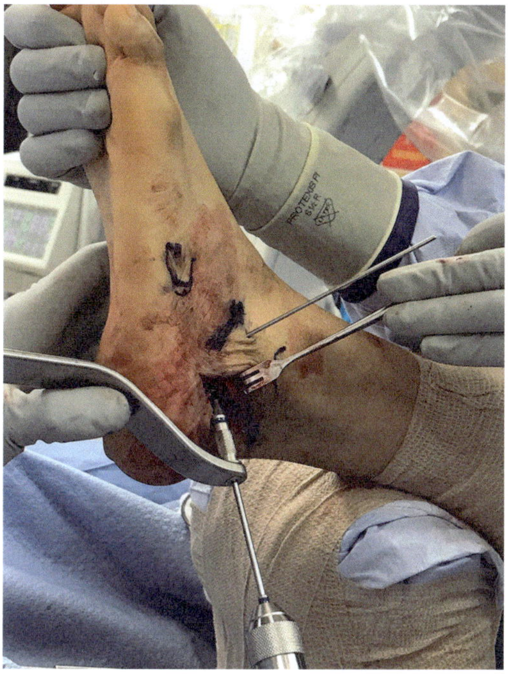

Fig. 10.6 Temporary fixation is applied utilizing a K-wire. In the technique here, a plate is applied and a locking screw applied followed by an inter-fragmentary screw directed toward the sustentaculum tali. Note the angle of the drill for the sustentaculum screw

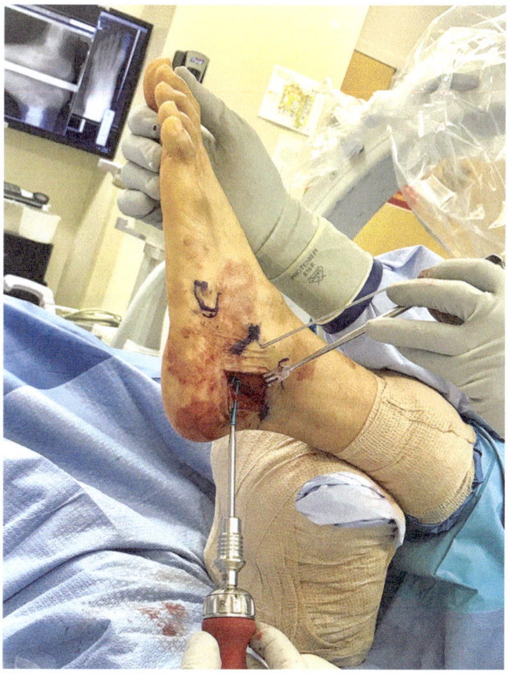

Fig. 10.7 Insertion of second (sustentaculum) screw. C-arm is used to check position

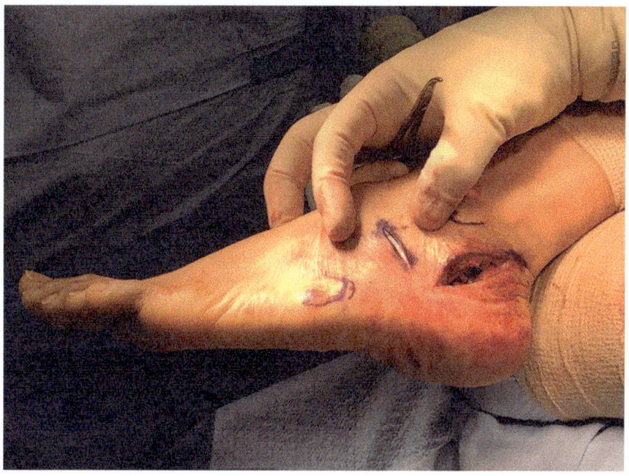

Fig. 10.8 Oblique incision for the Evans osteotomy placed within the relaxed skin tension lines

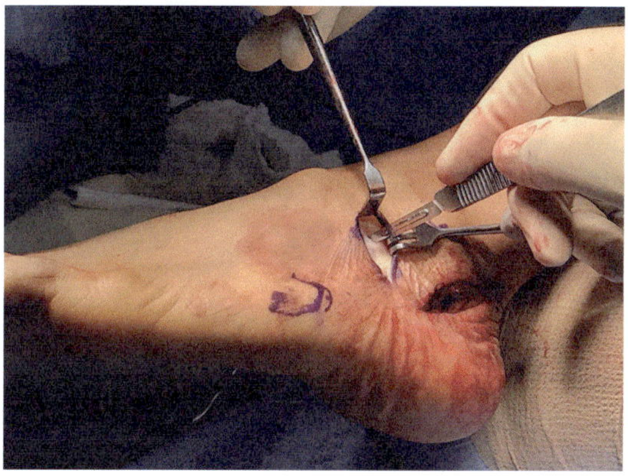

Fig. 10.9 Evans osteotomy incision through the extensor digitorum muscle belly

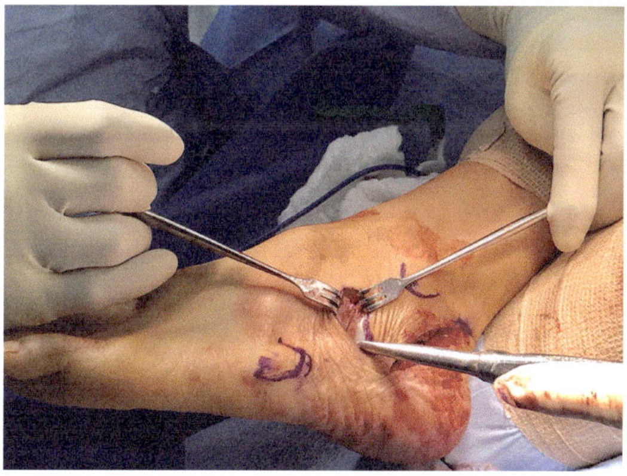

Fig. 10.10 Exposed calcaneus with inferior thin Crego retractor protecting the peroneal tendons and sural nerve

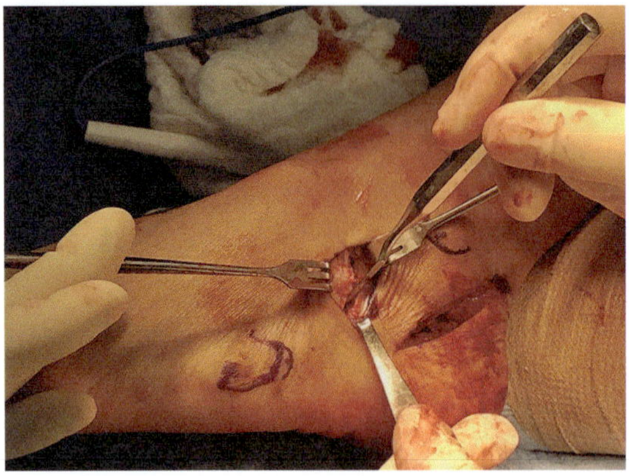

Fig. 10.11 Osteotome separating the osteotomy

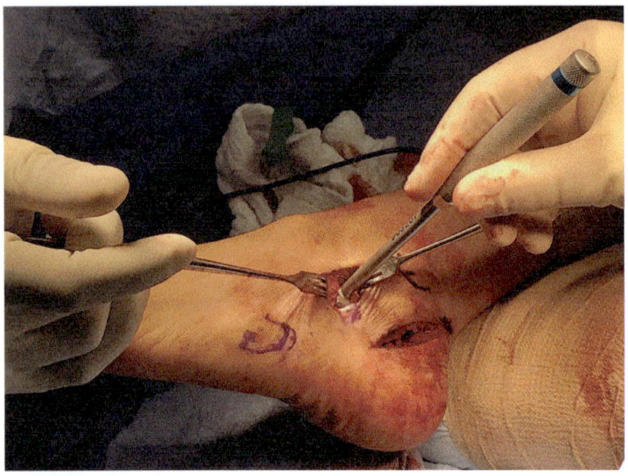

Fig. 10.12 Using a sizer to estimate the required bone graft

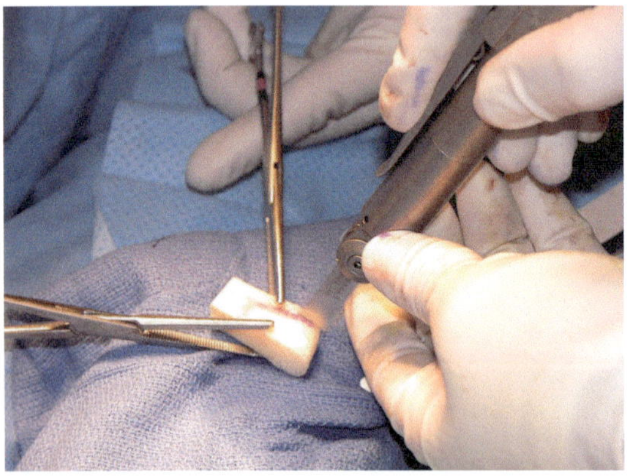

Fig. 10.13 Cutting an Evans bone graft wedge from a freeze-dried iliac crest graft

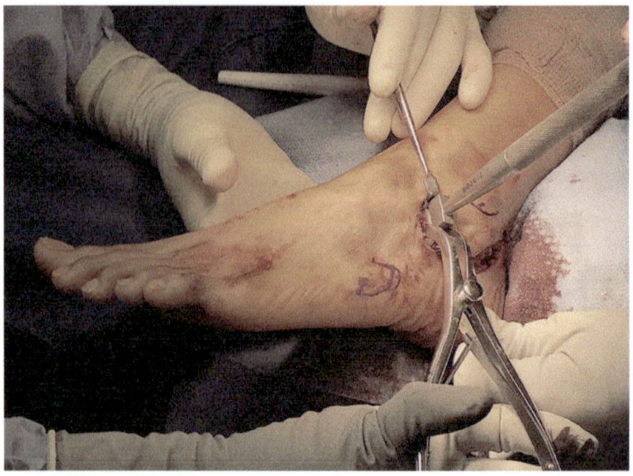

Fig. 10.14 Utilization of a smooth lamina spreader and tamp to apply the bone graft to Evans osteotomy site

tendons are retracted anteriorly and should not be invaded by the approach. An intraoperative x-ray can be performed to confirm the location and direction of the osteotomy. This helps to prevent the osteotomy from being performed too proximal or less commonly, more distal, which could threaten the posterior facet of the subtalar joint. Crego elevators can be used to protect the superior and inferior sides of the osteotomy. The osteotomy is performed with power instrumentation. Any incomplete areas can be checked with an osteotome. The osteotomy will not shift until the Crego elevators have been removed. The shift is usually performed about 6–10 mm, temporarily fixated with a pin, and then the position is checked with an intraoperative x-ray, including a calcaneal axial and lateral view. Care should be taken to ensure that the posterior portion of the calcaneus does not displace superiorly.

Final fixation can be achieved in a variety of ways. The calcaneus heals quite well, so it is not clear that one technique will have any advantage over another in terms of bone healing. One or two (vertically stacked) screws can be inserted from posterior to anterior. The authors' preference is for larger (6.5 mm) headless cannulated screws although smaller screws or headed screws, well countersunk, can also be used. It is important that the screw heads should not be prominent in order to avoid the necessity of screw removal. However, should future reconstruction be necessary through the calcaneus, headless screws can be difficult to locate. Lateral plating can be performed with a variety of systems. One preferable system utilizes a locking screw directed through the plate perpendicular to the calcaneus with a second lag screw directed toward the sustentaculum tali. Intraoperative x-rays confirm both the final position and fixation.

If the lateral side of the calcaneus is prominent after the shift, it can be tamped down flat. Good closure of the superficial fascia is critical to cover a lateral plate and to promote good scar mobility.

The osteotomy has produced good improvement in symptomatic relief of patients with painful pes valgus [54–56].

Cotton Osteotomy

The Cotton osteotomy is an opening wedge plantarflexory osteotomy of the medial cuneiform. It is best indicated for structural elevation of the first ray. It does not address hypermobility at the navicular cuneiform joint or first metatarsal cuneiform joint, two areas that are frequently responsible for medial column elevation and insufficiency (Figs. 10.15, 10.16, 10.17, 10.18, and 10.19). Nonetheless, the procedure is popular because it is effective at creating structural plantarflexion, is technically simple, and is relatively quick.

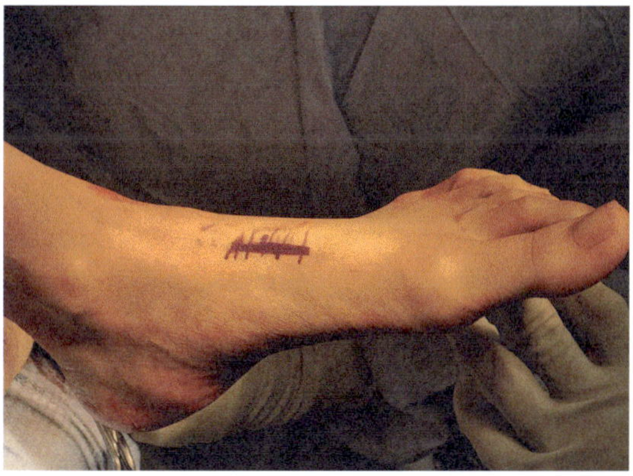

Fig. 10.15 Skin incision for a Cotton osteotomy

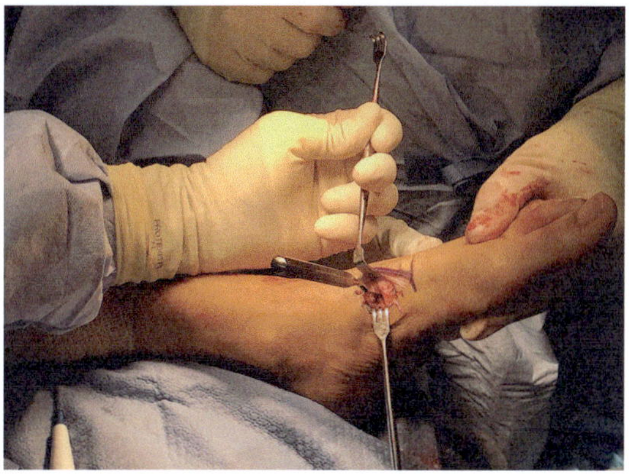

Fig. 10.16 Osteotome placement after saw cut to feather plantarly and wedge open the osteotomy

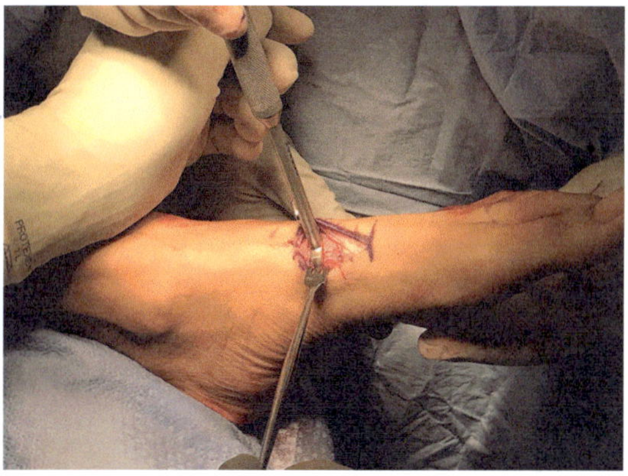

Fig. 10.17 Sizer placement for the Cotton osteotomy

The procedure relies on an understanding of the location of the proximal and distal joints of the medial cuneiform to avoid destabilizing those joints with dissection. Intraoperative x-ray can be used to check these as well as with range of motion for the first metatarsal cuneiform joint, in particular. The incision is centered over the medial cuneiform, parallel to the extensor hallucis longus (EHL) tendon, and carried down through the superficial fascia. The EHL must be properly protected so that the saw does not cut it during

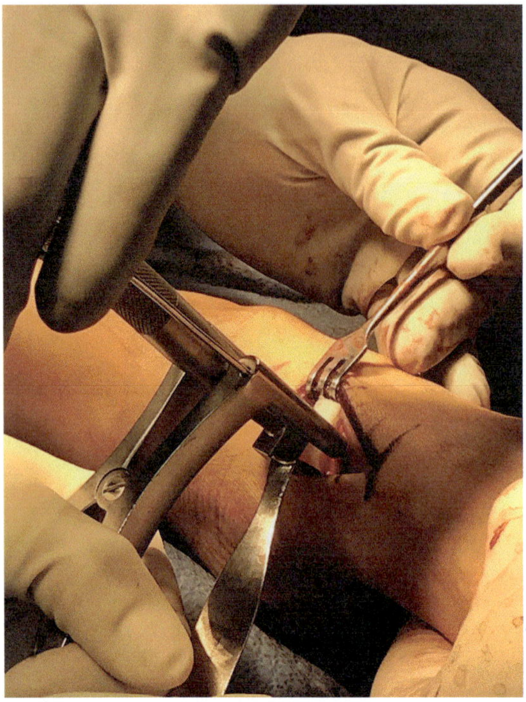

Fig. 10.18 Weinraub retractor opens the osteotomy to allow the placement of the graft

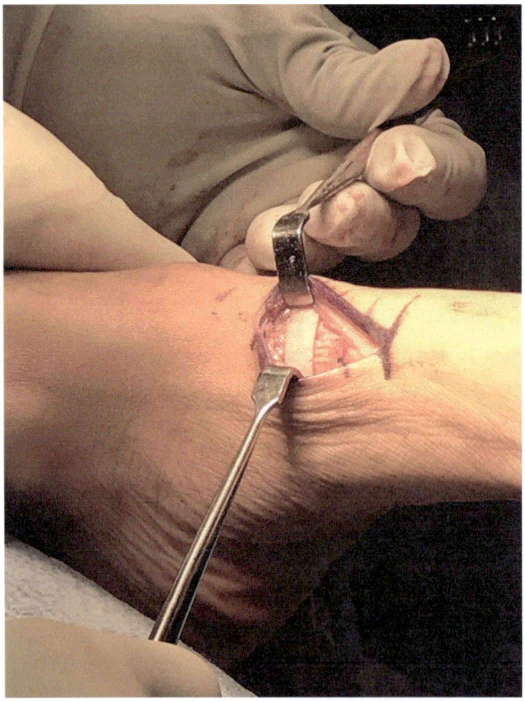

Fig. 10.19 Placement of the graft in the Cotton osteotomy

the osteotomy. Once the joint locations are confirmed, the periosteal incision can be performed transversely in the same direction as the osteotomy. The osteotomy is typically performed at the area of the distal two-thirds of the cuneiform. It is executed with a power saw and checked with an osteotome. The objective is to leave the plantar hinge intact, although if it cracks it is unlikely to displace. On the other hand, if the osteotomy is pried open before the plantar cortex is sufficiently thinned, it may cause the propagation of an intra-articular fracture line into the first metatarsal cuneiform joint. Once the osteotomy is sufficiently free, sizers can be used to check for the appropriate graft. Typically, a graft of 4–6 mm is adequate for correction, but certainly this varies depending on the size of the foot and the amount of deformity. Generally, fixation is not necessary, but should there be a need, small plates can be applied. Care should be taken not to excessively plantarflex the first ray in order to avoid a painful tibial sesamoiditis.

Medial Arch Suspension

Young, in 1939, first described the procedure of using a transfer of the tibialis anterior through a slot in the navicular, along with a tendoachillis lengthening. Young felt that the creation of the plantar ligament below the navicular cuneiform joint helped to reinforce the action of tibialis posterior. McGlamry and Beck modified the procedure by adding a transfer of the flexor digitorum longus, plication of the spring ligament, and other modifications [57]. For the decade of the 1970s, the medial arch suspension was the mainstay of flatfoot reconstruction. Although there was no fundamental structural reconstruction with the procedure, patients did surprisingly well. Looking at a group of Dr. E. Dalton McGlamry's patients in 1983, it was found that the subjective sense of improvement was the same in groups of patients who only had the medial arch suspension as compared to those patients who had both the Evans calcaneal osteotomy and the medial arch suspension, although those with structural correction had significantly improved radiographic findings. The principle behind the procedure is to remove the influence of the tibialis anterior on dorsiflexion of the first ray while effectively increasing the power of the peroneus longus to plantarflex the first ray. The procedure relies on a keyhole slot in the navicular to slide the tibialis anterior into place. The insertion into the first metatarsal cuneiform joint is left intact, but the functional insertion becomes the dorsal portion of the navicular. The tendon creates a plantar ligament between the navicular cuneiform joints, which helps to stabilize an area that is typically hypermobile. Shortening of the thick spring ligament is a powerful adjunct to the procedure.

Although the procedure is ideal for hypermobility of the medial column in conjunction with either an Evans calcaneal osteotomy or a calcaneal slide osteotomy, it is much less commonly performed now than the Cotton medial cuneiform osteotomy for addressing medial column issues. Typically, the medial arch suspension is more time consuming, requires more dissection, and is more technique dependent than the relatively simple Cotton osteotomy.

The Kidner procedure is not truly an effective procedure for the adolescent pes valgus deformity, but it does have a place in the patient with a painful accessory navicular. In those situations, if the patient is not responsive to conservative care, then surgical removal of the accessory bone, remodeling of the navicular as necessary, and advancement of the tibialis posterior are effective. After the loss of the accessory navicular, it is important to reattach the portion of the posterior tibialis tendon that had inserted in the accessory bone into the plantar medial portion of the navicular.

Sequencing

When combining procedures, the sequence can be an important element to make the procedure technically simpler. The authors prefer to perform the equinus lengthening first to avoid putting pressure on grafts or osteotomies later. The need for equinus release can be determined by placing the subtalar joint in the expected position of correction and then performing the Silfverskiold test.

When performing a double calcaneal osteotomy, the incisions should be mapped out in order to ensure that there is an adequate skin bridge between the two osteotomies. The posterior calcaneal slide osteotomy is typically performed first including fixation after confirming position on x-ray. Next, the dissection for the Evans osteotomy is performed through an oblique incision. The osteotomy is made taking care to preserve the middle facet and using sizers to determine the size of the graft needed. If the sizers are not available, then the osteotomy is opened and a ruler is used to measure the size of the gap when the talar head is covered by the navicular. At this point, with the subtalar joint placed in neutral position and the foot loaded, the medial column position is evaluated. If there is structural elevation of the medial column, then dissection proceeds for the Cotton osteotomy. The graft size is again determined by sizers, examining the medial column position with various sizes of wedges. The graft is then inserted.

If navicular cuneiform instability is present, then either a medial arch suspension or navicular cuneiform arthrodesis is performed. It is not possible to manipulate the foot adequately for a medial arch suspension once the Evans graft has been inserted. Therefore, if either of those procedures is necessary, they are performed before the final Evans graft positioning.

Other Osteotomies

The triple C osteotomy was described by Rathjen and Mubarak in 1998 consisting of sliding and medial closing wedge osteotomies of the posterior calcaneus, medial cuneiform osteotomy with a plantar-based closing wedge osteotomy, and an opening wedge osteotomy of the cuboid [58]. Moraleda et al.'s study compared the combination to the Evans procedure and determined somewhat higher complications with the Evans and somewhat less correction with the triple-C [59].

A Dwyer opening wedge osteotomy can be utilized to correct frontal plane heel valgus [60].

Arthroereisis

For the pes valgus deformity that is truly flexible, arthroereisis is a viable option to restrict abnormal subtalar motion. The commonly held theory is that the subtalar implant blocks abnormal motion of the talus, allowing inversion while preventing excessive eversion [61]. Several studies have demonstrated improvement in plantar pressure distribution after this procedure in the pediatric population [61]. Radiographic improvement has also been seen in the pediatric and adult populations [62] [63, 64]. Arthroereisis is generally held to have a low complication rate and is less invasive than other techniques. Many types of devices have been utilized as implants. Currently arthroereisis devices fall into five main material categories: stainless steel, titanium, polyethylene, combined construction, or bioresorbable [64]. These are often available in a set that contains sizers and insertional tools specific for the device.

Types of devices were classified by Vogler [65] and can be described as self-locking wedges where the surfaces of the talus and calcaneus are separated by a block of material. The axis of the subtalar joint is not restricted in these devices. The second type of device is an axis-altering device such as the STA-peg device that redirects the subtalar axis. This device goes back to 1975 when Smith and Miller described the device. Lundeen (1985) did a follow-up study on patients with these devices and identified that navicular cuneiform instability could result in recurrence [66]. Oloff et al. reported on the complications (1987) [67]. In addition, untreated equinus was identified as a possible source of recurrence. The third type, direct impaction devices, impinges on the anterior margin of the talus to restrict pronation past the desired range. A newer device, the extraosseous talotarsal stabilization device, occupies both the sinus tarsi and the tarsal canal with a threaded device that obtains an interference grip in the anteroposterior direction and is "unlikely to be constantly bearing body weight" according to Bali et al. in 2013 and has been demonstrated to decrease peak pressures over the entire foot [68, 69].

Surgical Technique

The patient is placed supine, although if adjunct procedures are planned a small bump may be placed under the hip for external rotation. A 27-gauge needle is used to identify the sinus tarsi from the lateral aspect, approximately 1 cm anterior and inferior from the tip of the lateral malleolus. Once identified, a small 1.5 cm incision is made over the sinus tarsi, following relaxed skin tension lines. This incision should avoid both the sural nerve and the intermediate dorsal cutaneous nerve. Using a mosquito hemostat, blunt dissection is performed through the subcutaneous tissue and deep fascia. The cannula rod for the implant sizer is then placed into and across the sinus tarsi. Tenting of the medial skin may be noted as a sign that the rod has passed the entire distance. Some arthroereisis sets have a dilation device to allow for stretching of the sinus tarsi, which is placed over the cannula rod and inserted into the sinus tarsi with gentle twisting. The sizers are then trialed, with examination of subtalar eversion with each sizer and intraoperative dorsoplantar and lateral radiographs taken to ensure correct positioning. The correct sizer will limit eversion to 2–4 degrees, and on radiograph the medial edge will sit at the midline of the talus. Once the correct size is determined, the sizer is removed and the corresponding sized implant is placed over the cannula rod. A driver is used to insert it into the sinus tarsi, and intraoperative radiographs are used to check the positioning of the device. After removal of the driver and rod, the area is irrigated, and deep closure is performed of the fascia, followed by superficial closure. The patient is placed in a compressive dressing and posterior splint for 1 week and is allowed to weight bear as tolerated after the procedure.

Complications

Arthroereisis carries specific risks, including sinus tarsi pain, implant extrusion and possible need for device removal, and over- or under correction. Complications such as synovitis and peroneal spasm have also been reported

[63]. Continued or worsened pain can occur if the implant chosen is too small or too large. However, the implant placement is generally reversible, allowing for correction of this type of complication [70].

Equinus

The conventional wisdom is to perform a posterior group lengthening along with the vast majority of flatfoot procedures. Typically, these are gastrocnemius recessions for those with exclusive gastrocnemius tightness or tendoachillis lengthening for gastroc soleus equinus. Pes valgus deformity is closely linked with equinus. In some cases, the equinus may be corrected with stretching exercises; in others surgical treatment is necessary. The Silfverskiold test is typically performed to make this distinction. There certainly is a segment of the adolescent flatfoot population that has tendoachillis shortening as the primary etiology. For those patients, lengthening is mandatory or the reconstructive procedures will fail. There are a number of patients in whom the equinus may be more secondary, as a result of the heel valgus position creating shortening over time. In adolescents, if the equinus is more marginal, I try to avoid the lengthening in order to avoid weakening the posterior group (Fig. 10.20). Some of these children at least can be effectively stretched out postoperatively.

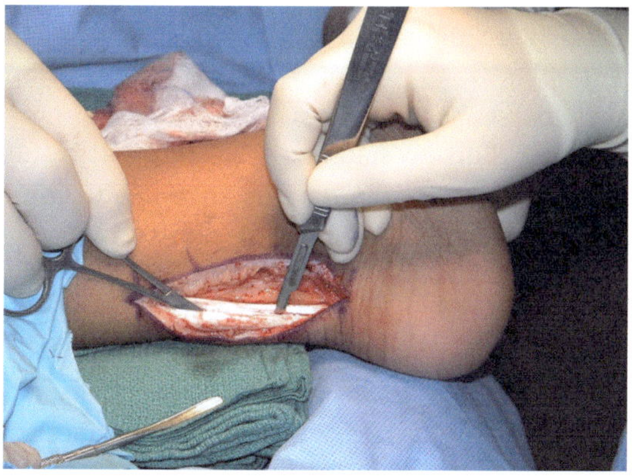

Fig. 10.20 An open frontal plane lengthening of the tendoachillis

If a Silfverskiold test reveals pure gastrocnemius equinus, an isolated gastrocnemius recession is indicated. If a gastrosoleal equinus is discovered, a tendo-Achilles lengthening (TAL) may be considered [71]. The TAL may be performed open or percutaneously. Similarly, a gastrocnemius recession may be performed open or endoscopic. Vulpius described a chevron cut through the gastrocnemius tendon and additionally incised the deep raphe of the soleus. Strayer described a transverse incision along the gastrocnemius tendon, just proximal to the aponeurosis, and sutured the tendon in its new lengthened position. The Baker variation to the Vulpius procedure, described below, uses a tongue-shaped incision in the tendon for lengthening [25].

Technique

The patient is placed prone or in the frog-leg position, depending on adjunct procedures. A 4 cm incision is made just medial to the posterior midline, at the level of the gastrocnemius-soleus musculotendinous junction, which can be palpated. The aponeurosis is identified, and care is taken to identify both lateral and medial borders before incisions are made. An incision is made through the paratenon longitudinally. With the ankle held in a neutral position, an incision is made from one-third of the width of the aponeurosis medially to the most medial edge, without cutting into the soleus muscle fibers, which lie deep. Next an incision is made of the lateral one-third of the aponeurosis in a similar fashion, watching for the sural nerve, which should be retracted. The final incision is then made approximately 2 cm distal to the two already made, in the middle one-third of the aponeurosis. The ankle is then dorsiflexed maximally, with the knee extended, to allow for the recession of the cut aponeurosis. If it does not lengthen, the incisions are reassessed to ensure all fibers have been cut. If further intervention is required, the median raphe of the soleus may be identified and cut. With the equinus properly resolved, the wound is irrigated, and closure of the paratenon and deep fascia is performed. A layered skin closure is performed, and a dressing of gauze and transparent adhesive is applied. For an isolated procedure, patients are kept immobilized for 4 weeks and are then transitioned to physical therapy and regular shoe gear.

For an endoscopic recession, the patient is placed supine, and a 1.5 cm incision is made posteromedially at the gastrosoleal junction. A cannula with a blunt trochar is inserted into the incision after dissection to the paratenon. The trochar is passed through laterally until the lateral skin is tented. Depending on the type of device used, a lateral incision may be necessary. The trochar is then removed. The slotted aspect of the cannula is swiveled to face the gastrocnemius aponeurosis. The endoscopic camera is placed into the cannula if the blade can be mounted on the camera, from the medial side, if not from the lateral side. The aponeurosis is visualized to ensure no other structures will be in danger of transection. With the ankle dorsiflexed, the hook blade is used (from medial, either attached to the camera or viewed with the camera via the lateral portal) to transect the gastrocnemius aponeurosis. The blade and camera are removed, and the ankle is again dorsiflexed to check adequate correction. The cannula is removed, and the skin is closed with simple sutures and dressed. Weightbearing is allowed postoperatively in a CAM boot with active and passive ankle range of motion daily.

For patients requiring a tendo-Achilles lengthening, Hoke described a triple hemisection of the Achilles, which has been adapted to a percutaneous method. Three stab incisions are marked out over the Achilles tendon – the most distal at the lateral one-third, the central at the medial one-third, and the most proximal at the lateral one-third. The distal incision is marked approximately 3 cm from the calcaneal insertion, with the central 6 cm from the insertion, and the proximal 11 cm from the insertion. A number 15 blade is used to create a longitudinal stab at the distal mark, and once the blade is advanced through the tendon, it is rotated 90 degrees so the cutting edge is lateral. In this fashion the lateral one-third of the tendon is transected. Care is taken to remove the blade from the skin in the same way it entered. This is repeated at the central mark, where the medial one-third of the Achilles tendon is transected. Finally, at the proximal mark, the lateral one-third of the tendon is transected. At this point the ankle is dorsiflexed and a release of the Achilles tendon should be felt. The incisions are irrigated and closed with simple sutures, and the sites are dressed. For an isolated procedure, the ankle is casted or splinted at a neutral 90 degrees of dorsiflexion, and the patient is kept non-weightbearing for 3–4 weeks.

Complications

Complications of all the above procedures include over-lengthening and rupture of either the gastrocnemius or Achilles tendon. Conversely, insufficient correction can also be a concern. Sural neuritis may also occur, particularly in gastrocnemius recessions as the sural nerve lies quite close to the surgical area. Adhesions of the gastrocnemius to the soleus, or of the Achilles tendon after an open procedure, have also been reported [25, 71]. Infection, postoperative muscle weakness, and recurrence of equinus have also been observed [72].

Arthrodesis

In the adolescent flexible flatfoot, arthrodesis has a more limited but still important role. In particular, in cases of hypermobility of the navicular cuneiform joint, fusion may be necessary. Failure to stabilize that joint will result in compensation through the medial column. Arthrodesis is indicated in some neuromuscular deformities [73]. Indications would include patients with ligamentous laxity such as Ehlers-Danlos syndrome. Generally, this would be performed in somewhat older adolescents. Degenerative joint disease would be another indication for fusion of a joint.

The navicular cuneiform fusion is particularly useful for patients with hypermobility at that joint. Failure to address hypermobility in that location will result in continued compensation, even when stabilization in the rearfoot has been achieved. Isolated fusion of the medial joint alone may be adequate in most cases, whereas fusion of all three joints may be performed in the event of more severe deformity or degenerative joint disease.

Fusion of the naviculocuneiform joint is critical when there is instability that cannot be addressed by a soft tissue procedure. The Cotton osteotomy does not create naviculocuneiform stability. The medial arch suspension does create stability at the naviculocuneiform joint, although not the rigidity that the arthrodesis creates. Nonetheless, it is important to remember that the goal of surgery is to create a pain-free, controllable foot, not necessarily one that looks perfect cosmetically or on radiographs. As with all arthrodesis procedures, the key elements are removal of all cartilage, correction of deformity, and stabilization until bone healing occurs. Screw or plate fixation can be used effectively here.

Midtarsal fusions and talonavicular fusions achieve significant correction but at the expense of loss of motion and adaptability of the foot. Nonetheless, there are patients in whom this type of correction is necessary.

Compensated Metatarsus Adductus

Demographics

The term *metatarsus adductus* describes a major feature of a group of pedal disorders. Focusing on isolated metatarsus adductus, which is reported to occur in 1 per 1000 live births, the deformity is characterized by adducted metatarsals in a single plane. Compensated metatarsus adductus occurs when the rearfoot pronates in response, in some cases creating an almost normal-appearing foot. There are differing theories on the root cause of metatarsus adductus. Some feel that increased intrauterine pressure causes the deformity, favored by the spontaneous resolution of many cases and the higher incidence in first-born children. Others believe that intrinsic causes such as muscle-tendon imbalances and soft tissue contractures lead to the deformity [74]. Abnormal positioning or growth of the medial cuneiform can also be a contributing factor.

Indications for Surgical Treatment

Given that the majority of metatarsus adductus cases will spontaneously resolve, there is some controversy regarding when to treat this condition. However, there is a great lack in data regarding how often this resolution occurs, and there is a general consensus that earlier treatment leads to better outcomes. Therefore, treatment is indicated in most cases, especially when seen early.

While most cases of metatarsus adductus can be resolved with conservative measures, there are those that require surgical intervention. Without correction, metatarsus adductus can lead to other foot deformities such as hallux valgus, contracted digits, and skewfoot [74]. Stretching, casting, and bracing are often successful, but for children where these have failed or for children older than 2 years of age, surgery may be indicated. For younger patients, soft tissue procedures are often attempted first, prior to osseous procedures that are more often used for adolescents and adults.

Summary

There are several surgical approaches that are successful in the pediatric flatfoot. The patient with the short tendoachillis will require lengthening. Multiple planes of stability must be achieved in the rearfoot and in the medial column. The goal of surgical correction is pain reduction and a controllable foot with reduction of deforming forces (Figs. 10.21, 10.22, 10.23, and 10.24). Approaches should be used that best balance the need for control of excess pronation with maintaining some flexibility and adaptability of the foot.

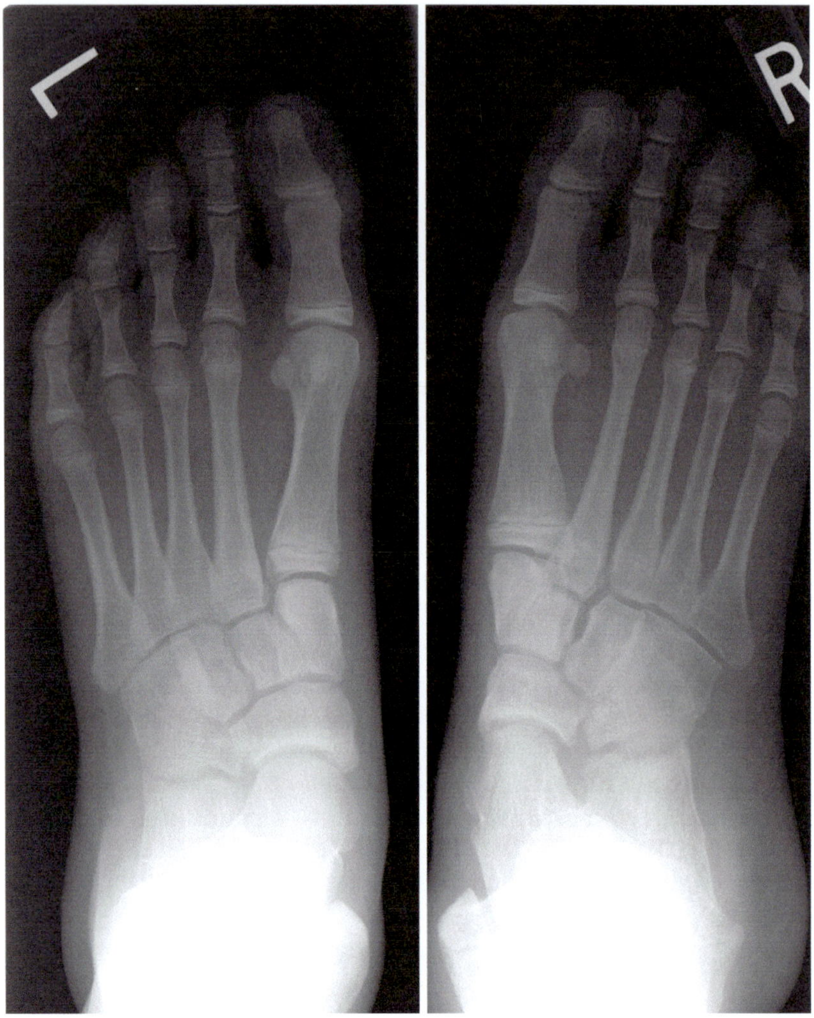

Fig. 10.21 DP preoperative radiograph. Significant deformity with increased talocalcaneal, talo-first metatarsal, and calcaneocuboid angles

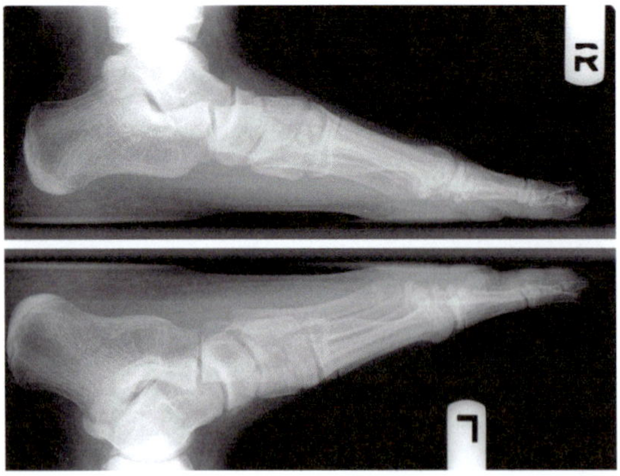

Fig. 10.22 Lateral preoperative radiograph. Significant deformity with decreased calcaneal inclination angle, increased talar declination angle, and an anterior break in the cyma line

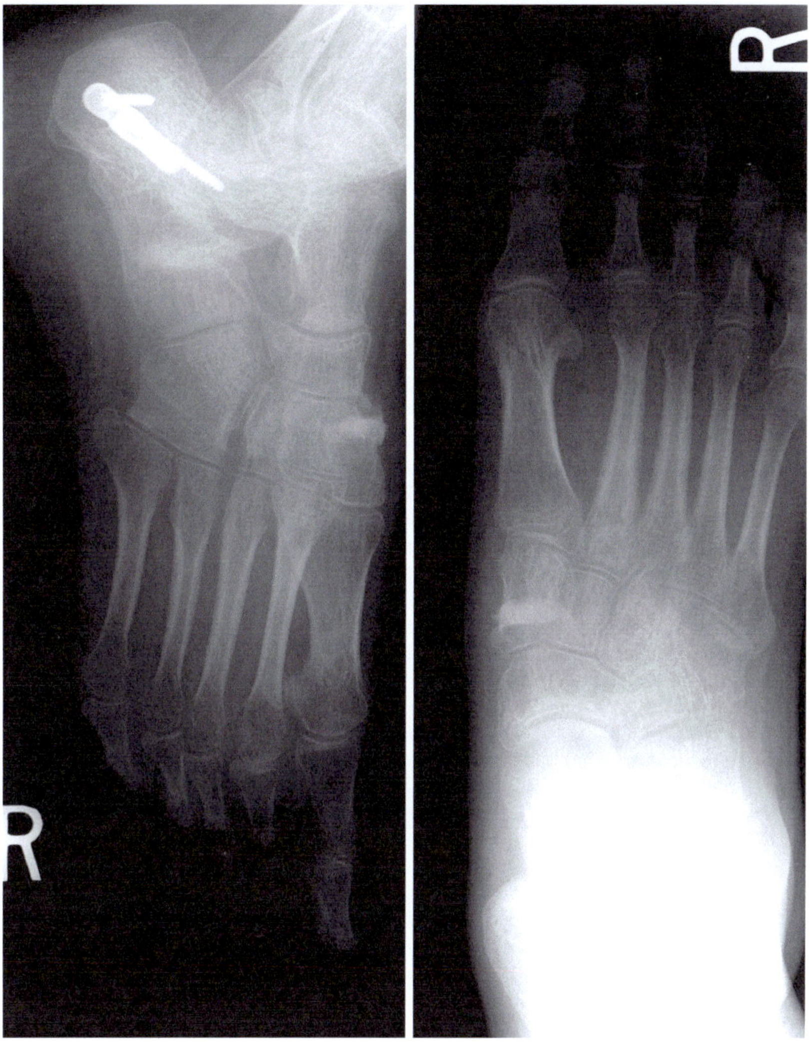

Fig. 10.23 Six-week postoperative DP and medial oblique radiographs. Procedures include an Evans osteotomy, medial calcaneal slide osteotomy, and Cotton osteotomy. Good joint realignment is noted

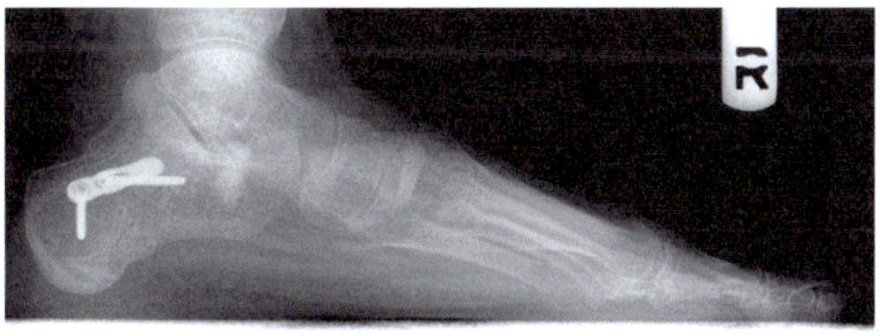

Fig. 10.24 Six-week postoperative lateral radiograph. Good deformity reduction and joint realignment is appreciated as well as healing of the osteotomy and graft sites

References

1. Toolan BC, Sangeorzan BJ, Hansen ST. Complex reconstruction for the treatment of dorsolateral peritalar subluxation of the foot. Early results after distraction arthrodesis of the calcaneocuboid joint in conjunction with stabilization of, and transfer of the flexor digitorum longus tendon to, the midfoot to treat acquired pes planovalgus in adults. J Bone Joint Surg Am. 1999;81(11):1545–60.
2. Basmajian JV, Stecko G. The role of muscles in arch support of the foot. J Bone Joint Surg Am. 1963;45:1184–90.

3. Gray EG, Basmajian JV. Electromyography and cinematography of leg and foot ("normal" and flat) during walking. Anat Rec. 1968;161(1):1–15.
4. Mann R, Inman V. Phasic activity of intrinsic muscles of the foot. J Bone Joint Surg Am. 1964;46:469–81.
5. Borton DC, Saxby TS. Tear of the plantar calcaneonavicular (spring) ligament causing flatfoot. A case report. J Bone Joint Surg Br. 1997;79(4):641–3.
6. Orr JD, Nunley JA. Isolated spring ligament failure as a cause of adult-acquired flatfoot deformity. Foot Ankle Int. 2013;34(6):818–23.
7. Kitaoka HB, Ahn TK, Luo ZP, An KN. Stability of the arch of the foot. Foot Ankle Int. 1997;18(10):644–8.
8. Staheli LT. Evaluation of planovalgus foot deformities with special reference to the natural history. J Am Podiatr Med Assoc. 1987;77(1):2–6.
9. Wearing SC, Hills AP, Byrne NM, Hennig EM, McDonald M. The arch index: a measure of flat or fat feet? Foot Ankle Int. 2004;25(8):575–81.
10. Napolitano C, Walsh S, Mahoney L, McCrea J. Risk factors that may adversely modify the natural history of the pediatric pronated foot. Clin Podiatr Med Surg. 2000;17(3):397–417.
11. Cowan DN, Robinson JR, Jones BH, Polly DW, Berrey BH. Consistency of visual assessments of arch height among clinicians. Foot Ankle Int. 1994;15(4):213–7.
12. Hillstrom HJ, Song J, Kraszewski AP, Hafer JF, Mootanah R, Dufour AB, et al. Foot type biomechanics part 1: structure and function of the asymptomatic foot. Gait Posture. 2013;37(3):445–51.
13. Ledoux WR, Hillstrom HJ. The distributed plantar vertical force of neutrally aligned and pes planus feet. Gait Posture. 2002;15(1):1–9.
14. Mootanah R, Song J, Lenhoff MW, Hafer JF, Backus SI, Gagnon D, et al. Foot type biomechanics part 2: are structure and anthropometrics related to function? Gait Posture. 2013;37(3):452–6.
15. Menz H, Dufour A, Riskowski J, Hillstrom H. Association of planus foot posture and pronated foot function with foot pain: the Framingham study. Arthritis Care Res. 2013;65(12):1991–9.
16. HARRIS RI, BEATH T. Hypermobile flat-foot with short tendo achillis. J Bone Joint Surg Am. 1948;30A(1):116–40.
17. Chen KC, Yeh CJ, Tung LC, Yang JF, Yang SF, Wang CH. Relevant factors influencing flatfoot in preschool-aged children. Eur J Pediatr. 2011;170(7):931–6.
18. Pourghasem M, Kamali N, Farsi M, Soltanpour N. Prevalence of flatfoot among school students and its relationship with BMI. Acta Orthop Traumatol Turc. 2016;50(5):554–7.
19. Stolzman S, Irby MB, Callahan AB, Skelton JA. Pes planus and paediatric obesity: a systematic review of the literature. Clin Obes. 2015;5(2):52–9.
20. Mahan KT, Diamond E, Brown D. Podiatric profile of the Down's syndrome individual. J Am Podiatry Assoc. 1983;73(4):173–9.
21. Em S, Oktayoglu P, Bozkurt M, Caglayan M, Karakoc M, Ucar D, et al. Serum relaxin levels in benign hypermobility syndrome. J Back Musculoskelet Rehabil. 2015;28(3):473–9.
22. Jack EA. Naviculo-cuneiform fusion in the treatment of flat foot. J Bone Joint Surg Br. 1953;35-B(1):75–82.
23. Benedetti MG, Ceccarelli F, Berti L, Luciani D, Catani F, Boschi M, et al. Diagnosis of flexible flatfoot in children: a systematic clinical approach. Orthopedics. 2011;34(2):94.
24. Grady JF, Kelly C. Endoscopic gastrocnemius recession for treating equinus in pediatric patients. Clin Orthop Relat Res. 2010;468(4):1033–8.
25. Blitz NM, Stabile RJ, Giorgini RJ, DiDomenico LA. Flexible pediatric and adolescent pes planovalgus: conservative and surgical treatment options. Clin Podiatr Med Surg. 2010;27(1):59–77.
26. Jane MacKenzie A, Rome K, Evans AM. The efficacy of nonsurgical interventions for pediatric flexible flat foot: a critical review. J Pediatr Orthop. 2012;32(8):830–4.
27. Evans D. Calcaneo-valgus deformity. J Bone Joint Surg Br. 1975;57(3):270–8.
28. Dollard MD, Marcinko DE, Lazerson A, Elleby DH. The Evans calcaneal osteotomy for correction of flexible flatfoot syndrome. J Foot Surg. 1984;23(4):291–301.
29. Dumontier TA, Falicov A, Mosca V, Sangeorzan B. Calcaneal lengthening: investigation of deformity correction in a cadaver flatfoot model. Foot Ankle Int. 2005;26(2):166–70.
30. Raines RA, Brage ME. Evans osteotomy in the adult foot: an anatomic study of structures at risk. Foot Ankle Int. 1998;19(11):743–7.
31. Mosca VS. Ragab AA, Stewart SL, Cooperman DR. Implications of Subtalar joint anatomic variation in calcaneal lengthening osteotomy. J Pediatr Orthop. 2003;23:79–83. J Pediatr Orthop. 2009;29(3):315–6.
32. Laidlaw PP. The Os calcis: part II. J Anat Physiol. 1905;39(Pt 2):161–77.
33. Bunning P, Barnett C. Variations in the talocalcaneal articulations. J Anat. 1963;97(5):636–43.
34. Bussewitz BW, DeVries JG, Hyer CF. Evans osteotomy and risk to subtalar joint articular facets and sustentaculum tali: a cadaver study. J Foot Ankle Surg. 2013;52(5):594–7.
35. Canavese F, Dimeglio A, Bonnel F. Postoperative CT-scan 3D reconstruction of the calcaneus following lateral calcaneal lengthening osteotomy for flatfoot deformity in children. Is the surgical procedure potentially associated with subtalar joint damage? Foot Ankle Surg. 2018;24(5):453–9.
36. Mahan KT, Hillstrom HJ. Bone grafting in foot and ankle surgery. A review of 300 cases. J Am Podiatr Med Assoc. 1998;88(3):109–18.
37. Foster JR, McAlister JE, Peterson KS, Hyer CF. Union rates and complications of lateral column lengthening using the interposition plating technique: a radiographic and medical record review. J Foot Ankle Surg. 2017;56(2):247–51.

38. Dunn SP, Meyer J. Displacement of the anterior process of the calcaneus after Evans calcaneal osteotomy. J Foot Ankle Surg. 2011;50(4):402–6.
39. Marengo L, Canavese F, Mansour M, Dimeglio A, Bonnel F. Clinical and radiological outcome of calcaneal lengthening osteotomy for flatfoot deformity in skeletally immature patients. Eur J Orthop Surg Traumatol. 2017;27:989.
40. Prissel MA, Roukis TS. Incidence of nonunion of the unfixated, isolated evans calcaneal osteotomy: a systematic review. J Foot Ankle Surg. 2012;51(3):323–5.
41. Mosca VS. Calcaneal lengthening for valgus deformity of the hindfoot. Results in children who had severe, symptomatic flatfoot and skewfoot. J Bone Joint Surg Am. 1995;77(4):500–12.
42. Sangeorzan BJ, Mosca V, Hansen ST. Effect of calcaneal lengthening on relationships among the hindfoot, midfoot, and forefoot. Foot Ankle. 1993;14(3):136–41.
43. Mahan KT, McGlamry ED. Evans calcaneal osteotomy for flexible pes valgus deformity. A preliminary study. Clin Podiatr Med Surg. 1987;4(1):137–51.
44. Brim SP, Hecker R. The Evans calcaneal osteotomy: postoperative care and an evaluation on the metatarsus adductus angle. J Foot Ankle Surg. 1994;33(1):2–5.
45. McCrea JD. The Evans procedure for treatment of severe pes planovalgus. J Am Podiatr Med Assoc. 1987;77(1):35–8.
46. Xia J, Zhang P, Yang YF, Zhou JQ, Li QM, Yu GR. Biomechanical analysis of the calcaneocuboid joint pressure after sequential lengthening of the lateral column. Foot Ankle Int. 2013;34(2):261–6.
47. Cooper PS, Nowak MD, Shaer J. Calcaneocuboid joint pressures with lateral column lengthening (Evans) procedure. Foot Ankle Int. 1997;18(4):199–205.
48. Jara ME. Evans osteotomy complications. Foot Ankle Clin. 2017;22(3):573–85.
49. Davitt JS, Morgan JM. Stress fracture of the fifth metatarsal after Evans' calcaneal osteotomy: a report of two cases. Foot Ankle Int. 1998;19(10):710–2.
50. Weil LS, Roukis TS. The calcaneal scarf osteotomy: operative technique. J Foot Ankle Surg. 2001;40(3):178–82.
51. Xu Y, Li XC, Xu XY. Calcaneal Z lengthening osteotomy combined with subtalar arthroereisis for severe adolescent flexible flatfoot reconstruction. Foot Ankle Int. 2016;37(11):1225–31.
52. Patrick N, Lewis GS, Roush EP, Kunselman AR, Cain JD. Effects of medial displacement calcaneal osteotomy and calcaneal Z osteotomy on subtalar joint pressures: a cadaveric flatfoot model. J Foot Ankle Surg. 2016;55(6):1175–9.
53. Scott RT, Berlet GC. Calcaneal Z osteotomy for extra-articular correction of hindfoot valgus. J Foot Ankle Surg. 2013;52(3):406–8.
54. Arangio GA, Salathé EP. Medial displacement calcaneal osteotomy reduces the excess forces in the medial longitudinal arch of the flat foot. Clin Biomech (Bristol, Avon). 2001;16(6):535–9.
55. Greenfield S, Cohen B. Calcaneal osteotomies: pearls and pitfalls. Foot Ankle Clin. 2017;22(3):563–71.
56. Weinfeld SB. Medial slide calcaneal osteotomy. Technique, patient selection, and results. Foot Ankle Clin. 2001;6(1):89–94.. vii
57. Beck EL, McGlamry ED. Modified young tendosuspension technique for flexible flatfoot. Analysis of rationale and results: a preliminary report on 20 operations. J Am Podiatry Assoc. 1973;63(11): 582–604.
58. Moraleda L, Salcedo M, Bastrom TP, Wenger DR, Albiñana J, Mubarak SJ. Comparison of the calcaneo-cuboid-cuneiform osteotomies and the calcaneal lengthening osteotomy in the surgical treatment of symptomatic flexible flatfoot. J Pediatr Orthop. 2012;32(8):821–9.
59. Moraleda L, Salcedo M, Bastrom TP, Wenger DR, Albinana J, Mubarak SJ. Comparison of the calcaneo-cuboid-cuneiform osteotomies and the calcaneal lengthening osteotomy in the surgical treatment of symptomatic flexible flatfoot. J Pediatr Orthop. 2012;32(8):821–9.
60. Dall G. Open lateral wedge osteotomy of the calcaneum for severe postural pes valgus in children. S Afr Med J. 1978;53(14):531–8.
61. Pavone V, Costarella L, Testa G, Conte G, Riccioli M, Sessa G. Calcaneo-stop procedure in the treatment of the juvenile symptomatic flatfoot. J Foot Ankle Surg. 2013;52(4):444–7.
62. De Pellegrin M, Moharamzadeh D, Strobl WM, Biedermann R, Tschauner C, Wirth T. Subtalar extra-articular screw arthroereisis (SESA) for the treatment of flexible flatfoot in children. J Child Orthop. 2014;8(6):479–87.
63. Needleman RL. Current topic review: subtalar arthroereisis for the correction of flexible flatfoot. Foot Ankle Int. 2005;26(4):336–46.
64. Metcalfe SA, Bowling FL, Reeves ND. Subtalar joint arthroereisis in the management of pediatric flexible flatfoot: a critical review of the literature. Foot Ankle Int. 2011;32(12):1127–39.
65. Vogler HW. Subtalar blocking operations for pathological pronation syndromes. In: McGlamry ED, editor. Comprehensive textbook of foot surgery. William and Wilkins: Baltimore; 1987.
66. Lundeen RO. The Smith STA-peg operation for hypermobile pes planovalgus in children. J Am Podiatr Med Assoc. 1985;75(4):177–83.
67. Oloff LM, Naylor BL, Jacobs AM. Complications of subtalar arthroereisis. J Foot Surg. 1987;26(2):136–40.
68. Bali N, Theivendran K, Prem H. Computed tomography review of tarsal canal anatomy with reference to the fitting of sinus tarsi implants in the tarsal canal. J Foot Ankle Surg. 2013;52(6):714–6.
69. Fitzgerald RH, Vedpathak A. Plantar pressure distribution in a hyperpronated foot before and after intervention with an extraosseous talotarsal stabilization device- a retrospective study. J Foot Ankle Surg. 2013;52:432–43.

70. Soomekh DJ, Baravarian B. Pediatric and adult flatfoot reconstruction: subtalar arthroereisis versus realignment osteotomy surgical options. Clin Podiatr Med Surg. 2006;23(4):695–708.. v
71. Lamm BM, Paley D, Herzenberg JE. Gastrocnemius soleus recession: a simpler, more limited approach. J Am Podiatr Med Assoc. 2005;95(1):18–25.
72. Hui HE, Beals TC, Brown NA. Influence of tendon transfer site on moment arms of the flexor digitorum longus muscle. Foot Ankle Int. 2007;28(4):441–7.
73. de Coulon G, Turcot K, Canavese F, Dayer R, Kaelin A, Ceroni D. Talonavicular arthrodesis for the treatment of neurological flat foot deformity in pediatric patients: clinical and radiographic evaluation of 29 feet. J Pediatr Orthop. 2011;31(5):557–63.
74. Connors JF, Wernick E, Lowy LJ, Falcone J, Volpe RG. Guidelines for evaluation and management of five common podopediatric conditions. J Am Podiatr Med Assoc. 1998;88(5):206–22.

Pediatric Tarsal Coalition and Pes Planovalgus

11

Craig A. Camasta and Timothy A. Graeser

Introduction/Etiology

Many aspects of tarsal coalitions, as well as the pediatric pes planovalgus deformity, have been previously addressed in the literature including the etiology, clinical presentation, diagnostic imaging, as well as conservative and surgical treatment. The authors believe that a large number of patients encountered fall somewhere between the flexible deformity (collapsing pes planovalgus) with no arthritic changes and the pes planovalgus deformity secondary to frank osseous coalition. For clarity, we will refer to this patient as falling into the "gray zone." Patients may present with a symptomatic, arthritic, non-coalesced foot or symptomatic incomplete osseous coalition. Patients may present with peroneal spasm from an etiology other than tarsal coalition, or conversely, they may demonstrate asymptomatic coalition with a rectus foot type.

There are several proposed theories related to the etiology of tarsal coalitions. Of these, the most widely accepted is LeBouq's theory of failure of differentiation of embryonic mesenchymal tissue believed to be a heritable autosomal dominant defect or an insult sustained in the first trimester of pregnancy [1, 2]. On the other hand, Pfitzner believed that coalitions occurred from ossification of accessory bones into the adjacent tarsal bones [3]. When Harris found evidence of tarsal coalitions in fetuses, it seemed to disprove Pfitzner's theory [4]. There have been reports of accessory bones mimicking tarsal coalitions, even though they are not incorporated into the adjacent bones [5]. Less commonly, coalitions can be acquired from arthritis, infection, neoplasm, or trauma [1].

The incidence of coalition has been reported from 0.04% to as high as 14.54%, although authors' experience would be in line with an incidence of around 1% of the general population [1, 6]. It is bilateral 50–80% of the time [1, 7]. There does not appear to be a sex predilection of tarsal coalitions, which is consistent with an autosomal dominant inheritance theory. Calcaneonavicular (CN) and talocalcaneal (TC) coalitions make up 90% of coalitions.

Patients with a CN coalition generally present at age 8 to 12, while patients with a TC coalition present around age 12–16 [1]. Although the

Electronic Supplementary Material The online version of this chapter (https://doi.org/10.1007/978-3-030-29788-6_11) contains supplementary material, which is available to authorized users.

C. A. Camasta (✉)
Pediatric and Adult Reconstructive Foot & Ankle Surgery Fellowship, Atlanta, GA, USA

Department of Surgery, Emory St. Joseph's Hospital, Atlanta, GA, USA

Faculty, The Podiatry Institute, Decatur, GA, USA

T. A. Graeser
Private Practice, Motio Foot and Ankle Specialists, Winter Springs, FL, USA
e-mail: DrGraeser@MotioFootAnkle.com

M. L. Butterworth, J. T. Marcoux (eds.), *The Pediatric Foot and Ankle*,
https://doi.org/10.1007/978-3-030-29788-6_11

majority of TC coalitions occur in the middle facet, posterior and anterior facet coalitions have also been reported [8, 9]. In this paper, TC coalitions will refer to the coalition specifically of the middle facet of the STJ. It has also been reported that concomitant TN and TC coalitions can occur in the same foot [10]. A talonavicular coalition is the third most common coalition, with less than 50 cases reported in the literature [1]. Although extremely rare, instances of naviculocuboid coalition have also been reported [67, 68].

Flexible Pediatric Pes Planovalgus Deformity

Clinical Examination

While the clinical presentation and diagnostic imaging findings of the osseous TC coalition have been discussed, the more commonly encountered deformity is the collapsing pes planovalgus foot type, which remains flexible and is free of any arthritic changes. These two conditions differ dramatically with regard to clinical and radiographic findings. Collapsing pes planovalgus patients rarely complain of "ankle pain," as seen in children with coalitions, and more commonly complain of pain along the medial longitudinal arch and sinus tarsi.

In stance phase of the gait cycle, the flexible pes planovalgus foot may appear similar to the coalesced pes planovalgus. Both may have a valgus heel position, abducted forefoot, collapse of the medial longitudinal arch, and a floating heel secondary to equinus. In open kinetics, however, the flexible pes planovalgus foot presents much differently. There is generally normal to increased motion in the hindfoot joints, as well as hypermobility in the medial column. These feet readily circumduct with active range of motion, unlike the rigid coalition foot (Video 11.1). The "step-forward" Hubscher maneuver, if performed as mentioned above, recreates the medial longitudinal arch through the windlass mechanism and confirms that the foot is flexibly reducible and not a rigid coalition foot type (Fig. 11.12). The ability to reduce the severe pes planovalgus foot in stance examination however does not indicate that this foot will be sufficiently corrected with joint-preserving surgical procedures. In the authors' experience, the severe pes planovalgus foot, especially in the obese adolescent patient, often requires a combination of arthrodesis procedures (single to multilevel) in combination with adjunctive joint-sparing corrective procedures to adequately correct the deformity.

Standard Radiographic Examination

Radiographically, the same parameters can be assessed in both the flexible pes planovalgus and coalition flatfoot patients. Among the abnormalities seen include decreased TN congruity, increased cuboid abduction angle, increased talar declination, and decreased calcaneal inclination angles on the weight-bearing DP and lateral radiographs, similar to the coalition foot. The difference resides in the absence of the signs of coalition, such as the "halo" sign, talar beaking, broadening of the lateral talar process, and other radiographic findings suggestive of coalition.

Pes Planovalgus Secondary to Osseous Talocalcaneal Coalition

Clinical Examination

The patient with a frank osseous coalition commonly presents with a rigid pes planovalgus foot type, with or without peroneal spasm. This condition generally starts as a painless decrease in the range of motion of a joint and progresses to a symptomatic rigid deformity. Patients often complain of "ankle pain" that is aggravated with activity or have a history of recent or recurrent ankle sprains [7]. Talocalcaneal (TC) coalitions usually become symptomatic around the ages of 12–16, which correlates with the time they begin to ossify [11]. Since the absence of inflammatory cells has been reported in histopathological studies, it is believed that pain is secondary to mechanical stress arising from the periosteum surrounding the ossifying coalition [12, 13].

Occasionally, coalition patients do not have the commonly associated pes planovalgus foot type, making the diagnosis more difficult [14].

On clinical examination patients generally have a mild to deep pain within the subtalar joint with limitation of passive range of motion of this joint. During open kinetic chain examination, these patients have a valgus position of the rearfoot, as well as an equinus position at the level of the ankle, forefoot pronation, and loss of medial longitudinal arch height. If the coalition is unilateral, this position is easily observed relative to the contralateral limb [11] (Fig. 11.1). Bilateral coalitions can also present in a similar fashion; however, when both feet are involved, the deformity is not so obvious. Circumduction of the feet will not be possible in the coalesced foot but is easily accomplished in the uninvolved side.

Pes Planovalgus with Peroneal Spasm

On occasion, a patient will present with a peroneal spasm on the affected side. Spasm occurs from a biomechanical "splinting" of the STJ, effectively reducing the pressure of this joint [15]. The result is secondary adaptive shortening of the peroneal musculature in response to heel valgus. Electromyography (EMG) studies have shown spasticity of the peroneus longus muscle in patients with a coalition, as well as the soleus and gastrocnemius muscles [16]. The "triad" of peroneal spastic pes planovalgus has been reported as spasms of the peroneal muscles, painful pes planovalgus deformity, and a tarsal coalition [17]. It is important to remember that although peroneal spasm most commonly occurs in association with a tarsal coalition, it is not pathognomonic and it does occur in the non-coalesced foot [14]. A pes planovalgus deformity without coalition can lead to peroneal spasm, especially after degenerative joint changes have developed. Rare causes of peroneal spasm have also been reported to include talar osteochondral lesions, rheumatoid arthritis, a slipped upper femoral epiphysis, dysplasia epiphysealis hemimelica (Trevor disease), tuberculosis of the talus, and many others [15, 18–24]. Any circumstance that might restrict movement around the ankle or STJ, as well as any cause of pain in these areas, can lead to peroneal spasm [15]. In these cases, a common peroneal nerve block may be a beneficial diagnostic modality. A rigid foot secondary to peroneal spasm may become flexible following a nerve block, leading the clinician to exclude an osseous coalition from the differential diagnoses [15].

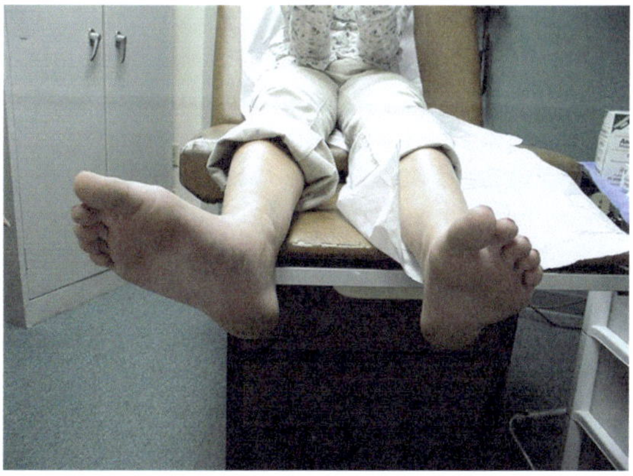

Fig. 11.1 Unilateral right foot coalition with peroneal spasm in resting position of dorsiflexion and eversion. Note the appearance of the non-involved left foot, which gravity-rests in plantarflexion

During stance examination, it is often difficult to distinguish the coalition foot from the flexible collapsing pes planovalgus foot. Both may demonstrate varying degrees of heel valgus with an abducted forefoot. They may have a floating heel if an equinus component is present (Fig. 11.2a). Several tests can be employed to assess the mobility of the rearfoot. A toe-raise test can be performed, where the patient is asked to rise on the toes of both feet simultaneously. In a flexible foot, the heel will invert and reduce because the equinus component is negated, allowing the extrinsic musculature to realign the foot (Fig. 11.2b). In the coalition foot, the heel remains everted or vertical due to the rigid nature of the condition (Fig. 11.3). Another test to identify coalition is the "heel-tip test." In a flexible foot, the patient attempts to actively raise the medial border of the foot. This would result in supination of the subtalar joint and subsequently internal rotation of the tibia and external rotation of the patella. In a coalition foot, raising the

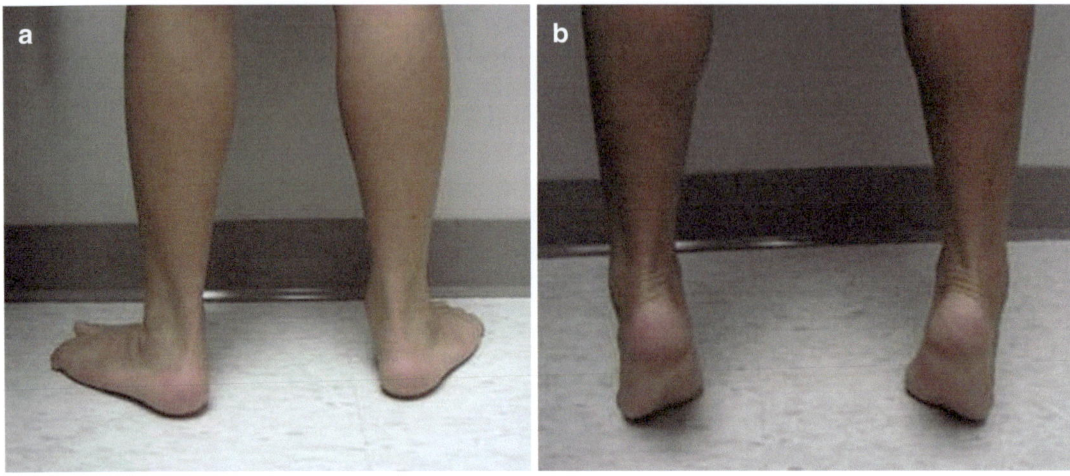

Fig. 11.2 Equinus-compensated pes valgus with floating heel (**a**). Reduction of pes valgus with toe-raise test (**b**), demonstrating arch reduction and heel inversion, indicating a reducible deformity secondary to primary equinus contracture

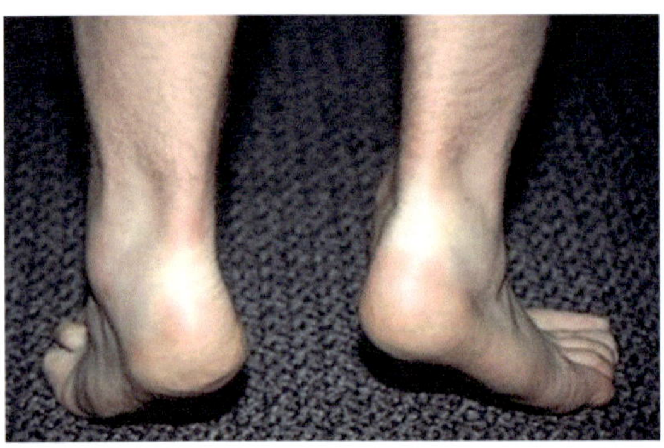

Fig. 11.3 Rigid pes valgus of the right foot secondary to a tarsal coalition, which fails to reduce the deformity with the toe-raise test. Note comparison to the left foot, which demonstrates normal heel inversion with toe-raise test

medial border of the foot fails to externally rotate the patella because of the loss of motion of the subtalar joint [7].

The Hubscher maneuver is also an effective way to examine the flexibility and reducibility of a pes planovalgus deformity, when performed correctly. In stance, the hallux is manually dorsiflexed and the leg externally rotated, which will demonstrate a restored arch in the flexible/reducible foot, via windlass loading of the plantar fascia. Conversely, this maneuver will fail to restore the arch in a rigid/coalesced foot. Radiographic assessment of this maneuver is also useful from a diagnostic and surgical planning standpoint. However, this maneuver may fail to demonstrate arch restoration in flexible patients who have significant concomitant equinus contracture. Equinus contracture precludes the ability to reduce the arch and is often the primary deforming force that leads to and propagates its development. Having the patient stand and then step forward with the involved extremity can negate the effects of equinus. With the foot plantarflexed on the leg, the gastrosoleal complex is relaxed, and a flexible deformity will reduce, and likewise captured on radiographic examination during this "step-forward" Hubscher maneuver (Figs. 11.4).

Another important component of the clinical examination is gait analysis. In a patient with a coalition, the heel will strike the ground in a vertical to everted position and will not re-supinate in late midstance, effectively remaining everted throughout the gait cycle. As a coalition becomes more painful, compensatory external rotation of the hip occurs, which serves to shorten the length of the lever arm over the foot (Video 11.2). Also, the gliding motion at the midtarsal joint (MTJ) becomes more of a hinge motion. During dorsiflexion, the MTJ becomes narrow superiorly and widens inferiorly [3]. It has been shown that the contact area in the midfoot in patients with a coalition is twice that of the non-coalesced foot [16].

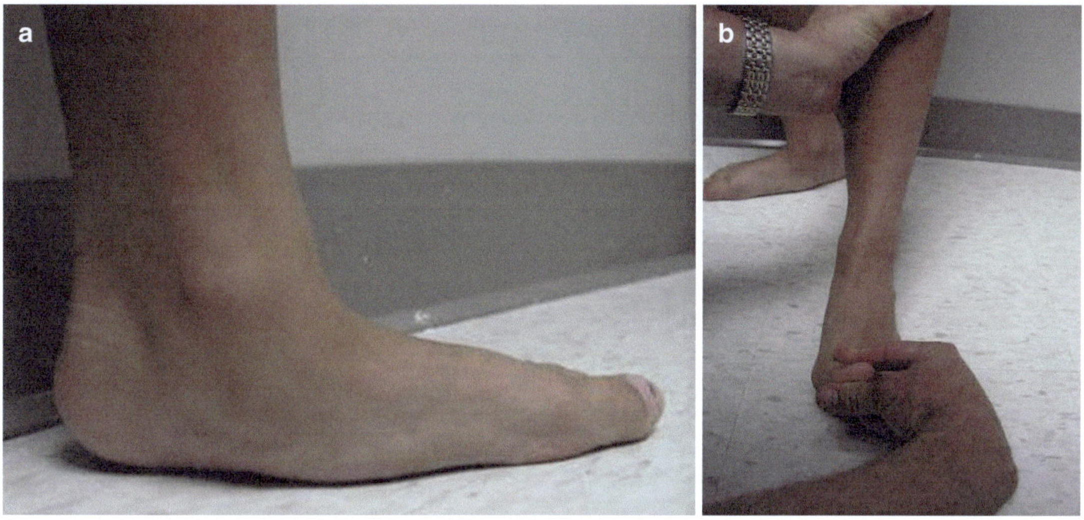

Fig. 11.4 Standing view of pes valgus foot with collapsed medial arch and floating heel secondary to equinus contracture (**a**). "Step-forward" Hubscher maneuver demonstrating reduction of the pes valgus deformity (**b**), which eliminates the effect of equinus by plantarflexing the foot on the leg

Patients with significant equinus contracture also demonstrate compensatory stance and gait postural effects. Pes planovalgus deformities that occur secondary to fully compensated equinus contracture translate forces upward through the extremity, causing genu recurvatum and genu valgum, internal rotation of the limb, forward pelvic tilt, lumbar lordosis, and forward shift of the center of balance [25] (Fig. 11.5). The center of balance is displaced such that a plumb line from the ear to the foot falls in front of the ankle joint, often as far as the metatarsophalangeal joint level. The patient's arms and shoulders may also be seen leaning forward compared to the rest of the body (Fig. 11.6a). In the authors' experience, correction of the pes planovalgus and equinus deformities is effective in realigning this postural misalignment (Fig. 11.6b). Gait analysis in patients with a partially to fully compensated equinus ("equinus-compensated pes planovalgus") deformity also reveals an interesting compensatory lack of full knee extension, whereby they fail to fully extend the knee in the limb-bearing phase of gait, causing a vertical "bouncing" gait pattern which is evident by watching the patient's head and torso while walking. Therefore the "equinus-compensated pes planovalgus" foot type leads to proximal compensations including genu recurvatum, lumbar lordosis, a shift of the center of balance in stance, and lack of full knee extension in gait (Video 11.3).

Distal compensation occurs at various levels of the foot secondary to ankle joint equinus. A wide range of compensation can occur, from little to no compensation, partial compensation, or full distal compensation [25]. Patients who demonstrate little or no pronatory compensation in the STJ and MTJ usually have some component of a neuromuscular disease. In contrast, full distal compensation may occur. This is the patient with a hypermobile pes planovalgus with the rearfoot and forefoot maximally everted. And, between these two exist the patients with partial distal compensation, who present with some degree of STJ pronation. These patients often have early heel off due to the insufficient dorsiflexory motion [25].

Standard Radiographic Evaluation

Plain-film radiographs are very helpful in the evaluation of a patient with a pes planovalgus foot type. According to Crim, TC coalitions had an 88% diagnostic specificity radiographically,

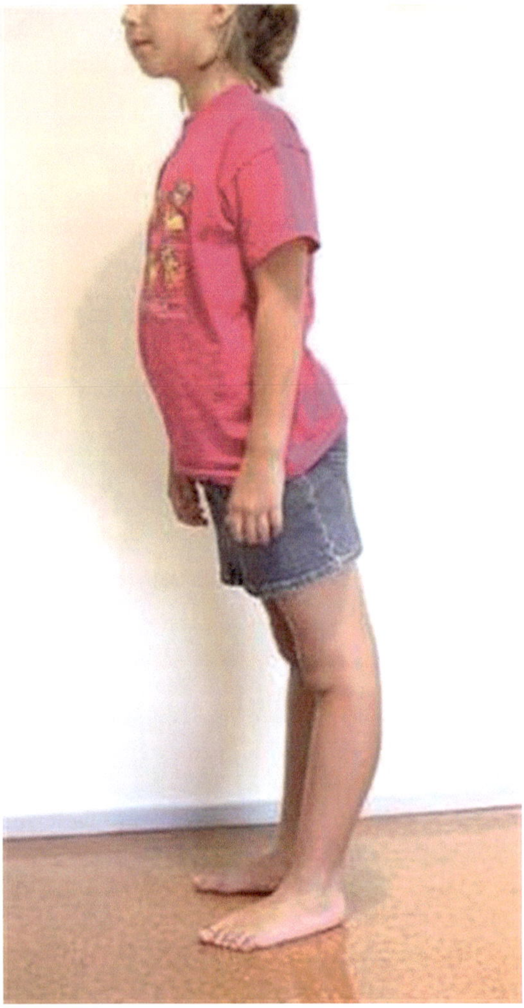

Fig. 11.5 Equinus-compensated pes valgus deformity demonstrating genu recurvatum, lumbar lordosis, and forward shift of center of balance

while CN coalitions had a 97% diagnostic specificity [26]. On the dorsoplantar (DP) radiograph, the talonavicular congruity would demonstrate an increase in uncovering of the medial talar head in a pes planovalgus deformity. The calcaneal abduction angle may also be increased in this foot type. The lateral radiograph may demonstrate a decreased calcaneal inclination angle and an increased talar declination angle. The talar-first metatarsal angle will also increase as the subtalar joint (STJ) pronates and the talus plantarflexes. These parameters can be compared to the values found in the normal foot [27, 28]. Once the initial radiographic evaluation is completed, other signs of TC coalition are assessed.

In a frank osseous TC coalition, there is frequently STJ sclerosis, narrowing of the posterior facet, and absence of the middle facet on the lateral radiograph, although these can be absent in up to 50% of patients with a coalition [29]. Irregularity of the middle facet and hypertrophy of the sustentaculum may also be seen. The lateral radiograph may also show evidence of the "C" sign formed from the medial talar dome and posteroinferior border of the sustentaculum tali [11, 29]. It has also been noted that, from an anatomic-pathologic basis, the "C" sign is a bony bridge between the talar dome and sustentaculum tali, in combination with a prominent inferior border of the sustentaculum tali [11, 29], although the biomechanical implications extend beyond this. The authors believe that the "C" sign actually completes more of a "halo" appearance when the TN joint is factored in (Fig. 11.7). This "halo" sign occurs from spherical diffusion of pressure forces between the ankle, subtalar, and talonavicular joints. A middle facet coalition results in uneven medial forces through the middle facet, rather than the posterior facet, which normally bears the load of these forces. In 1 study with 16 coalitions, the "C" sign was 86.6% sensitive and 93.3% specific, higher than any other radiographic sign of tarsal coalition [29]. Although it has been called the most reliable sign of a coalition [30], Brown has shown that the "C" sign may be more indicative of collapsing pes planovalgus deformity than coalition [14].

Another common radiographic finding in a patient with a coalition is beaking of the talus (Fig. 11.8). During the gait of a coalition foot, the proximal edge of the navicular impinges on and overrides the anterior aspect of the talar head to compensate for lack of STJ motion. This causes elevation of the TN ligament and periosteum off the head of talus, resulting in a periosteal reaction [3, 31]. It is important to understand that this is a traction spur, not an osteophyte of degeneration [7].

One may also observe rounding or flattening of the lateral talar process along with narrowing of the posterior facet. As the rotary motion of the STJ is lost, there is a decrease in the inter-

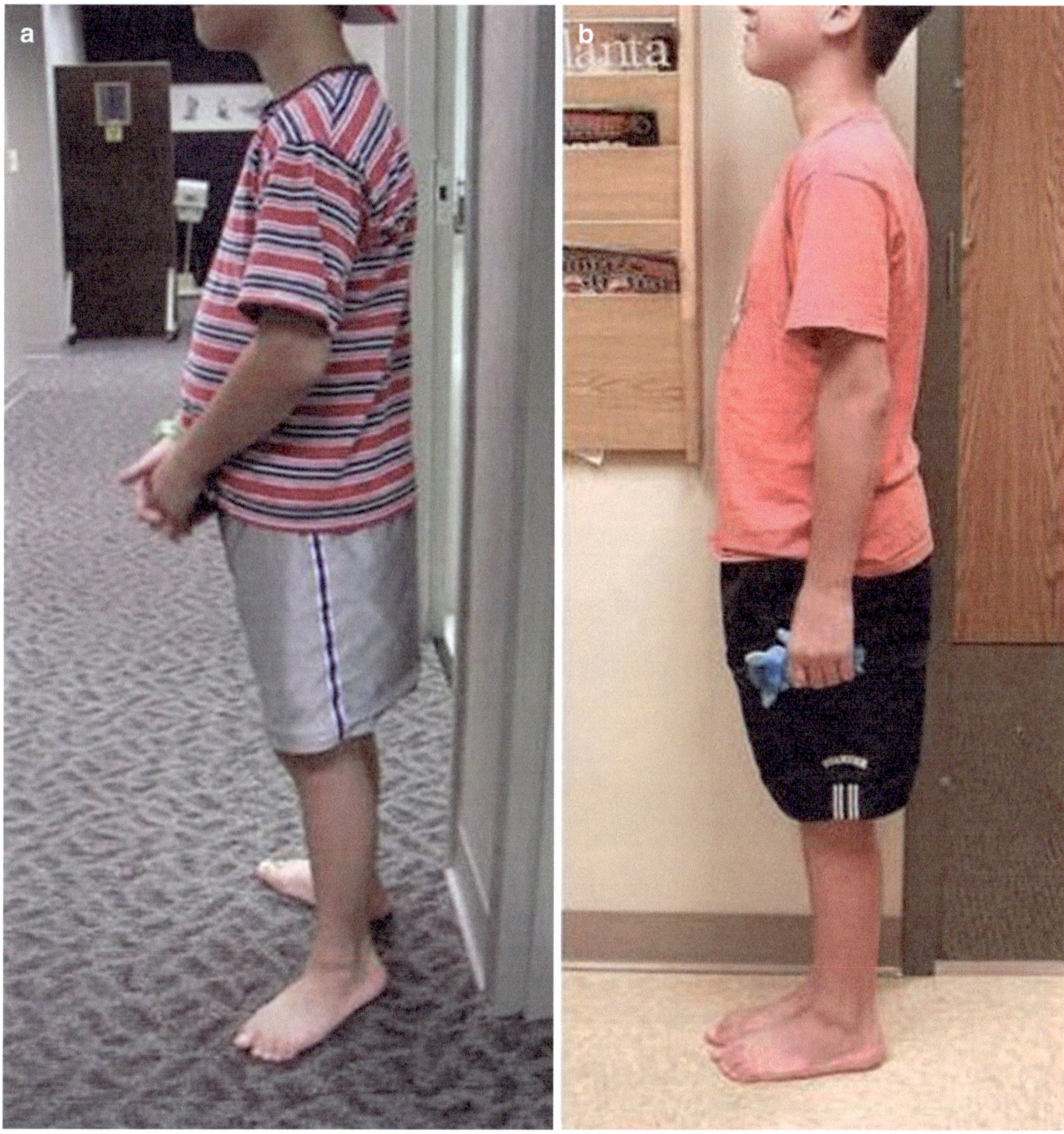

Fig. 11.6 Equinus-compensated pes valgus with plumb line of center of balance forward of the ankle joint (**a**) and postoperative correction of pes valgus and equinus release demonstrating normalization of posture and center of balance (**b**)

nal rotation of the STJ. In addition to loss of the longitudinal arch and adaptive shortening of the peroneal tendons, impingement of the talus on the lateral aspect of the calcaneus also occurs. This leads to broadening and flattening of the lateral talar process and narrowing of the posterior facet [3].

A calcaneal axial radiograph may also reveal findings consistent with a TC coalition. This image allows the clinician to look at the congruency of the posterior and middle facets, which normally have a parallel relationship. Aberrations of this relationship occur with middle facet coalitions, and there exists more angulation between these two facets, often upward of 45 degrees (Fig. 11.9).

A radiographic "step-forward" Hubscher maneuver can also be performed, utilizing the

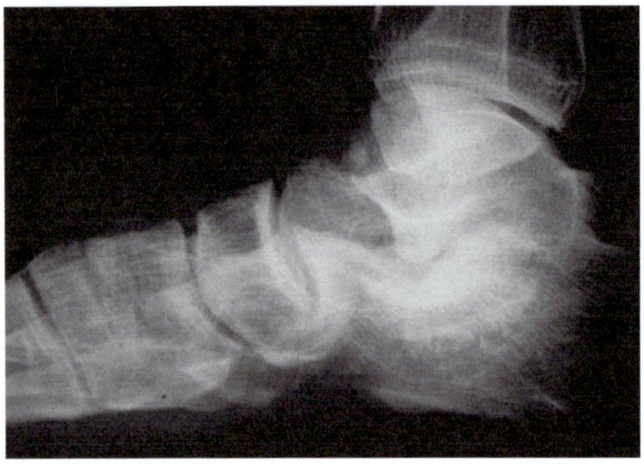

Fig. 11.7 Middle facet coalition demonstrating radiographic sclerosis of the subtalar joint and the "halo" effect of spherical diffusion of ankle and hindfoot forces

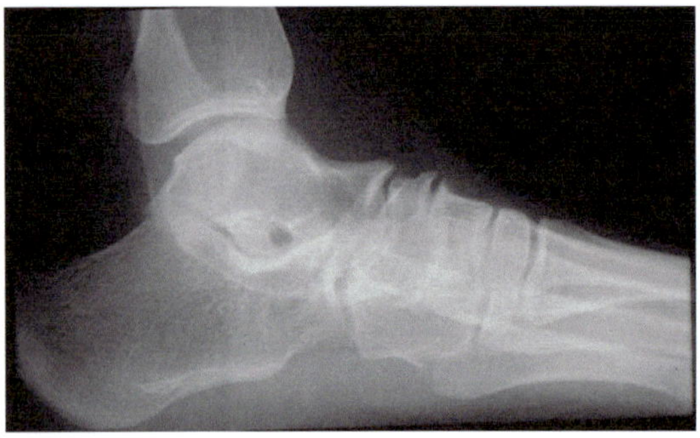

Fig. 11.8 Talar neck and navicular-cuneiform "beaking" in a patient with middle facet and calcaneal-navicular bar coalitions

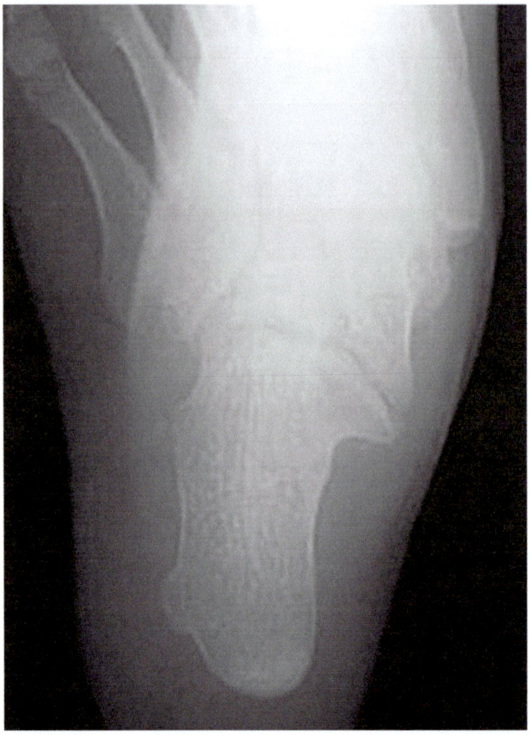

Fig. 11.9 Calcaneal axial radiograph in a patient with a middle facet coalition demonstrating oblique posterior and middle facets

aforementioned technique. This is compared to the normal weight-bearing lateral radiograph to determine the amount of reducibility of the deformity. The osseous TC coalition foot will not reduce with this technique, while the flexible pes planovalgus will.

If a CN coalition is suspected, a 45-degree lateral oblique projection/medial oblique view radiograph is the best position to demonstrate the bridge from the calcaneus to the navicular [3]. A true osseous bridge may not be seen, but a close proximity of these two bones may be observed, as well as flattening of the lateral navicular as it approaches the calcaneus (Fig. 11.10) [3]. There may also be loss of the dense cortical rim at the junction of these two bones [11] or indistinct, irregular juxtaposed cortical bone [3]. The lateral radiograph may demonstrate the "anteater" sign, which is the extension of the anterior process of the calcaneus as it extends beyond the calcaneo-cuboid joint. This normally triangular-shaped area of the calcaneus becomes elongated, and its tip is squared and abuts the lateral margin of the navicular [32]. Hypoplasia of the talar head, as well as talar beaking, may also accompany the CN coalition [11].

Computerized Tomographic and Magnetic Resonance Imaging

If a coalition is suspected on radiographic evaluation, further imaging studies are helpful. The authors believe that computerized tomography (CT) is the superior diagnostic modality for evaluating TC coalitions. CT is the gold standard of imaging because of its ability to demonstrate osseous anatomy better than other modalities and its usefulness in surgical planning [33]. It

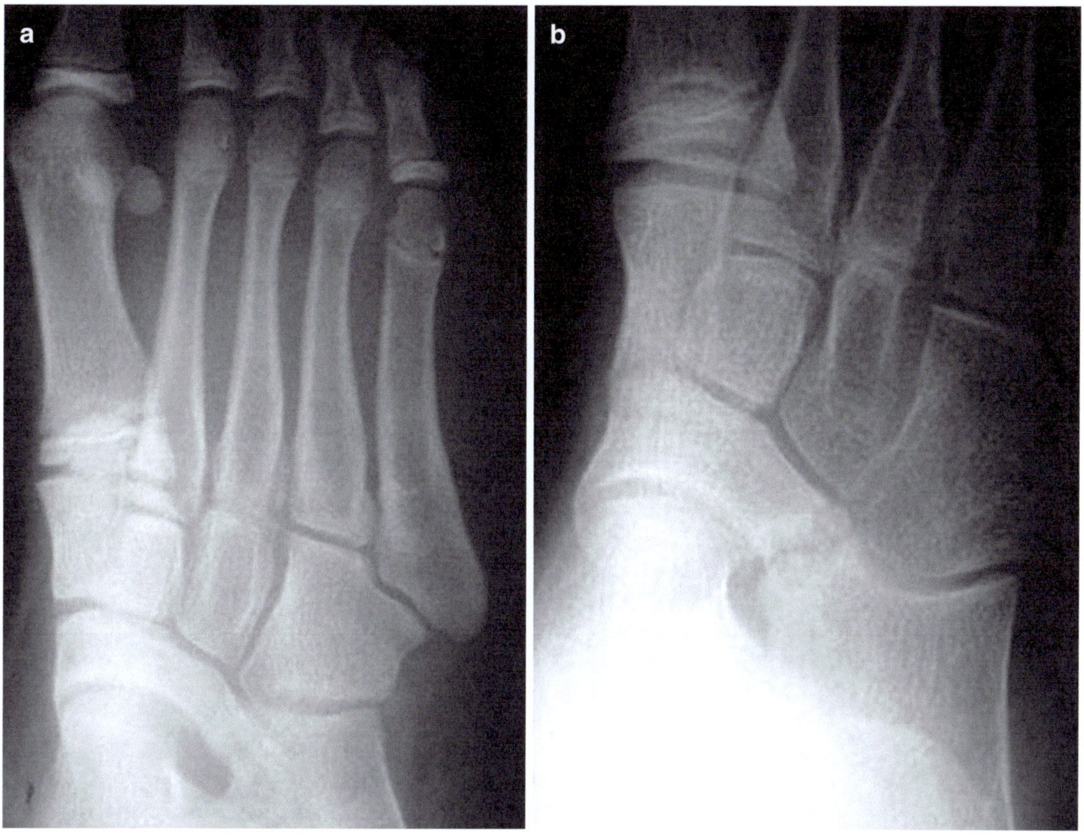

Fig. 11.10 Calcaneonavicular bar with a complete bone bridge (**a**) and with an incomplete bone bridge (**b**)

has been shown in numerous studies that CT is better than magnetic resonance imaging (MRI) [32–36], although others have favored the use of MRI over CT [31, 37].

The argument is often made that MRI is better at detecting nonosseous coalitions than CT, and differentiating the fibrous from cartilaginous coalition is only possible with MRI [31, 33, 37]. The authors agree that making this differentiation is impossible with CT; however, whether or not a coalition is fibrous or cartilaginous often has little implication in making the diagnosis and even less influence on the patient's symptoms. There are subtle findings on CT that can be diagnostic of nonosseous coalitions that are not visible on MRI, and the clinician trained to recognize these findings will do so more accurately with a CT [30–36]. These will be discussed in detail with nonosseous coalitions.

The authors have found that a CT of the hindfoot, if ordered in 1 mm × 1 mm sections, is the preferred way of evaluating the subtalar joint. This type of imaging of 1 mm sections, with no gap between the slices obtained perpendicular to the subtalar joint, is easily attainable. This provides true axial images (Fig. 11.11). This "coalition-specific axial plane" is not a true axial but is more accurate in its ability to visualize the posterior and middle facets of the STJ. Sagittal reconstructions are generally also performed, but axial images are the most reliable for determining the extent of joint involvement [34]. CT images will also be able to reveal any subtle arthritic changes of the subtalar and other surrounding joints. This information is most useful for surgical planning.

Because of the high specificity of radiographs in identifying CN coalitions, CTs are generally only useful in ascertaining if any arthritic

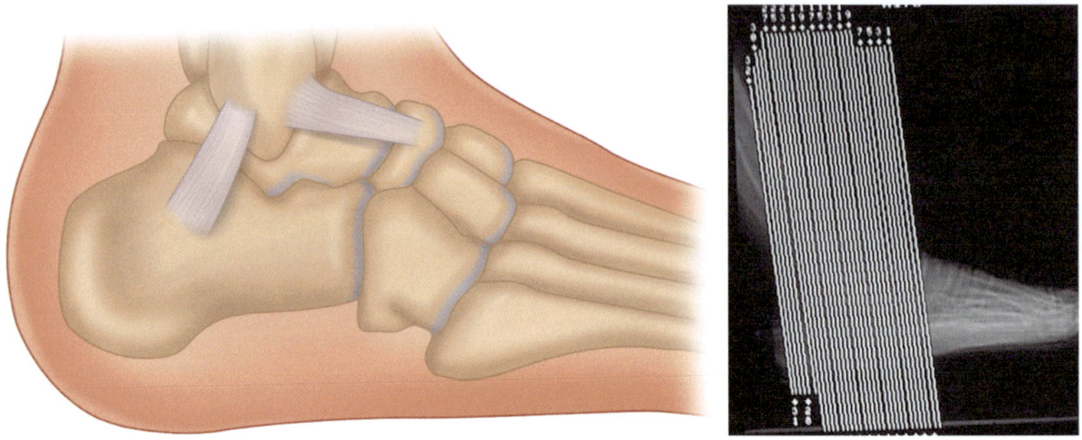

Fig. 11.11 Scout film with a coalition-specific axial protocol. Orientation of computerized tomographic area of interest and angle of study, ordered as a 1.0 × 1.0 mm slices

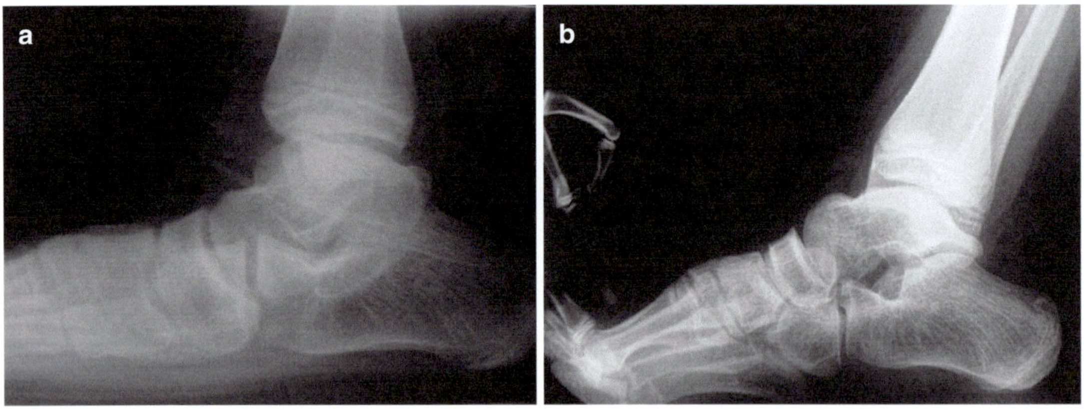

Fig. 11.12 Severe pes valgus lateral radiograph mimicking a middle facet coalition (**a**) and "step-forward" Hubscher maneuver demonstrating reduction of arch and restoration of the normal alignment of the subtalar joint (**b**)

changes are present in the STJ [26]. It should also be mentioned that on occasion a patient will have a coexisting CN and TC coalition [8], and a CT effectively images all possible areas of coalition and/or arthritic involvement (Fig. 11.12).

The "Gray Zone"

The two types of patients discussed thus far, the rigid coalition flatfoot and the flexible pes planovalgus foot, represent opposing ends of the spectrum of painful pediatric flatfoot deformities, and the diagnoses are readily discernible with routine clinical and radiographic examinations. However, many patients have signs and symptoms that lie somewhere in between these two extremes, making an accurate diagnosis more challenging. There are patients with coalitions that have not yet ossified and may still have some motion in the hindfoot joints. Some, but not all, of these nonosseous coalitions have arthritic changes. There are also patients with a stiff pes planovalgus foot that does not have a coalition, but demonstrates significant radiographic arthritic changes. These stiff, poorly reducible deformities generally begin as a flexible pes planovalgus foot type that develops adaptive osseous changes over time, secondary to the severity and duration of the deformity.

In the authors' experience, a majority of these patients are overweight /obese adolescents, and the increasing frequency of this phenomenon appears to parallel societal statistics regarding obesity. Numerous reports have shown a positive correlation between increased body mass index (BMI) and pes planovalgus [38–43]. The increased biomechanical stress on these feet is more difficult to compensate for in the overweight or obese child. Subsequently, there is an accelerated arthritic process that otherwise might not have manifested until after skeletal maturity. Focused clinical and radiographic examinations are needed to differentiate the coalition foot from the arthritic pes planovalgus foot, which will play an important role in determining an appropriate treatment strategy for these patients.

Peroneal Spasm in the Non-coalesced Pes Planovalgus Foot

Patients may present with an apparent peroneal spastic pes planovalgus without evidence of a tarsal coalition. The paucity of radiographic and CT findings of a coalition in these patients suggests that peroneal spasm is not pathognomonic for a tarsal coalition. As previously mentioned, peroneal spasm can occur secondary to multiple conditions other than a tarsal coalition. Four children in one report presented with true spasm of the peroneal muscles and extensors secondary to trauma or ligamentous strain [23]. Jack was the first to report that peroneal spasm can occur in the non-coalesced foot that is rigid secondary to osteoarthritis of the tarsal joints [23]. In these cases, a common peroneal nerve block may be a beneficial diagnostic modality. A rigid foot secondary to peroneal spasm may become flexible with a diagnostic nerve block, leading the clinician to exclude an osseous coalition from the differential diagnoses [15]. Rest, physical therapy, and casting have also been shown in some cases to relieve the spasticity of the peroneal muscles [23, 44]. In the author's experience, there are few patients who respond positively to conservative treatment, especially over an extended period of time. In general, younger patients will respond more positively to conservative measures than their older counterparts, especially in the absence of arthritic changes. More commonly, conservative treatment will help reduce symptoms temporarily until surgical correction is performed.

Any circumstance that restricts movement in the tarsal joints, as well as any cause of pain in these areas, can lead to these abnormal muscle responses [15]. It has been demonstrated by electromyography (EMG) that a "peroneal spastic" lower extremity actually lacks spasm of these peronei in most cases and is more accurately an organic shortening of the muscles that have adapted to a long-standing deformity [24]. When Blockey performed EMG studies on patients with peroneal spasm, he found that there was increased tension on the peroneus brevis tendon, but no increase in the motor unit activity that would be seen in a classic reflex muscle spasm. He attributed this to an increase in tone in the muscle produced by chemical changes within the muscle, independent of its nerve supply [44]. Jack also discounted Harris' theory and believed that if there was a lack of spasm of the peroneal muscles, and it was truly only an adaptive shortening, then an anesthetic block would not allow relaxation of the deformity [23]. This is especially true of younger children who have not had years of fixed eversion and chronic symptoms seen in patients 17 years and older [23].

Despite their extensive research on tarsal coalitions, Harris and Beath believed that "the term peroneal spastic flat foot should be abandoned in favor of more precisely descriptive designations of the different varieties of the deformity" [24]. When a peroneal spastic pes planovalgus is evaluated in a systematic fashion, an anatomic cause usually can be elucidated [22].

Case Reports

Case 1

Idiopathic spasticity of the extensor tendons (peroneus tertius and extensor digitorum longus) has been observed by the authors in an

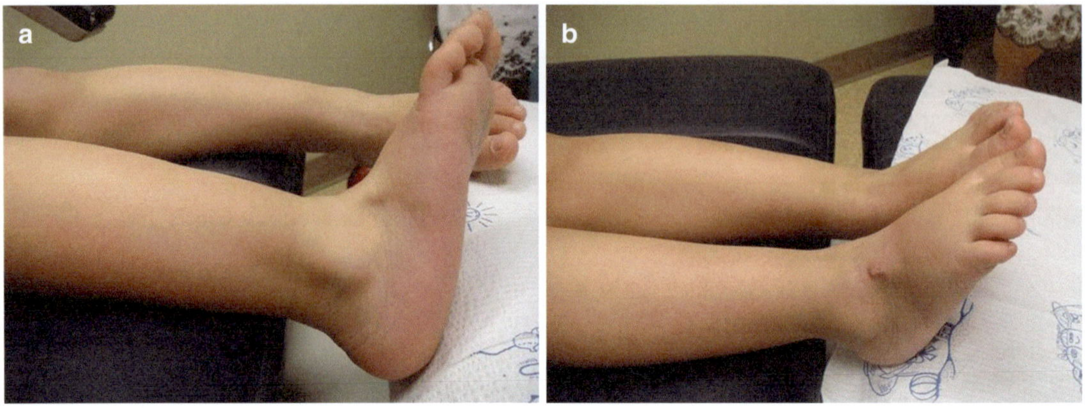

Fig. 11.13 Four-year-old female patient with idiopathic apparent peroneal spastic flatfoot with no evidence of coalition (**a**) and 1 year following the lengthening of peroneus tertius and extensor digitorum longus tendons (**b**)

asymptomatic 4-year-old female patient with a severe unilateral pes planovalgus deformity with no equinus contracture. After a neurological consultation revealed no identifiable source or etiology for the muscle spasm (including an MRI of the spine), this patient was treated by lengthening of the extensor tendons. She is managed with custom orthoses and will remain under observation through osseous maturity (Fig. 11.13). Of interest in this case was that general anesthesia failed to relax the contracted tendons, suggesting that the deformity was a fixed contracture rather than true muscle spasm.

Case 2

A 14-year-old patient presented with a painful severe pes planovalgus deformity with peroneal spasm in open kinetic, stance, and gait examinations (Fig. 11.14a). She was treated for neonatal clubfoot with surgery at 1 year, and her parents reported progressive collapse of the medial arch beginning at age 7. The foot was stiff but manually reducible (Fig. 11.14b), and the equinus contracture was profound. Toe-raise demonstrated heel inversion with near-complete reduction of the medial longitudinal arch (Fig. 11.14c, d). Peroneal spasm developed in this case due to adaptive shortening of the tendons, as their position of advantage was far lateral to the axis of the STJ and MTJ. This patient demonstrated an apparent tarsal “halo” sign and subtalar and midtarsal arthritis, suggestive of a middle facet coalition (Fig. 11.14e). However, a “step-forward” Hubscher lateral radiograph demonstrated complete reduction of the hindfoot alignment and a reducible arch (Fig. 11.14f). In this case, the severity of STJ and MTJ subluxation distorted the normal appearance of the joints suggesting a bony coalition. Medial and plantar subluxation of the talus on the calcaneus rotated the subtalar joint such that radiographically the talus was in front of the calcaneus and not resting upon it, thereby making the subtalar joint appear non-existent, falsely suggestive of a coalition. This patient was treated with an Achilles tendon lengthening and triple arthrodesis (Fig. 11.14g).

Case 3

A 32-year-old female patient presented with gradual, progressive increased unilateral pain in the sinus tarsi with no history of injury. Within a year of symptom onset, the patient developed unilateral peroneal spasm. Plain films failed to demonstrate significant findings; however, CT examination revealed a subchondral bone cyst at the anterior margin of the posterior facet of the calcaneus (Fig. 11.15a). MRI revealed bony edema (Fig. 11.15b), and the patient was treated by curettage of the bone cyst with allogeneic bone grafting.

Asymptomatic Tarsal Coalitions

Not all coalitions result in a pes planovalgus foot type and not all coalitions are painful. Asymptomatic coalitions can be found incidentally when imaging a patient for other purposes. In this situation, the coalition is presumed to be asymptomatic because the foot is in a rectus position with no deformity [17] (Fig. 11.16). This situation is analogous to a patient who undergoes

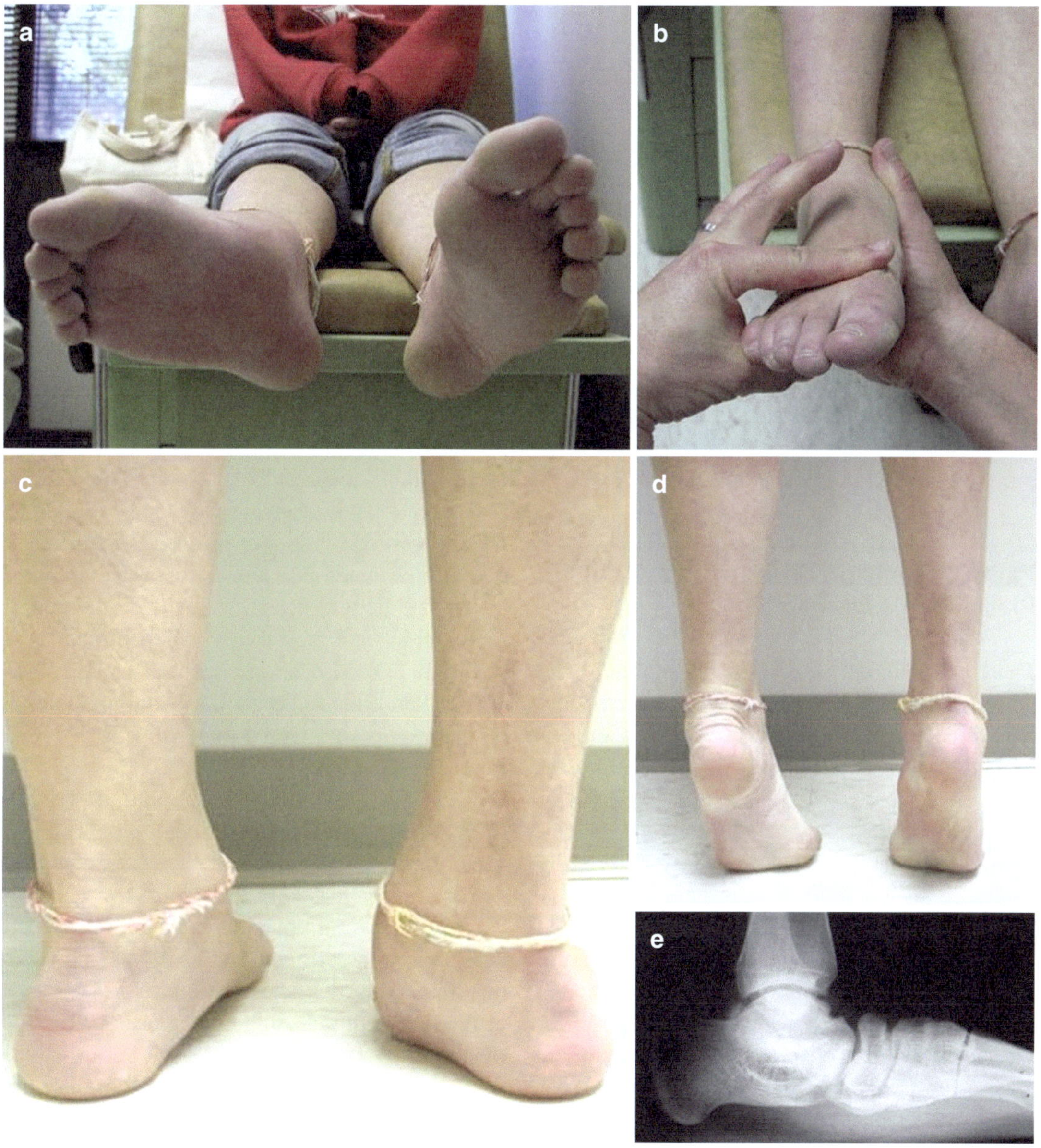

Fig. 11.14 Fourteen-year-old female patient with apparent peroneal spastic flatfoot who had clubfoot correction at 1 year of age and developed progressive collapse of the arch due to recurrent equinus contracture (**a**), but the foot was manually reducible (**b**). Stance examination demonstrated severe collapsing pes valgus (**c**), but toe-raise test demonstrated complete arch restoration (**d**). Lateral foot radiograph appeared consistent with a subtalar joint coalition (**e**); however, the "step-forward" Hubscher maneuver revealed a reducible hindfoot with no coalition (**f**). The patient underwent a triple arthrodesis and Achilles tendon lengthening (**g**)

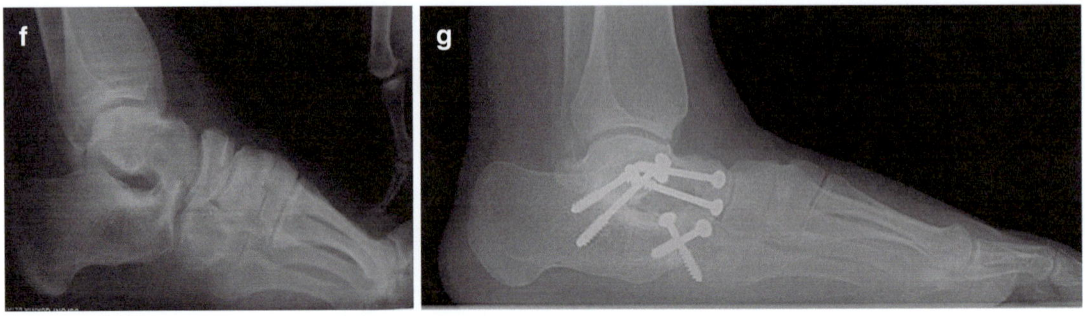

Fig. 11.14 (continued)

an isolated hindfoot fusion to address arthritis or misalignment. A neutral position of an isolated hindfoot fusion can render the foot stable and pain-free, and there is no long-term evidence to suggest that adjacent joints will undergo degenerative arthritis. Much to the contrary, the authors believe that creating a stable neutral position of an isolated hindfoot fusion can be beneficial in preventing adjacent joint arthritis (Fig. 11.17).

Painful Coalition Without Pes Planovalgus Deformity

There exists another group of patients that present with a painful coalition, but have a rectus foot type (no pes planovalgus). In the authors' experience, this is usually seen in patients with a calcaneonavicular bar (either fibrous/cartilaginous or bony) or in patients with a coalition of the subtalar joint. Middle facet coalitions are either rigidly coalesced with a solid bone bridge or obliquely angulated and arthritic [33, 36, 45]. When the middle facet is arthritic but not bone-bridged, pain is located medially, inferior to the medial malleolus, at the site of coalition. The posterior facet can also demonstrate arthritic changes in addition to the middle facet, which manifests as pain in the sinus tarsi. When the middle facet has a solid bone bridge, the posterior facet can also become painfully arthritic. Differential weight distribution on the smaller middle facet leads to a stress reaction within the bone and can be characterized on MRI evaluation as medullary edema at the site of bony coalition (Fig. 11.18).

The Role of Diagnostic Imaging

Both plain-film radiographs and CT will help to delineate the etiology in the rigid painful foot. Most importantly, this information will help guide the surgical treatment plan. With the exception of the CN coalition, radiographs are primarily valuable as a screening tool and are rarely totally diagnostic. A severely arthritic pes planovalgus foot may have changes similar to those observed in the foot with a TC coalition. A severely pronated STJ can obscure the visibility of the middle and posterior facets on the lateral radiographs and mistakenly be identified as a coalition. Likewise, some coalitions lack obvious changes on plain radiograph evaluation and may be mistakenly interpreted as negative for a coalition [7, 9, 14, 26, 29].

The authors have found that radiology reports can be misleading or incomplete at times in describing potential pathologic changes. According to Solomon, CT has a low sensitivity for diagnosing nonosseous coalitions, which is related to the difficulty in distinguishing these disorders from the osteoarthritic STJ [6]. Much of the literature that supports the use of MRI for identification of coalition has been published by radiologists [26, 29, 31, 36, 37]. Of note, one study published by Emery et al. concluded that while MRI had a high rate of agreement with CT with regard to detecting tarsal coalition, CT remains the gold standard when clinical suspicion for coalition is high. MRI might be of more value when more broad evaluation for other possible causes of foot or ankle pain is desired [35].

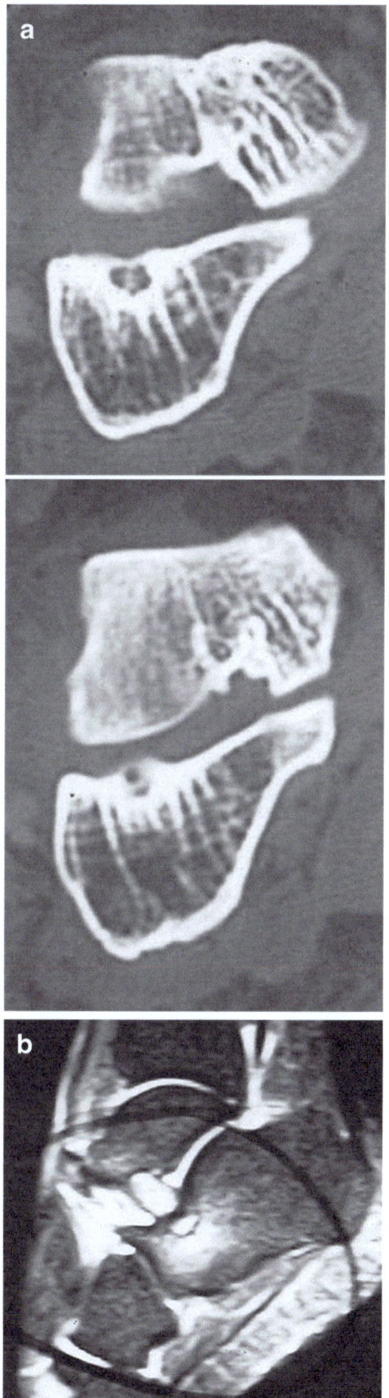

Fig. 11.15 Axial computerized tomographic images of a 32-year-old female patient with peroneal spasm secondary to a subchondral bone cyst of the posterior facet of the subtalar joint (**a**) and sagittal T2 magnetic resonance image revealing fluid-filled cyst with adjacent bony edema (**b**)

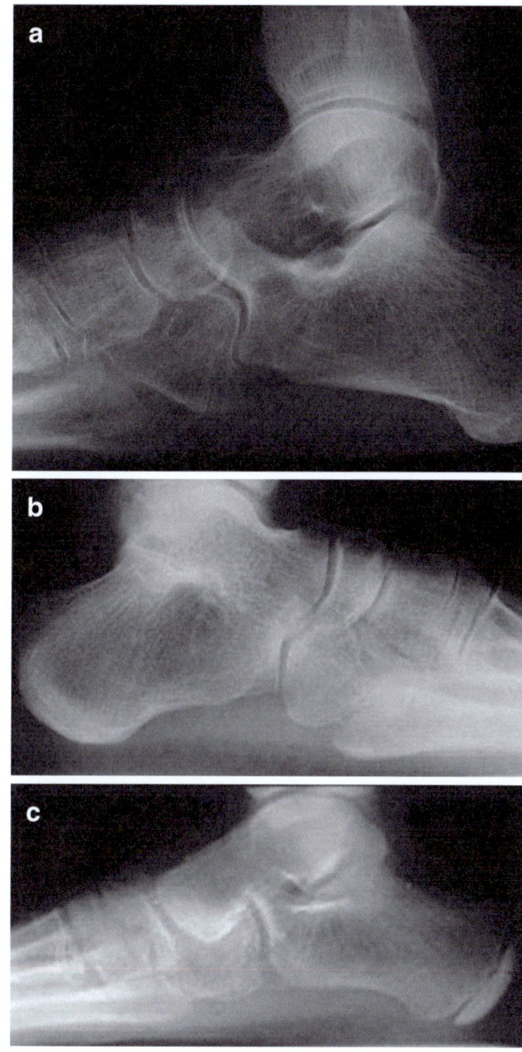

Fig. 11.16 Asymptomatic coalitions: calcaneonavicular bar in a 56-year-old female patient (**a**), subtalar joint coalition in a 48-year-old male patient (**b**), and a talonavicular coalition in an adolescent female patient (**c**). Note the neutral alignment arch position and complete bone bridge coalition in each of these cases

In a case series published by Guignand et al., the authors evaluated 19 symptomatic feet without evidence of synchondrosis on plain X-ray. They concluded that MRI was the most effective means of diagnosis for these predominantly fibrous or cartilaginous CN coalitions [63]. MRI has been shown to be more sensitive to nonosseous coalition and differentiate a fibrous coalition

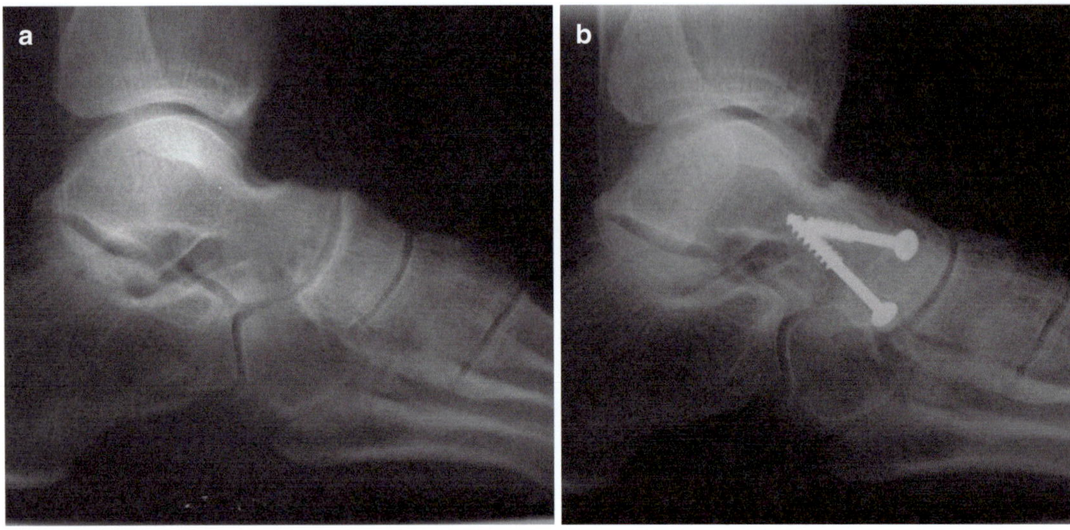

Fig. 11.17 Preoperative (**a**) and 6-year postoperative (**b**) isolated talonavicular arthrodesis with no evidence of adjacent joint arthritis

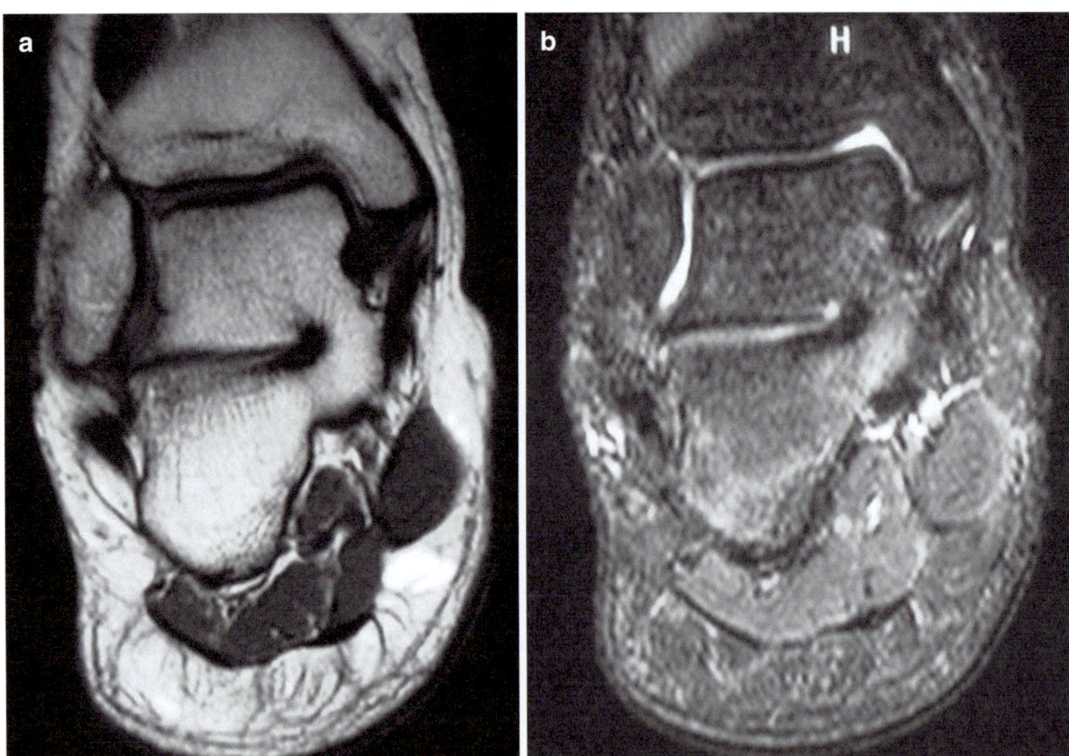

Fig. 11.18 MRI of a 15-year-old patient with a symptomatic middle facet coalition with a complete bone bridge on T1 magnetic resonance images (**a**), demonstrating bony edema on T2 images due to uneven stress loading of the medial aspect of the subtalar joint (**b**)

from a cartilaginous coalition [60]. Ultimately the authors feel that the decision-making process around advanced imaging should include both the level of clinical suspicion for tarsal coalition and the anatomic location of symptoms.

With regard to nonosseous STJ coalition, subtle findings on CT may actually support the diagnosis more readily than MRI and accentuate the same findings found on plain-film radiography. Talar beaking and flattening of the lateral talar process are readily identifiable on the sagittal sections. Narrowing of the middle and posterior facets are seen in the sagittal plane, as well as other arthritic changes (Fig. 11.19). The most important plane to closely scrutinize in a CT is the previously mentioned "coalition-specific axial plane." This view of the subtalar joint enhances visualization of the middle and posterior facets and more accurately identifies secondary arthritic changes that may exist. In this view, the posterior and middle facets are normally parallel. In a nonosseous coalition, an obvious planar abnormality may exist between these two facets. The middle facet may have the "drunken waiter" appearance [37]. This appearance of a superior-lateral- to inferior-medial-directed middle facet occurs from a dysplastic sustentaculum tali in a coalition. It appears that an unsteady waiter is tipping his tray (the middle facet), when normally it would be straight [37] (Fig. 11.20). The middle facet may also show changes of the subchondral bone. This appears as irregularity of the calcaneal and talar borders of this facet, which are normally smooth. Narrowing of the middle and posterior facet joint spaces is commonly observed. There is often a medial lipping of the middle facet seen in this plane. Broadening of the middle facet and sustentaculum tali also occurs not only from medial to lateral but also from anterior to posterior, as the biomechanical stresses of the coalition lead to hypertrophy of the surrounding bony surfaces. These osseous changes of the calcaneus and talus surrounding the middle and posterior facets correlate to the appearance of the "halo" sign on plain-film radiographs.

Once the above two planes have been evaluated, and evidence of a coalition exists, the clinician should then focus on the frontal plane

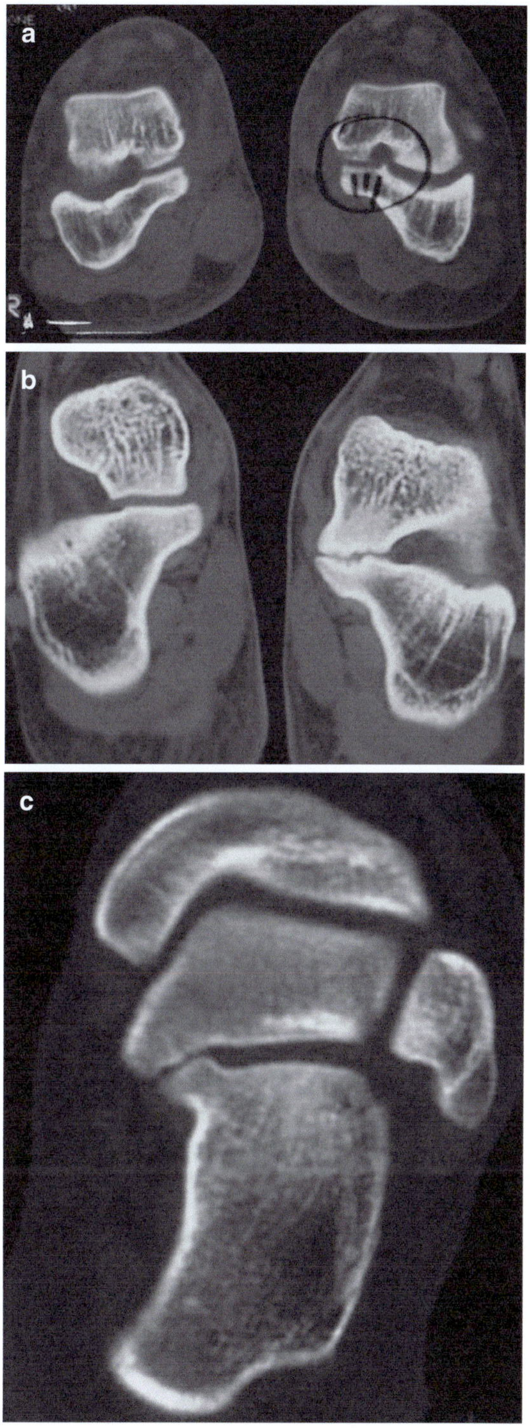

Fig. 11.19 Subtle computerized tomogram findings of middle facet coalitions as viewed on axial plane imaging. Subtle medial spurring (**a**) and joint space arthritic narrowing (**b**, **c**) may be reported as negative for coalition due to lack of frank osseous bridging

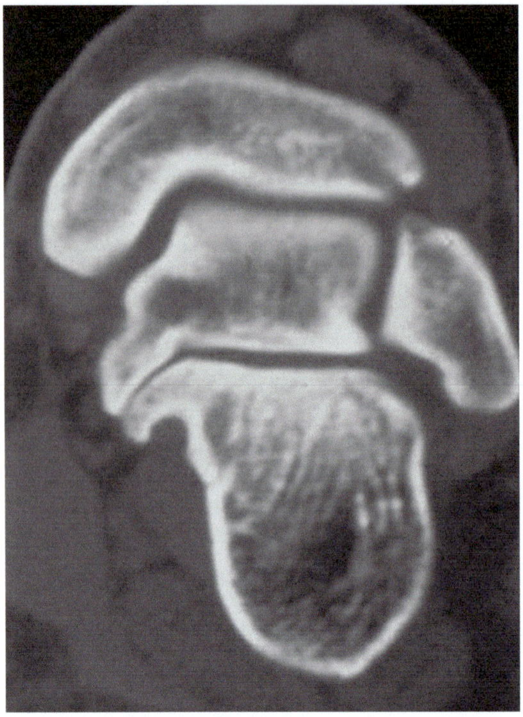

Fig. 11.20 Oblique middle facet coalition, described as a "drunken waiter" sign

images. The most important findings in this plane are the secondary positional changes that exist as a result of the coalition. It is not uncommon to have a neutral heel that exists with a coalition, and this linear relationship between the tibia, talus, and calcaneus is appreciated on the frontal plane CT images (Fig. 11.21a). These patients lack the heel valgus alignment and will rarely have peroneal spasm. More commonly, though, the calcaneus is in an everted or valgus position, relative to the tibia (Fig. 11.21b). The amount of eversion can be assessed, as well as the shape of the talus in the frontal plane. In some severe coalition cases, "lateral tarsal wedging" occurs. The authors interpret this to be an adaptive change in the long-standing coalition foot that results in wedging of the talus or calcaneus between the tibia and the severely everted calcaneus. Normally in the frontal plane, the talus will have a rectangular appearance. As the heel rotates into the valgus, there becomes an increased stress on the lateral side of the talus or calcaneus. With severe deformi-

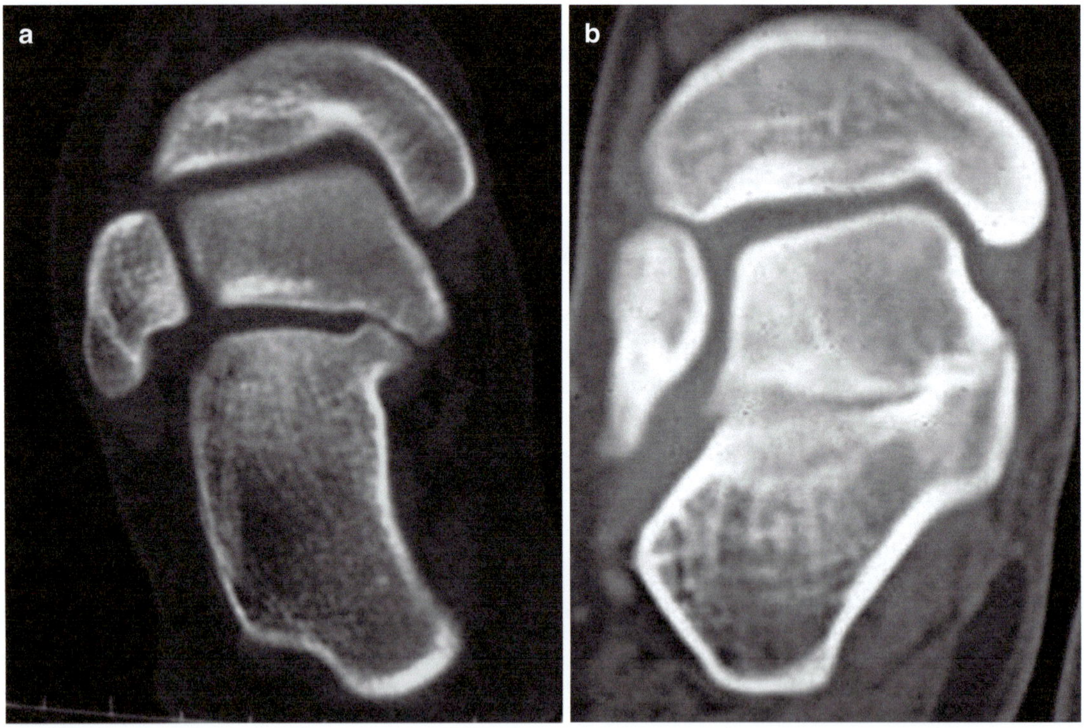

Fig. 11.21 Axial computerized tomogram of a middle facet coalition with a vertical calcaneus, which is perpendicular to the distal tibial plafond, with no pes valgus or peroneal spasm (**a**), and middle facet coalition with valgus alignment of calcaneus relative to the tibial plafond and significant pes valgus and peroneal spasm (**b**)

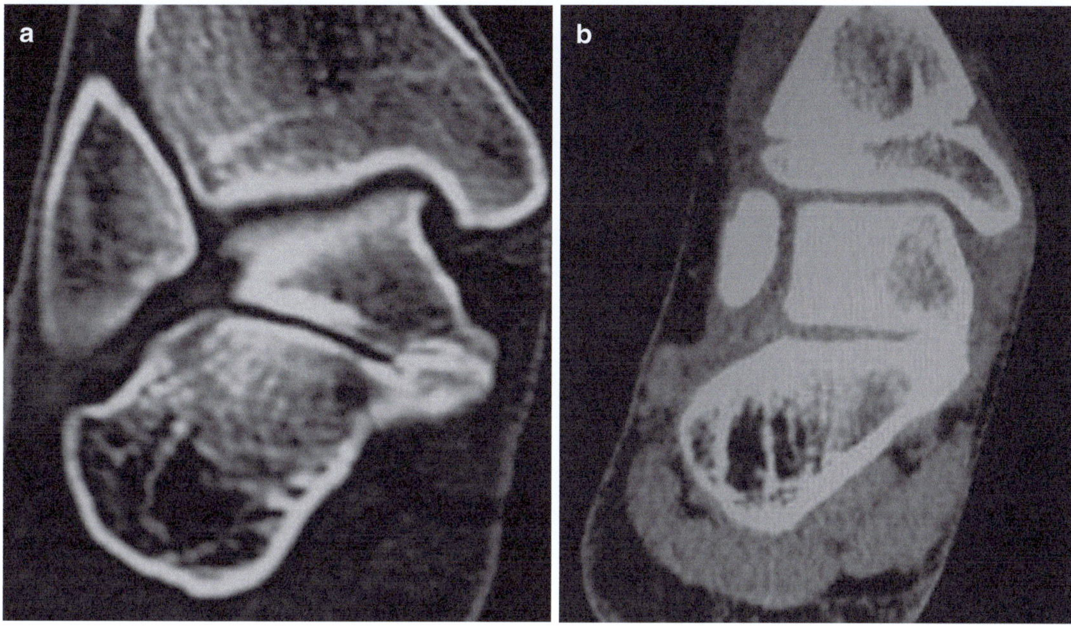

Fig. 11.22 "Lateral tarsal wedging." Adaptive changes within the subtalar joint in patients with peroneal spastic pes valgus may demonstrate either lateral wedging of the talus (**a**) or lateral wedging of the calcaneus (**b**)

ties, the authors believe that this increased stress changes the shape of the talus (Fig. 11.22a) or the calcaneus (Fig. 11.22b) by wedging it laterally. This wedging occurs in varying degrees, depending of the severity of the deformity. In the author's experience, there appears to be a positive correlation between lateral tarsal wedging and peroneal spasm. An understanding of this relationship is important as it can change the choice of surgical procedure for correction and will be discussed below.

The frontal plane CT view may also show evidence of calcaneal fibular remodeling [46]. Cystic changes may be seen in the calcaneus and fibular malleolus. A "cup-like" pseudoarticulation may be present between the calcaneus and fibula, which may be present secondary to a fixed heel valgus, resulting in an abnormal contact between these two bones [46]. With the proper clinical examination and image interpretation, the clinician can better differentiate between the pes planovalgus deformity that has become rigid secondary to arthritic changes and the rigid foot with a coalition, with or without arthritic changes.

Surgical Planning for Tarsal Coalition

The information gained in diagnostic imaging of coalitions assists in developing a surgical plan that is individualized to the patient based on age, clinical findings, and imaging characteristics. A recent innovation even brings patient-specific coalition resection guides based off of CT images, akin to the tibial and talar cutting guides used in some total ankle arthroplasty systems [63]. Two main surgical options are coalition resection and fusion, with or without adjunctive reconstructive procedures to address pes planovalgus and/or equinus. In the authors' experience, a CN coalition responds better to resection than a TC coalition, and, in general, a coalition resection, regardless of location, fares better long term in younger patients. This is generally supported by the existing literature. Giannini found that patients 14 years and younger responded better to resection than their older counterparts [47], although successful outcomes have also been shown after coalition resection in adult patients [48].

Various surgical techniques may be employed for resection of a CN coalition [1, 11]. Interpositional fat, extensor digitorum brevis muscle belly, or bone wax are inserted at the discretion of the surgeon. There is evidence that supports interposition to prevent recurrence, but the evidence is conflicting with regard to the particular type of material used for this purpose [45, 49, 50, 68]. In the author's experience, adequate resection of the margins of the coalition is imperative to prevent re-growth of the bony bridge, especially in CN coalitions. Adequate resection may be confirmed intraoperatively with clinical and radiographic examination (Fig. 11.23).

If a pes planovalgus deformity is seen in association with a CN coalition, an Evans or medializing calcaneal osteotomy can be performed with a CN coalition resection. Other associated deformities are also addressed, including ankle equinus and forefoot varus. It should be emphasized that adjunctive joint-sparing reconstructive procedures to correct a pes planovalgus concurrently with a coalition resection is primarily indicated in patients with no significant arthritic changes in the hindfoot joints. It is also possible to have a subtalar joint middle facet coalition in conjunction with a CN bar (Fig. 11.24).

A middle facet coalition may also be amenable to treatment with resection alone or in combination with other procedures [64]. Generally, an incision is placed over the middle facet to allow full visualization of the bony bridge and to allow for adequate resection. Resection has also been described with arthroscopic and endoscopic guidance [51, 66]. A study by Hetsroni showed no difference in the kinematics of the subtalar joint during stance after resection of the coalition compared to the preoperative kinematics [52]. Another study demonstrated that plantar pressures during gait are close to normal after coalition resection, although normal plantar pressures are not recreated during running after resection of the coalition [53]. Similarly, Lyon found that there were significant differences in measurements of plantar pressures even after coalition resection, as compared to the normal foot [16]. There is no widely held consensus when it comes to the efficacy of isolated coalition resection versus resection combined with correction of coexisting hindfoot deformity. Some studies have reported poorer outcomes associated with larger degrees of hindfoot values treated with isolated resection [50], while recent studies by Mahan et al. and Khoshbin et al. found no difference

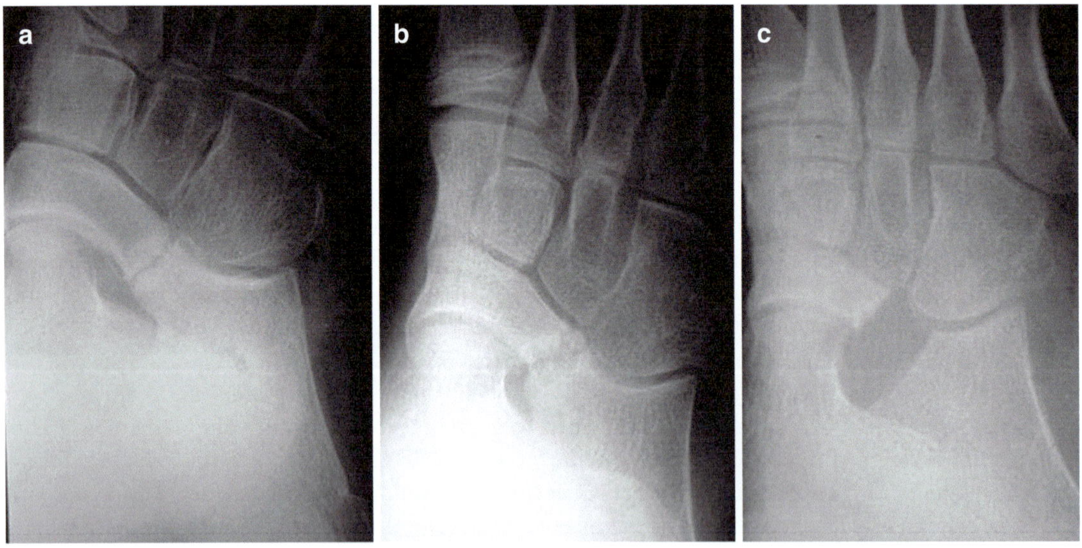

Fig. 11.23 Calcaneonavicular bar with incomplete bone bridge (**a**), recurrence after inadequate resection (**b**), and adequate resection with clear margins of bony separation (**c**)

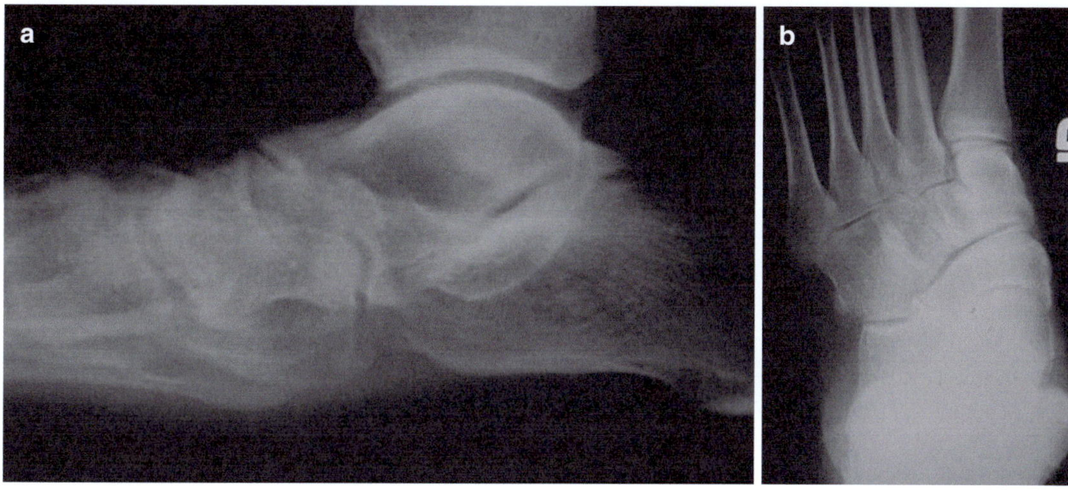

Fig. 11.24 Patient with both a middle facet coalition (**a**) and a calcaneonavicular bar coalition (**b**) in the same foot, emphasizing the need for comprehensive imaging evaluation in order to formulate an appropriate surgical treatment plan

in outcomes for patient treated largely with isolated resection, including patients with coalitions greater than 50% of the posterior facet and heel values over 16 degrees [65, 69]. Giannini found an 85.7% improvement in postoperative pain and 92.8% increase in range of motion in 14 patients who underwent middle facet coalition resection in combination with a poly-L-lactic acid bioabsorbable implant in the sinus tarsi [48].

In the absence of arthritic changes in the posterior facet, middle facet coalition resection can be performed with various combinations of an Evans calcaneal osteotomy, medializing calcaneal osteotomy, medial column osteotomy or fusion, and lengthening of the Achilles tendon or gastrocnemius aponeurosis. At surgeon discretion, these adjunctive procedures are performed concurrently with resection or in a staged second procedure. Mosca et al. reported good results with the treatment of 13 coalitions in 8 patients who underwent calcaneal lengthening osteotomy for hindfoot valgus deformity correction both with and without coalition resection [61]. In another report of 6 feet with coalition resection in combination with pes planovalgus repair without a rearfoot fusion, the AOFAS Ankle-Hindfoot Scores were all excellent postoperatively [54]. There was also significant improvement radiographically of the calcaneal inclination, Meary's angle, and DP talar-first metatarsal angles [54].

Patients with arthritic changes of the subtalar or surrounding joints are usually not amenable to coalition resection alone. Resection of a middle facet coalition in a patient who demonstrates arthritic changes in the posterior facet can accelerate the progression of arthritis, fail to relieve their pain, and necessitate performing a subtalar joint arthrodesis (Fig. 11.25). Likewise, patients with significant arthritis involving the posterior and middle facets, regardless of age, require primary arthrodesis in order to alleviate symptoms. The foot without significant misalignment is generally amenable to isolated arthrodesis of the subtalar joint (Fig. 11.26).

On occasion, an osseous middle facet coalition is found to be associated with a normal positioned rearfoot and isolated pain in the subtalar joint. The authors perform an "in situ" fusion of the subtalar joint in this situation by resecting the remaining cartilage and subchondral bone of the posterior facet and interpose cancellous bone, without disruption of the already fused middle facet. The authors do not employ fixation across this type of fusion, since stabilization is afforded by the solid middle facet coalition (Fig. 11.27).

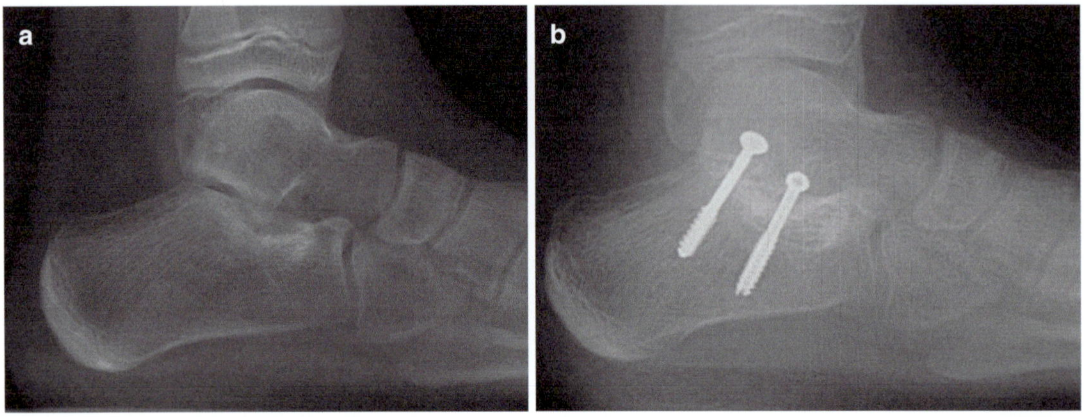

Fig. 11.25 Twelve-year-old female patient 7 months following middle facet coalition resection with exacerbated medial and lateral subtalar joint pain and arthrosis (**a**) and 1 year following isolated subtalar joint arthrodesis (**b**)

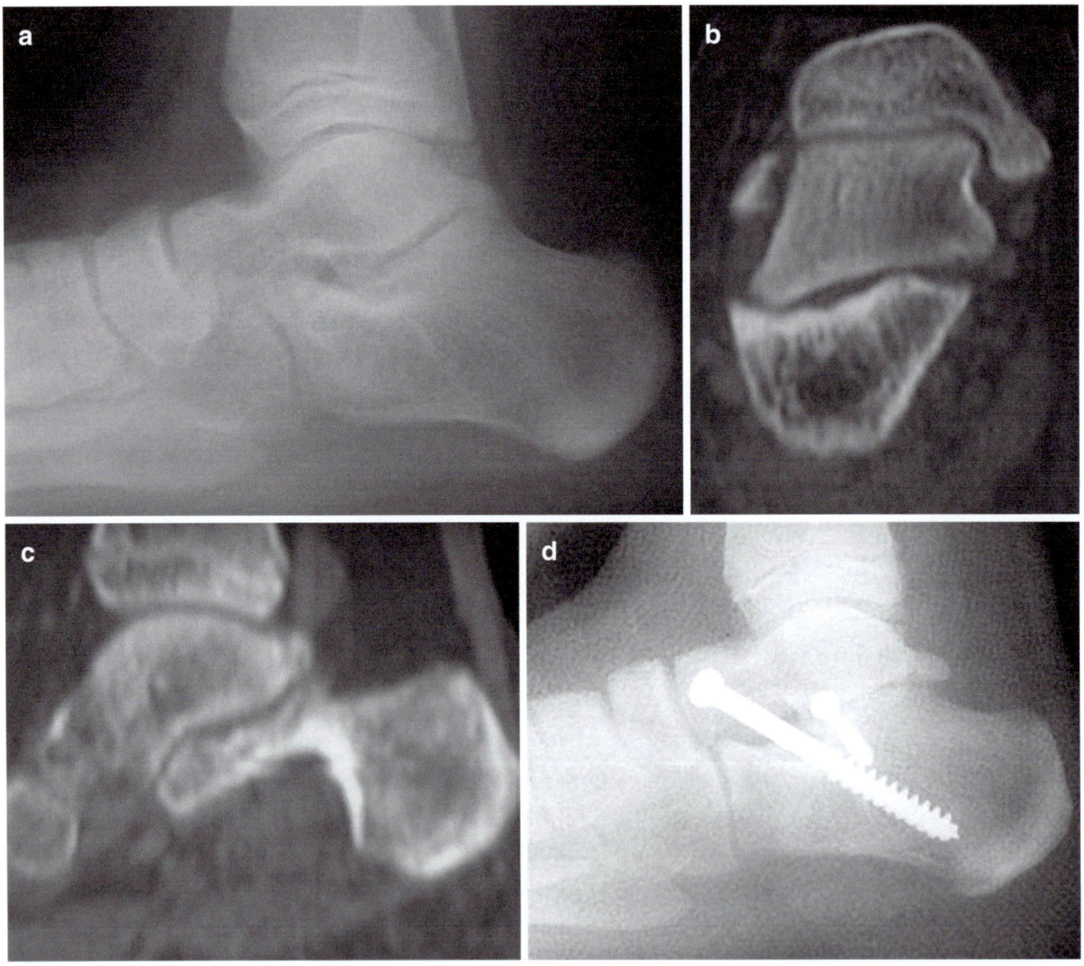

Fig. 11.26 Eight-year-old female patient with painful arthritic subtalar joint arthritis, plain radiograph (**a**), axial computerized tomogram demonstrating significant posterior facet degenerative changes (**b**), sagittal computerized tomogram revealing middle facet involvement (**c**), treated with isolated subtalar joint arthrodesis (**d**)

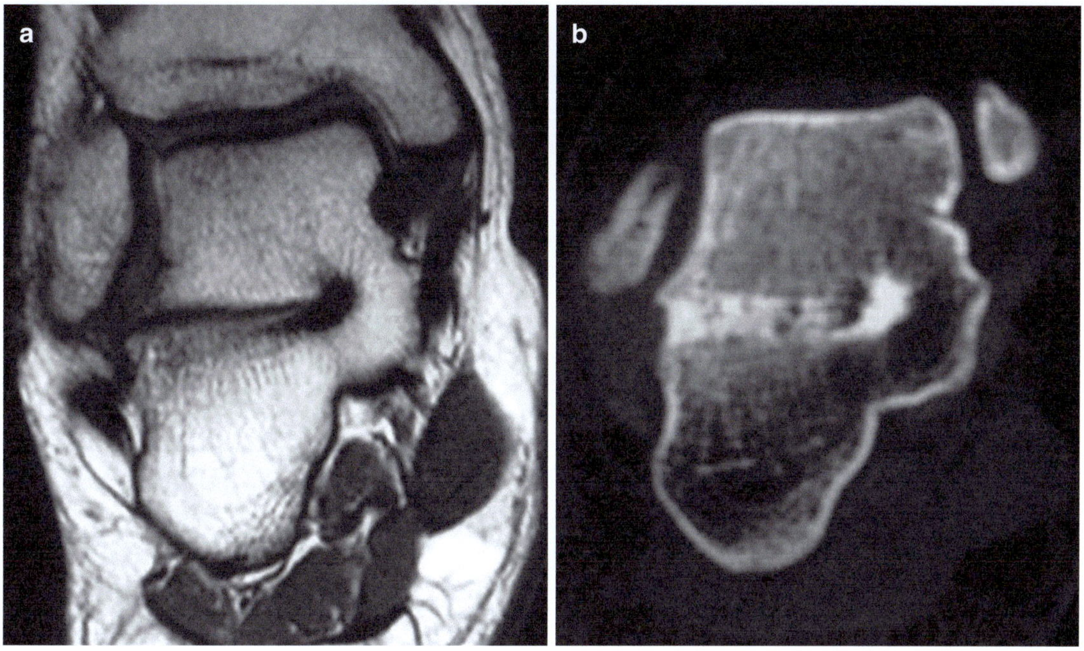

Fig. 11.27 Axial T1 magnetic resonance image of a 15-year-old female with a painful, complete bone bridge of a middle facet coalition with no valgus heel alignment (**a**) and 8 month post in situ arthrodesis axial computerized tomogram demonstrating bone consolidation of allograft, without cut-down of the middle facet coalition (**b**)

More commonly, a valgus position of the calcaneus relative to the tibia exists in patients with a tarsal coalition (Fig. 11.28). An "in situ" fusion would not correct the positional deformity of the rearfoot, and a more extensive approach is necessary to fuse the subtalar joint. If a nonosseous coalition exists in the middle facet, the joint is opened, thus separating the coalition, in order to resect the joint surfaces in preparation for arthrodesis. If an osseous coalition is present with valgus heel alignment, it is also necessary to separate the coalition to aid in joint resection and adequate repositioning of the subtalar joint. Once the joint surfaces are adequately resected and alignment corrected, fixation is necessary for compression and stabilization across the arthrodesis site.

The more severe or long-standing deformity will also develop adaptive changes in the forefoot to compensate for the valgus alignment of the heel. Repositioning of the STJ into a rectus position will accentuate the varus alignment of the forefoot. In this situation, the midfoot/forefoot will also need to be surgically addressed in order to pronate the forefoot to allow the medial column to purchase the ground. A modified

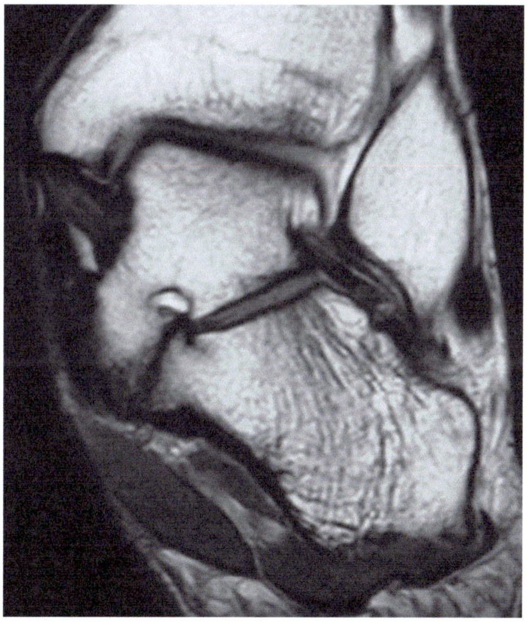

Fig. 11.28 Axial T1 magnetic resonance image of a patient with a middle facet coalition with peroneal spasm and significant heel valgus (lateral tarsal wedging) and articulating calcaneal and fibular segments. This foot is not amenable to coalition resection and will require multi-level arthrodesis in order to address the coalition and correct the valgus foot alignment

Young's tenosuspension, osteotomy of the medial cuneiform with bone graft (Cotton osteotomy), naviculocuneiform arthrodesis, or talonavicular arthrodesis can be performed to plantarflex the medial column, in addition to arthrodesis of the subtalar joint. A double arthrodesis, consisting of the talonavicular and subtalar joints, can be performed in the patient with moderate-severe positional deformities of the forefoot, without involvement of the calcaneocuboid joint [55–57].

Adaptive Changes with Lateral Tarsal Wedging

Patients with lateral tarsal wedging, either talar or calcaneal, generally require even more positional correction due to the hypoplastic nature of the lateral aspect of the talus (and/or calcaneus). This generally involves the use of an opening bone graft or wedge resection of the subtalar joint, depending on the degree of deformity. The authors published a case series describing a technique using a press-fit femoral head or tricortical iliac crest allograft fashioned into laterally based wedge in the subtalar joint that achieved satisfactory outcomes in 9 patients with a mean follow up of 25.5 months [62]. The use of internal fixation in this situation is variable, as a compression-fit bone graft is usually stable enough for consolidation without the aid of compression devices. Thus, the need for screw fixation is based on stability of the fusion site, and this decision is made at the time of surgery (Fig. 11.29). Finally, a triple arthrodesis is typically necessary in the more severe deformity, whereby resection of the MTJ allows for multiplane correction (Fig. 11.30).

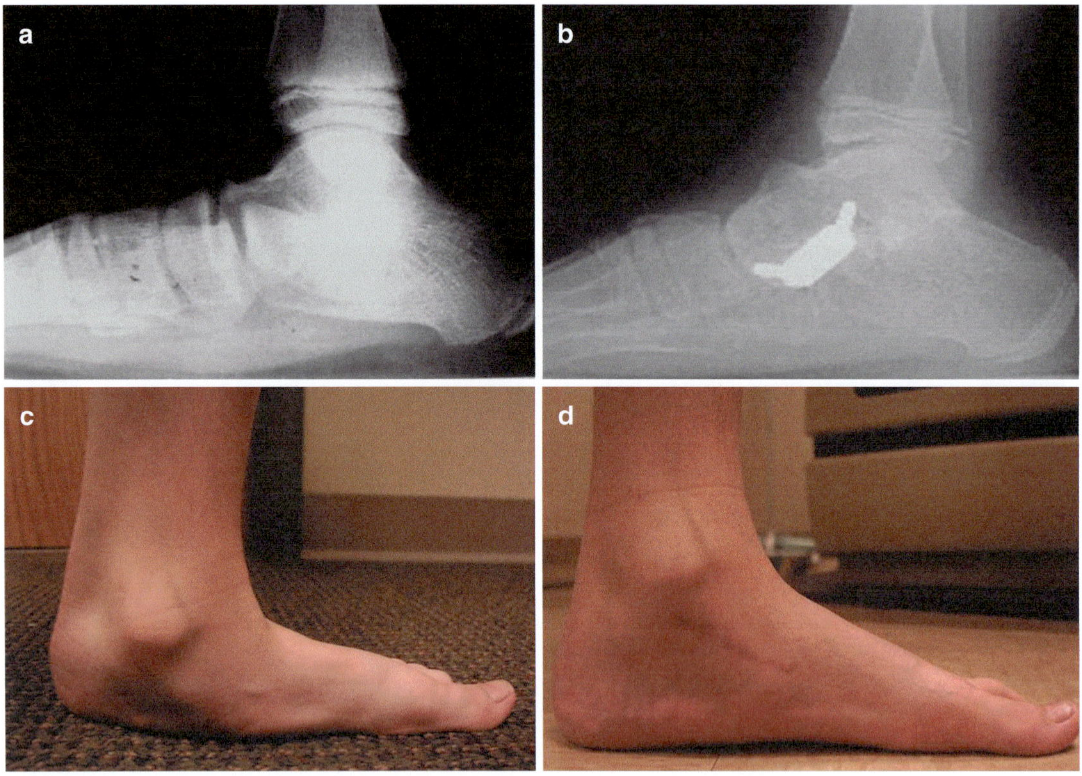

Fig. 11.29 Eleven-year-old patient with a painful middle facet coalition with severe pes valgus, before (**a**) and after (**b**) double arthrodesis, utilizing allograft iliac crest to reverse-wedge the subtalar joint fusion site. Before (**c**) and after (**d**) clinical appearance of the medial longitudinal arch. Computerized tomogram prior to surgery (**e**) demonstrating heel valgus alignment with lateral tarsal wedging and computerized tomogram 6 months following bone graft realignment arthrodesis of the subtalar joint demonstrating significant frontal plane correction (**f**)

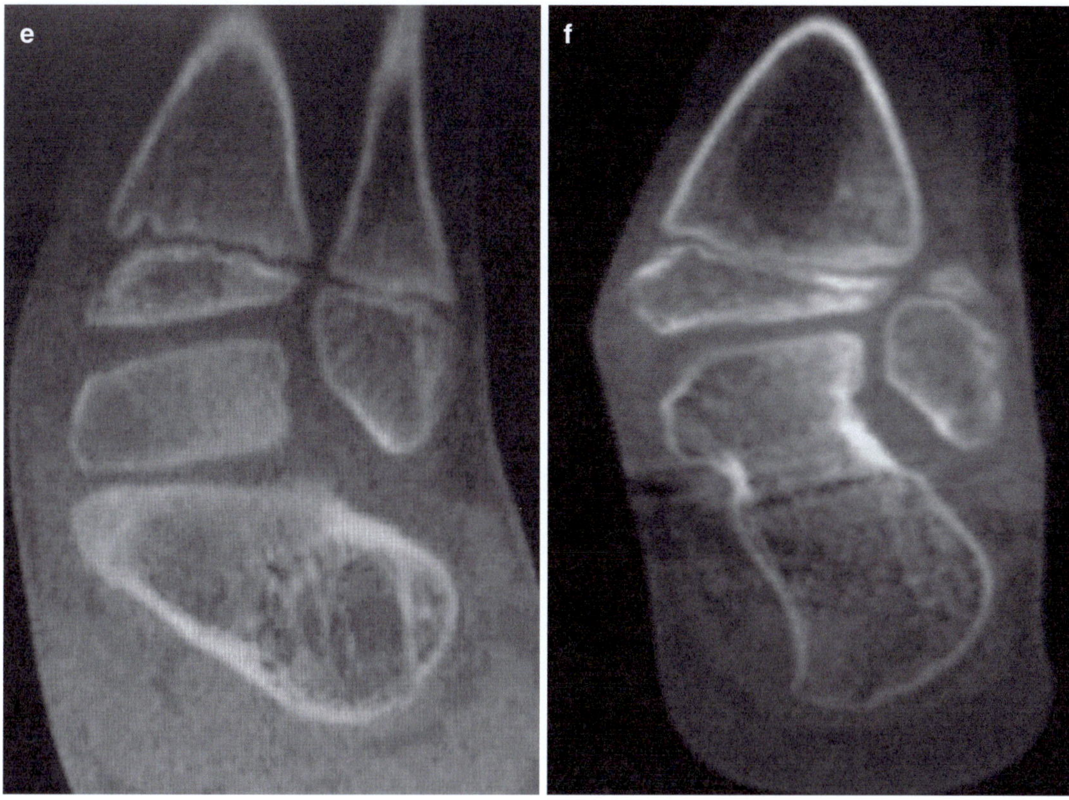

Fig. 11.29 (continued)

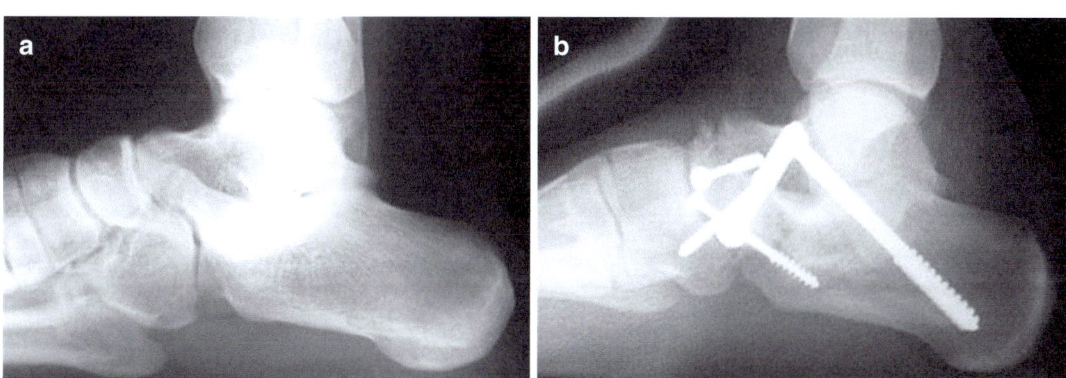

Fig. 11.30 Preoperative (**a**) and postoperative (**b**) lateral radiographs showing patient with middle facet and calcaneonavicular bar coalitions requiring triple arthrodesis to address arthritis

Conclusion

Pediatric pes planovalgus deformity encompasses a diverse range of clinical presentation: the flexible deformity, the osseous coalition, and everything in between. While algorithms do exist to establish some general guidelines for surgeons in the diagnosis and treatment of these disorders [1, 58, 59, 61], they offer limited guidance in the treatment of patients who present with symptoms and findings in the "gray zone" between painful flexible pes planovalgus and the frank osseous tarsal coalition. The authors believe that careful examination utilizing the full spectrum of available clinical evaluation techniques combined with an educated analysis of radiographic and CT findings is critical to accurately diagnose the etiology of the painful tarsal coalition and pes planovalgus deformity and subsequently perform the necessary surgical correction.

References

1. Downey MS. Tarsal coalition. In: Banks AS, Downey MS, Martin DE, Miller SJ, editors. McGlamry's comprehensive textbook of foot and ankle surgery. 3rd ed. Philadelphia: Lippincott Williams & Wilkins; 2001. p. 993–1031.
2. Leonard MA. The inheritance of tarsal coalition and it relationship to spastic flat foot. J Bone Joint Surg Br. 1974;56B(3):520–6.
3. Mosier KM, Asher M. Tarsal coalitions and peroneal spastic flat foot. J Bone Joint Surg Am. 1984;66-A(7):976–83.
4. Harris BJ. Anomalous structures in the developing human foot. Anat Rec. 1955;121:399.
5. Ceroni D, De Coulon G, Spadola L, De Rose V, Kaelin A. Calcaneus secundarius presenting as calcaneonavicular coalition: a case report. J Foot Ankle Surg. 2006;45(1):25–7.
6. Solomon LB, Ruhli FJ, Taylor J, Ferris L, Pope R, Henneberg M. A dissection and computer tomography study of tarsal coalitions in 100 cadaver feet. J Orth Res. 2003;21:352–8.
7. Bohne WH. Tarsal coalition. Curr Opin Pediatr. 2001;13:29–35.
8. Jayakumar S, Cowell HR. Rigid flatfoot. Clin Orthop Relat Res. 1977;122:77–84.
9. Staser J, Karmazyn B, Lubicky J. Radiographic diagnosis of posterior facet talocalcaneal coalition. Pediatr Radiol. 2007;37:79–81.
10. Wheeler R, Guevera A, Bleck E. Tarsal coalitions: review of the literature and case report of bilateral dual calcaneonavicular and talocalcaneal coalitions. Clin Orthop Relat Res. 1981;156:175–7.
11. Blakemore LC, Cooperman DR, Thompson GH. The rigid flatfoot: tarsal coalitions. Clin Podiatr Med Surg. 2000;17(3):531–55.
12. Katayama T, Tanaka Y, Kadono K, Taniguchi A, Takakura Y. Talocalcaneal coalition: a case showing the ossification process. Foot Ankle Int. 2005;26(6):490–3.
13. Kumai T, Takahura Y, Akiyama K, Higashiyama I, Tamai S. Histopathological study of nonosseous tarsal coalition. Foot Ankle Int. 1998;19(8):525–31.
14. Brown RR, Rosenberg ZS, Thornhill BA. The C sign: more specific for flatfoot deformity that subtalar coalition. Skelet Radiol. 2001;30(2):84–7.
15. Lowy LJ. Pediatric peroneal spastic flatfoot in the absence of coalition: a suggested protocol. J Am Podiatr Med Assoc. 1998;88(4):181–91.
16. Lyon R, Liu X, Cho S. Effect of tarsal coalition resection on dynamic plantar pressures and electromyography of lower extremity muscles. J Foot Ankle Surg. 2005;44(4):252–8.
17. Yu GV. Asymptomatic tarsal coalitions. Reconstructive surgery of the foot and leg, update 1993. Tucker: The Podiatry Institute; 1993. p. 246–55.
18. Blair J, Perdios A, Reilly C. Peroneal spastic flatfoot caused by a talar osteochondral lesion: a case report. Foot Ankle Int. 2007;28(6):724–6.
19. Doig SG, Menelaus MB. Association of slipped upper femoral epiphysis and peroneal spastic flatfoot. J Pediatr Orthop. 1991;11(2):220–1.
20. Graves SC, Keuster DJ, Richardson EG. Dysplasia epiphysealis hemimelica (Trevor disease) presenting as peroneal spastic flatfoot deformity: a case report. Foot Ankle. 1991;12(1):55–8.
21. Glockenberg A, Weinreb A, Pevny J. Rheumatoid arthritis-induced peroneal spastic flatfoot. J Am Podiatr Med Assoc. 1987;77(4):185–7.
22. Cowell HR. Talocalcaneal coalition and new causes of peroneal spastic flatfoot. Clin Orthop Relat Res. 1972;85:16–22.
23. Jack FA. Bone anomalies of the tarsus in relation to "peroneal spastic flat foot". J Bone Joint Surg. 1954;36(4):530–42.
24. Harris RI, Beath T. Etiology of peroneal spastic flat foot. J Bone Joint Surg Br. 1948;30B(4):624–34.
25. Downey MS. Ankle equinus. In: Banks AS, Downey MS, Martin DE, Miller SJ, editors. McGlamry comprehensive textbook of foot and ankle surgery. 3rd ed. Philadelphia: Lippincott Williams & Wilkins; 2001. p. 715–60.
26. Crim JR, Kjeldsberg KM. Radiographic diagnosis of tarsal coalition. Am J Radiol. 2004;182:323–8.
27. Kricun ME. The normal foot. In: Forresster DM, Kricun ME, Kerr R, editors. Imaging of the foot and ankle. Rockville: Aspen Publishers; 1988. p. 25–43.
28. Berquist TH, Johnson KA. Anatomy, normal variants, and basic biomechanics. In: Berquist TH, editor. Radiology of the foot and ankle. New York: Raven Press; 1989. p. 1–34.
29. Lateur LM, Van Hoe LR, Van Ghillewe KV, Gryspeerdt SS, Baert AL, Dereymaeker GE. Subtalar coalition: diagnosis with the C sign on lateral radiographs of the ankle. Radiol. 1994;193:847–51.
30. Wright EM, Lieberman R, Brekke M, Reicher M, Green D. Tarsal coalition. In: Reconstructive surgery of the foot and ankle, update 1997. Tucker: The Podiatry Institute; 1997.
31. Wechsler RJ, Schweitzer ME, Deely DM, Horn BD, Pizzutillo PD. Tarsal coalition: depiction and char-

acterization with CT and MR imaging. Radiology. 1994;193:447–52.
32. Crim J. Imaging of tarsal coalition. Radiol Clin North Am. 2008;46:1017–26.
33. Kulik SA, Clanton TO. Tarsal coalition. Foot Ankle Int. 1996;17(5):286–96.
34. Saxena A, Erickson S. Tarsal coalitions: activity levels with and without surgery. J Podiatr Med Assoc. 2003;93(4):259–63.
35. Emery KH, Bisset GS, Johnson ND, Nunan PJ. Tarsal coalition: a blinded comparison of MRI and CT. Pediatr Radiol. 1998;28:612–6.
36. Newman JS, Newberg AH. Congenital tarsal coalition: multimodality evaluation with emphasis on CT and MR imaging. Radiographics. 2000;20: 321–32.
37. Nalaboff KM, Schweitzer ME. MRI of tarsal coalition: frequency, distribution and innovative signs. Bull NYU Hosp Joint Dis. 2008;66(1):14–21.
38. Napolitano C, Walsh S, Mahoney L, McCrea J. Risk factors that may adversely modify the natural history of the pediatric pronated foot. Clin Podiatr Med Surg. 2000;17(3):397–417.
39. Pfeiffer M, Kotz R, Ledl T, Hauser G, Sluga M. Prevalence of flat foot in preschool-aged children. Pediatrics. 2006;118(2):634–9.
40. Wearing SC, Hills AP, Byrne NM, Hennig EM, McDonald M. The arch index: a measure of flat or fat feet? Foot Ankle Int. 2004;25(8):575–81.
41. Mickle KJ, Steele JR, Munro BJ. The feet of overweight and obese young children: are they flat or fat? Obesity. 2006;14(11):1949–53.
42. Villarroya MA, Esquivel JM, Tomas C, Moreno LA, Buenafe A, Bueno G. Assessment of the medial longitudinal arch in children and adolescents with obesity: footprints and radiographic study. Eur J Pediatr. 2009;168(5):559–67.
43. Chen JP, Chung MJ, Wang MJ. Flatfoot prevalence and foot dimensions of 5- to 13-year-old children in Taiwan. Foot Ankle Int. 2009;30(4):326–32.
44. Blockey NJ. Peroneal spastic flat foot. J Bone Joint Surg Br. 1955;37B(2):191–202.
45. Thometz J. Tarsal coalition. Foot Ankle Clin. 2000;5(1):103–18.
46. Kernbach KJ, Blitz NM. The presence of calcaneal fibular remodeling associated with middle facet coalition: a retrospective CT review of 35 feet. Investigation involving middle facet coalitions-Part II. J Foot Ankle Surg. 2008;47(4):288–94.
47. Giannini S, Ceccarelli F, Vannini F, Baldi E. Operative treatment of flatfoot with talocalcaneal coalition. Clin Orthop Rel Res. 2003;411:178–87.
48. Scott AT, Tuten HR. Calcaneonavicular coalition resection with extensor digitorum brevis interposition in adults. Foot Ankle Int. 2007;28(8):890–5.
49. Cowell HR, Elener V. Rigid painful flatfoot secondary to tarsal coalition. Clin Orthop Relat Res. 1983;177:54–60.
50. Lemley F, Berlet G, Hill K, Philbin T, Isaac B, Lee T. Current concepts review: tarsal coalition. Foot Ankle Int. 2006;27(12):1163–9.
51. Field C, Ng A. Resection of middle facet coalition with arthroscopic guidance. J Foot Ankle Surg. 2009;48(2):273–6.
52. Hetsroni I, Nyska M, Mann G, Rozenfeld G, Ayalon M. Subtalar kinematics following resection of tarsal coalition. Foot Ankle Int. 2008;29(11):1088–93.
53. Hetsroni I, Ayalon M, Mann G, Meyer G, Nyska M. Walking and running plantar pressure analysis before and after resection of tarsal coalition. Foot Ankle Int. 2007;28(5):575–80.
54. Kernbach KJ, Blitz NM, Rush SM. Bilateral single-stage middle facet talocalcaneal coalition resection combined with flatfoot reconstruction: a report of 3 cases and review of the literature. Investigations involving middle facet coalitions-Part I. J Foot Ankle Surg. 2008;47(3):180–90.
55. Sammarco VJ, Magur EG, Sammarco GJ, Bagwe MR. Arthrodesis of the subtalar and talonavicular joints for correction of symptomatic hindfoot malalignment. Foot Ankle Int. 2006;27(9): 661–6.
56. Beischer AD, Brodsky JW, Pollo FE, Peerebroom J. Functional outcome and gait analysis after triple or double arthrodesis. Foot Ankle Int. 1999;20(9):545–53.
57. Mann RA, Beaman DN. Double arthrodesis in the adult. Clin Orthop Relat Res. 1999;365:74–80.
58. Harris EJ, Vanore JV, Thomas JL, Kravitz SR, Mendelson SA, Mendicino RW, Silvani SH, Gassen SC. Diagnosis and treatment of pediatric flatfoot. J Foot Ankle Surg. 2004;43(6):341–73.
59. Downey MS. Tarsal coalitions: a surgical classification. J Am Podiatr Med Assoc. 1991;81(4):188–97.
60. Lawrence DA, Rolen MF, Haims AH, Zayour Z, Moukaddam HA. Tarsal coalitions: radiographic, CT, and MR imaging findings. HSS J. 2014;10: 153–66.
61. Mosca VS, Bevan WP. Talocalcaneal tarsal coalitions and the calcaneal lengthening osteotomy: the role of deformity correction. J Bone Joint Surg Am. 2012;94:1584–94.
62. Schwartz JM, Kihm CA, Camasta CA. Subtalar joint distraction arthrodesis to correct calcaneal valgus in pediatric patients with tarsal coalition: a case series. J Foot Ankle Surg. 2015;54(6):1151–7.
63. Guignand D, Journeau P, Mainard-Simard L, et al. Child calcaneonavicular coalitions: MRI diagnostic value in a 19-case series. Orthop Traumatol Surg Res. 2011;97:67–72.
64. Gantsoudes GD, Roocroft JH, Mubarak SJ. Treatment of talocalcaneal coaltions. J Pediatr Orthop. 2012;32(3):301–7.
65. Mahan ST, Spencer SA, Vezeridis PS, Kasser JR. Patient-reported outcomes of tarsal coalitions treated with surgical excision. J Pediatr Orthop. 2015;35(6):583–8.

66. Bonasia DE, Phistikul P, Amendola A. Endoscopic coalition resection. Foot Ankle Clin N Am. 2015;20:81–91.
67. Piqueres X, de Zabala S, Torrens C, Marin M. Cubonavicular coalition: a case report and literature review. Clin Orthop Relat Res. 2002;396:112–4.
68. Krief E, Ferraz L, Appy-Fedida B, Deroussen F, Plancq MC, Collet LM, Gouron R. Tarsal coalitions: preliminary results after operative excision and silicone sheet interposition in children. J Foot Ankle Surg. 2016;55(6):1264–70. https://doi.org/10.1053/j.jfas.2015.03.009. Epub 2015 May 16.
69. Khoshbin A, Law P, Caspi L, Wright J. Long-term functional outcomes of resected tarsal coalitions. Foot Ankle Int. 2013;34(10):1370–5.

12 Congenital Talipes Equinovarus

Daniel J. Hatch

One of the more common deformities of the foot and ankle present at birth is congenital talipes equinovarus (CTEV) or clubfoot. Clubfoot is a three-dimensional deformity that has an incidence of 1/1000 in the Caucasian population [1]. There is a higher incidence in South African blacks and Polynesians (6/1000) [2]. Males are more frequently affected at a ratio of three to one to females. Forty percent of cases are bilateral [3]. When untreated, clubfoot can be very disabling resulting in pain, severe deformity, inability to wear shoes, and inability to ambulate (Fig. 12.1).

Definition

CTEV is comprised of four components: equinus, varus, adductus, and cavus [4] (Fig. 12.2). Equinus is the foot in a plantarflexed position compared to the lower leg. Varus is in reference to the position of the calcaneus. Adduction is the relationship of the forefoot to the rearfoot. Cavus is the overall increase in height of the arch of the foot. There are four basic classifications of clubfoot: congenital (idiopathic), teratologic, syndromic, and positional [5]. Idiopathic is the most common and can present at birth as an isolated defect. It may be first diagnosed in utero by ultrasound at 15–16-weekgestation [6]. Sometimes this can be identified as early as 12-week gestation [7]. Aurell et al. evaluated the ultrasound anatomy of 30 untreated clubfeet in 22 children in their neonatal clubfoot study [8]. The authors found close proximity of the navicular and medial malleolus along with capsular thickening medially. Teratologic clubfoot types are associated with neuromuscular disease processes such as spina bifida and myelomeningocele. Syndromic clubfoot is associated with genetic abnormalities and other disease processes of which clubfoot commonly occurs. Examples of this type would include arthrogryposis, Larsen syndrome, and Moebius syndrome [2, 9, 10]. Positional (sometimes called postural) clubfoot is a relatively normal foot that was held in an abnormal position in utero. This type is more easily corrected and usually does not require treatment with an Achilles tenotomy or extensive bracing.

Etiology

The etiology of idiopathic clubfoot is multifactorial and involves several common theories. Idiopathic clubfoot results from in utero rather than embryonic conditions. The more frequently cited factors involved in the development of

D. J. Hatch (✉)
Medical Center of the Rockies, Loveland, CO, USA

North Colorado Podiatric Surgical Residency, Greeley, CO, USA
e-mail: dhatch@footandanklecolorado.com

M. L. Butterworth, J. T. Marcoux (eds.), *The Pediatric Foot and Ankle*,
https://doi.org/10.1007/978-3-030-29788-6_12

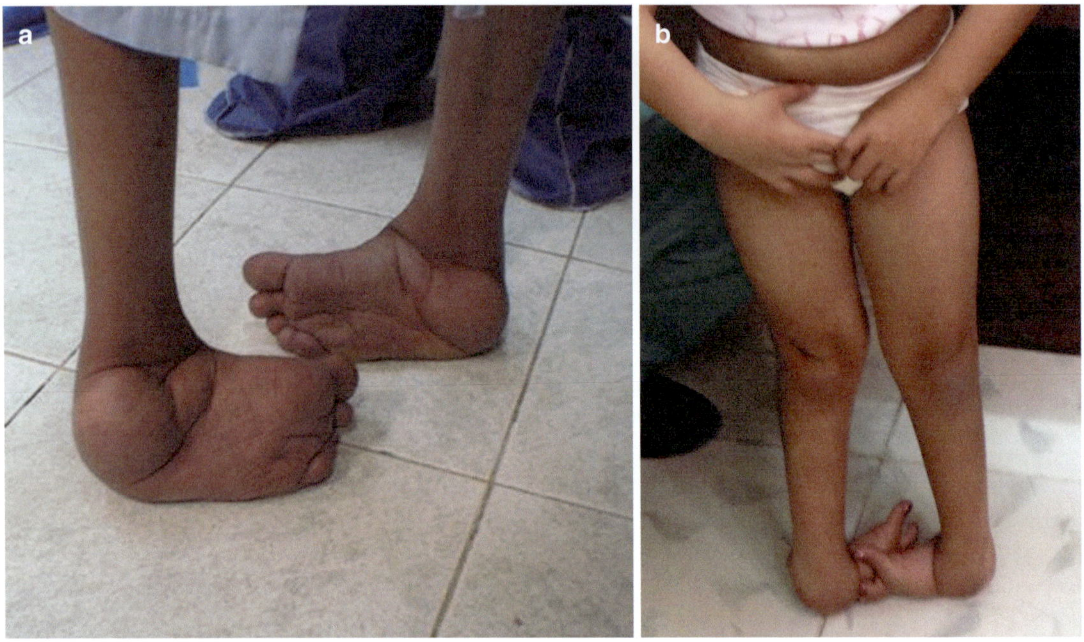

Fig. 12.1 Neglected clubfoot

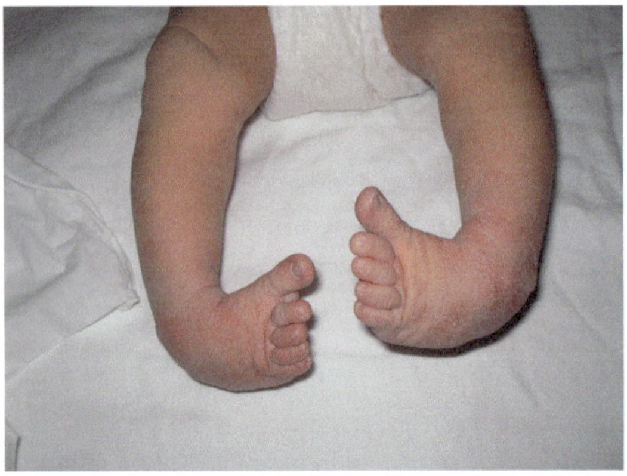

Fig. 12.2 Idiopathic clubfoot

clubfoot include in utero positioning, environmental factors, neuromuscular with increased collagen synthesis, and genetic origin. Some less frequently reported causes include intrauterine developmental arrest [11], a defect in the germ plasm of the talus [12, 13], hypoplastic dorsalis pedis artery [14], and neurological defects affecting muscles of the lower extremity [15].

In utero mal-positioning was identified by Hippocrates [16] and supported by Browne [17, 18]. Additionally it has been reported that there is a greater incidence of clubfoot after amniocentesis [19]. Farrell et al. found that amniocentesis at 12 weeks correlated with a 1.63% increased chance of clubfoot [20]. The authors found this timing correlated with a maximal amount of foot and ankle growth. It is believed that the loss of amniotic fluid contributes to the "crowding" of the uterine cavity [20].

Environmental factors are rare and would include drug exposures [21] and smoking [4, 22].

Ippolito and Ponseti's histological study of five clubfeet and three normal feet in aborted fetuses found shortening and thickening of the talonavicular and spring ligaments suggesting a possible etiology of clubfoot to be a "retracting fibrosis" [23]. The authors also found that the distal leg muscles showed a decrease in size and number of muscle fibers. Other studies have supported the theory of increase in fetal myosin and ensuing fibrosis [15, 24–26].

There is a high genetic influence in clubfoot [2, 27–32]. Idelberger in 1939 found a concordance of clubfoot in 32.5% of monozygotic twins and only 2.9% of dizygotic twins [33].

Wynne- Davies found that if one child in a family had clubfoot, then the second child's chance of clubfoot would be 1/35 [2]. In 2008 Gurnett et al. reported on a genetic variance of the gene PITX1 that was found to be associated with clubfoot deformity [34]. Additional gene factors have been identified including TBX4, RBM10, HOXA, and HOXD [22, 35]. Idiopathic clubfoot is an isolated condition without other musculoskeletal findings and accounts for the majority (80%) of congenital clubfoot. The idiopathic deformity is present with a polygenic threshold influence [22, 35, 36]. The genetic influence may not only determine the incidence of clubfoot, but it may also influence the severity and type of deformity.

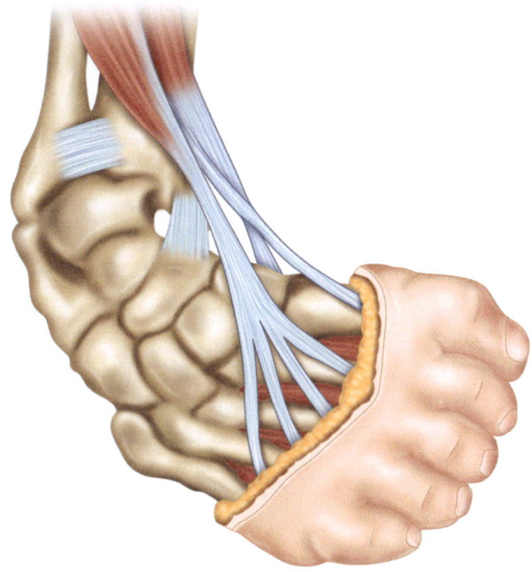

Fig. 12.3 Medially displaced tendons

Pathoanatomy

In 1803 Antonio Scarpa described the abnormal anatomy of congenital clubfoot recognizing that there was medial displacement of the navicular, cuboid, and calcaneus with respect to the talus [37]. Several studies have been performed on fetuses of varying ages [4, 38]. When unilaterally present, the clubbed foot is smaller both in length and girth, and the calf muscles are retracted and less developed compared to the contralateral side. The head and neck of the talus are deviated medially and plantarly, while the body of the talus is rotated laterally [12, 39, 40]. The navicular is subluxed medially and may at times even closely juxtapose the medial malleolus [4]. Ponseti would utilize his thumb as a method of measurement to document the distance between the talar head and the medial malleolus as an indicator of treatment progression [41]. The calcaneus is plantarflexed and inverted with tight medial ligaments and tendons. This gives the appearance of an "empty heel" where the calcaneal tuberosity is elevated. The extensor tendons are medially displaced due to the position of the foot in relation to the leg [4] (Fig. 12.3). The posterior muscle groups are tight and contracted with proximal migration of the posterior muscle bellies.

While Ponseti was not an advocate of radiographs in the infant due to lack of ossification and reliable measurements, it is noted that on the AP radiograph Kite's angle is decreased, occasionally, to zero along with increased forefoot adduction. On the lateral projection, the talus and calcaneus are in equinus.

Kinesiology

The understanding of clubfoot mechanics dates back to Farabeauf [42] and was further expanded by Huson [43, 44]. Farabeauf, a French anatomist, detailed his thoughts on foot mechanics in his *Precis de manual operative* first published in 1872. Huson wrote his doctoral dissertation in 1961 on "A Functional and Anatomical study of the Tarsus" and noted that the tarsal joints rotate about a moving axis rather than around a fixed hinge [43]. Ponseti attributes Huson with his understanding of foot mechanics that provided him the understanding to treat clubfoot successfully [4, 41]. Motion of the calcaneus is not simply inversion and eversion in the frontal plane. Farabeauf likened the motion to the keel of a ship in which it would pitch, roll, and yaw. This calcaneus' motion is in all three planes with the interosseous talocalcaneal ligament serving as the axis point. It is an interesting anatomic observation that this ligament lies within the same axis as the subtalar joint which has been described as being approximately 42 degrees from the transverse plane and 16 degrees from the sagittal plane [45–47]. The main tenant of the Ponseti's conservative treatment for clubfoot incorporates this overall understanding of subtalar joint mechanics. In order for the body of the calcaneus to evert, the anterior process of the calcaneus must first abduct [48] (Fig. 12.4). Abduction of the anterior process of the calcaneus is accomplished by abducting the forefoot as a single unit about the rearfoot by applying counterpressure against the lateral aspect of the talar head. This tri-plane maneuver initiated by the transverse plane abduction allows the heel to freely move under the talus into a more everted position with the anterior process of the calcaneus in a more abducted and dorsiflexed position.

Terminology

Clubfeet can be placed into five categories of clubfoot based upon treatment status including untreated, neglected, recurrent, resistant, and complex or atypical clubfoot [5, 49]. Untreated clubfoot is defined as a child under 2 years of age who has not been previously treated, whereas a neglected clubfoot occurs in a child over 2 years of age who has not been previously treated. A recurrent clubfoot, or relapse, presents in a child previously treated who has re-developed equinus and varus position of the heel. Recurrence of clubfoot deformity is most often due to lack of adherence to the treatment protocols and bracing (Fig. 12.5). A resistant clubfoot is more difficult to treat conservatively and usually involves an underlying neuromuscular disorder such as spina bifida. The complex or atypical clubfoot is a unique and challenging entity that is treated in a different fashion compared to typical idiopathic types. The complex clubfoot has a pronounced calcaneal equinus, a central crease in the arch, and a short first metatarsal due to forefoot equinus (Fig. 12.6).

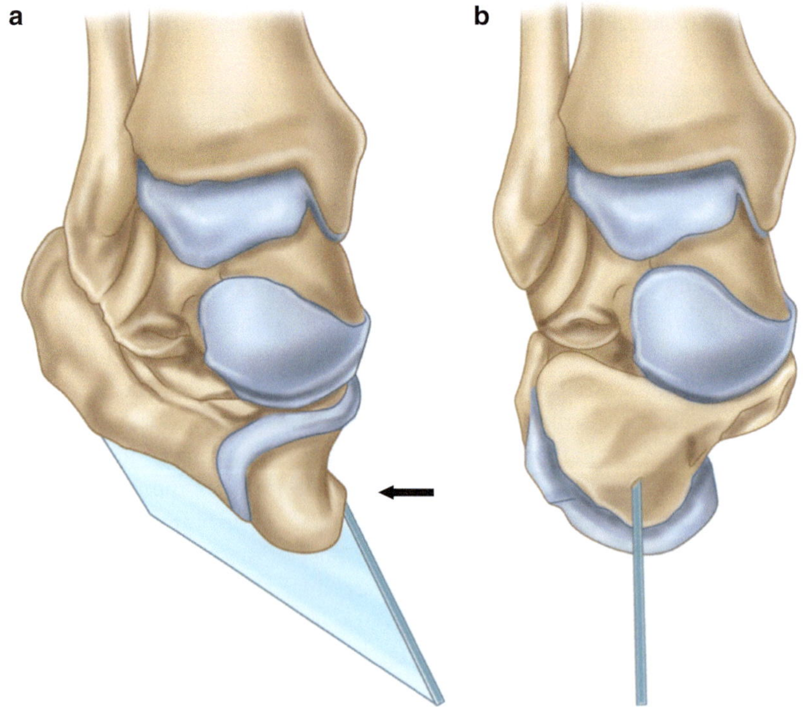

Fig. 12.4 Abduction of the calcaneal beak initiates eversion of the heel. (a) In clubfoot the anterior beak of the calcaneus is positioned under the head of the talus. (b) Abduction of the beak in relation to the talar head will allow correction of the heel varus

Clinical Assessment

When examining the neonate with a clubfoot deformity, care is first taken to reassure the parents that their child will be fine and most likely has clubfoot by chance and without fault. A gestational history and method of delivery should be known. A neuromuscular examination should be performed along with examination of the child's lower back (indentations/hair growth) and hips for signs of dislocation. Once the overall assessment is performed, attention is then directed to the lower legs and feet. Care is taken to identify any creases posteriorly or in the arch that would indicate severe contractures. Additionally, the rigidity of the deformity is assessed by evaluating the reducibility of the equinus and forefoot adductovarus. While there have been various classification schemes, the two more frequently cited are the Dimeglio and the Pirani systems. At times these schemas are even used concurrently [50]. Dimeglio et al. proposed a 20-point scoring system based upon 4 reduction of deformity attributes: equinus, heel varus, forefoot adduction about the hindfoot, and forefoot derotation about the talus. Each of the attributes was given up to four points for maximum reducibility with an additional point added for each of the following: presence of a posterior crease, presence of a medial crease, presence of cavus deformity, and muscle condition [51] (Table 12.1, Fig. 12.7). Dimeglio's classification emphasizes reducibility of the contracted deformity in the sagittal, frontal, and horizontal planes. Pirani et al. developed a 6-point scale giving 1 point for the presence of each of the following clinical signs: posterior

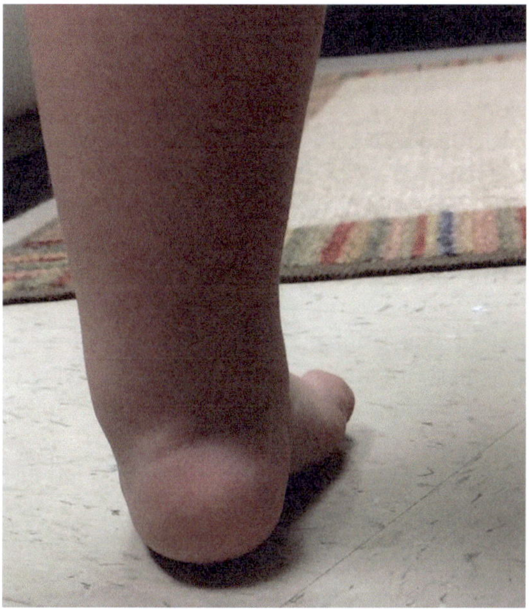

Fig. 12.5 Recurrent clubfoot. Recurrent clubfoot: note equinus and varus heel

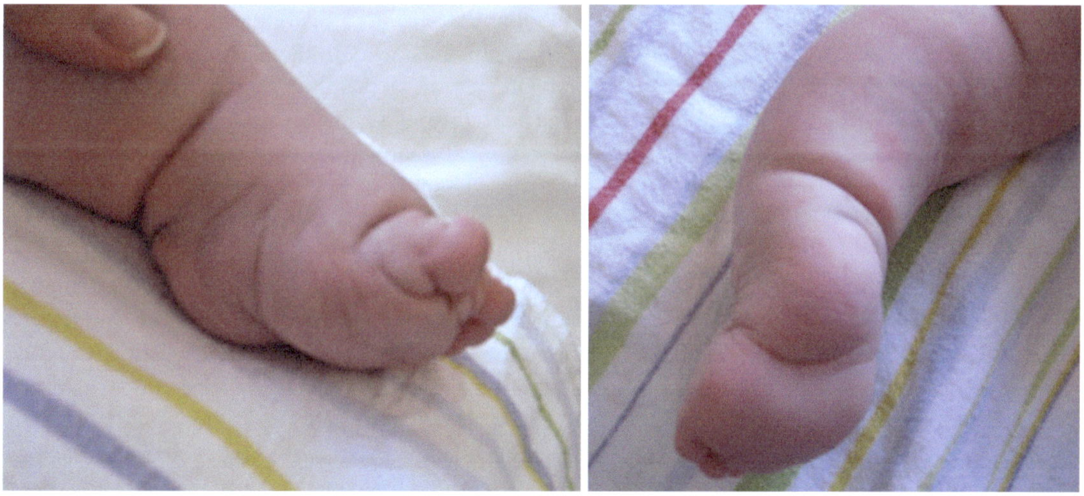

Fig. 12.6 Complex clubfoot. Complex: note equinus, plantar crease, and overall increased girth of foot and ankle along with short hallux

Table 12.1 Dimeglio scoring system

Reducibility is based upon the degree of contracted deformity at:		
90°–45° = 4 pts		
45°–20° = 3 pts		
20°–0° = 2 pts		
0°–(−20°) = 1 pt		
<−20° = 0		
Deformity	Range	Points
Equinus	0–4pts	
	4 = 90° P flexed	
Heel varus	0–4 pts	
	4 = 90° inverted	
Forefoot derotation	0–4 pts	
	4 = rigid internally	
Forefoot adduction	0–4 pts	
Posterior crease	1 point	
Medial crease	1 point	
Cavus	1 point	
Muscle condition	1 point	
Total points	20 max	0–20

crease, presence of an empty heel, rigid equinus, curvature of the lateral border of the foot, medial crease, and prominent of the lateral aspect of the talar head. The posterior crease sign implies a posterior contracture of the ankle joint. The emptiness of the heel refers to the inability to palpate the tuberosity of the calcaneus due to rigid equinus of the heel. The medial crease implies a more medial contracture of the foot (Fig. 12.8).

Each clinical sign is graded on a point scale with 0 as normal, 0.5 as mild, and 1.0 as severe [52, 53] (Table 12.2, Fig. 12.9). Pirani's classification emphasizes foot morphology as it correlates with severity of deformity; however, he added transverse plane reduction of the forefoot about the lateral talar head (prominent lateral aspect of the talar head) and rigidity of the equinus deformity. Attempts are being made to utilize these classifications as predictors of treatment types and success [54, 55].

Treatment History and Options

Plaster casts were first applied for the treatment of clubfoot in 1838 by Guerin [44]. Early treatment of clubfoot was attempted by forceful manipulations using the Thomas wrench [44]. In 1908 Robert Jones reported favorable results if treatment was initiated early [56]. He would first manipulate and cast the deformity followed by wedge resection of the tarsus only if needed. Kite published his method in 1930 [57]. He claimed a 95% success rate, and subsequently his treatment was popular in the orthopedic world for many years [57, 58]. Unfortunately, Kite's method could not be reproduced with outcomes comparable to his study. The treatment was a long process addressing each clubfoot component individually. Kite would first treat the forefoot adduction by abducting the forefoot against counterpressure at the cuboid. Heel varus was then corrected followed lastly by improving the ankle equinus. Repair of the heel varus was difficult, and Kite's method was met with frequent failures that resulted in a high incidence of surgical intervention. Recent literature has compared Kite's method to Ponseti's with more favorable outcomes in the Ponseti treatment [59–61].

There has been a paradigm shift in the surgical treatment of clubfoot since the early 1900s. This is due to an improved understanding of foot mechanics and the success of the Ponseti casting technique. Presently surgical repair is reserved for the most difficult deformities related to neglected, syndromic, and teratologic conditions. Initial surgical repair was performed due to the lack of improvement with conservative options at that time. From a historical perspective, surgical treatment started in the early 1900s by Codivilla and his medial approach [62, 63]. While there have been a variety of methods proposed in the surgical treatment of clubfoot, there appear to be several surgical approaches that are considered classic surgical treatments. These include the methods of Turco, Carroll, and Crawford. These various incisional approaches would attempt to alleviate structures under contracture and tighten the soft tissue present with laxity. Turco proposed a posterior to medial incision to isolate the contracted tissues [64, 65] (Fig. 12.10). Norris Carroll advocated a two incisional approach in 1990 [66]. This involved a medial incision and a posterior incision. He further explained his technique in an article in 1993 [67] (Fig. 12.11).

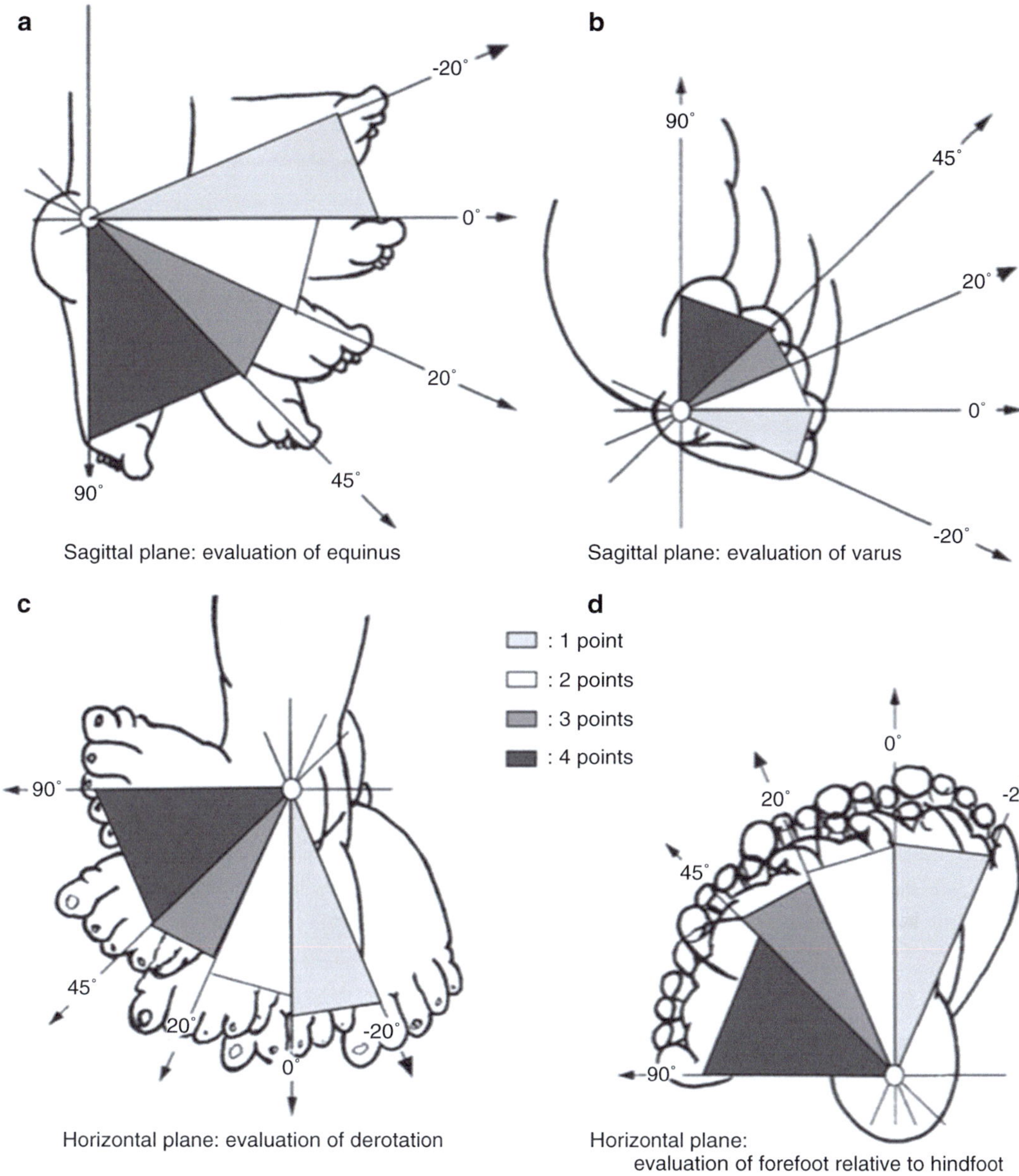

Fig. 12.7 Dimeglio's classification of clubfoot

Crawford popularized the "Cincinnati" incision for clubfoot advocating an improved exposure and surgical scar [68] (Fig. 12.12). All these approaches had the goal of a plantigrade foot and being able to wear shoes. Mahapatra and Abraham in 2016 found the Cincinnati approach to have less wound complications and better functional result than the Turco method in their study [69]. Subsequent soft tissue procedures have been described for realignment of the foot; however, problems with scarring, stiffness, and arthrosis have occurred [70–72]. These factors along with the surgical complications of over- and undercorrection have led most surgeons to reserve surgical repair to the most resistant recalcitrant deformities. In fact, Zionts compared a member survey of the Pediatric Orthopaedic Society of North America (POSNA) from 2001

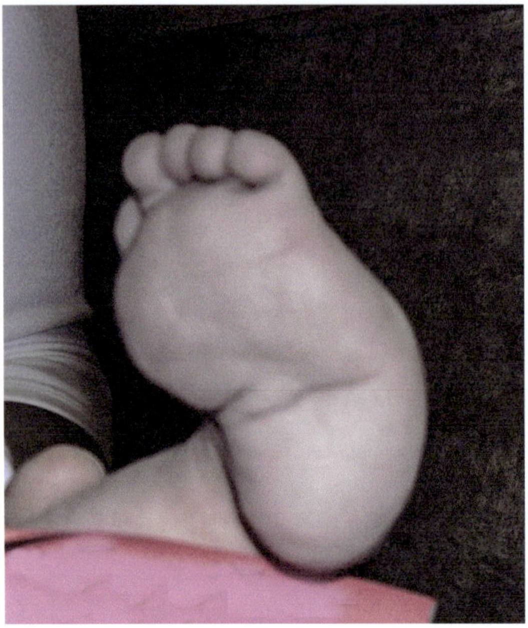

Fig. 12.8 Medial crease. A sign of medial contractures

Table 12.2 Pirani scoring system

	Rating	Points
Hindfoot contracture		
(a) Posterior crease	0, 0.5, 1	
(b) "Empty heel"	0,1	
(c) Rigidity of equinus	0, 0.5, 1	
Midfoot contracture		
(a) Curvature of lateral border of foot	0, 0.5, 1	
(b) Medial arch crease	0, 0.5, 1	
(c) Reduction of lateral talar head	0, 0.5, 1	
	Total points: Max = 6	0–6

to 2012 and found that member use of extensive surgical release fell from 54% to 7% [73]. Lastly, Švehlík et al. found in their long-term prospective trial with a minimum 10-year follow-up that the Ponseti-treated children had better outcomes than the surgical group [74].

In the most neglected and resistant deformities, talectomy may be employed. These would include rigid conditions seen in more syndromic and teratologic conditions. Menelaus in 1971 described his results and technique of talectomy

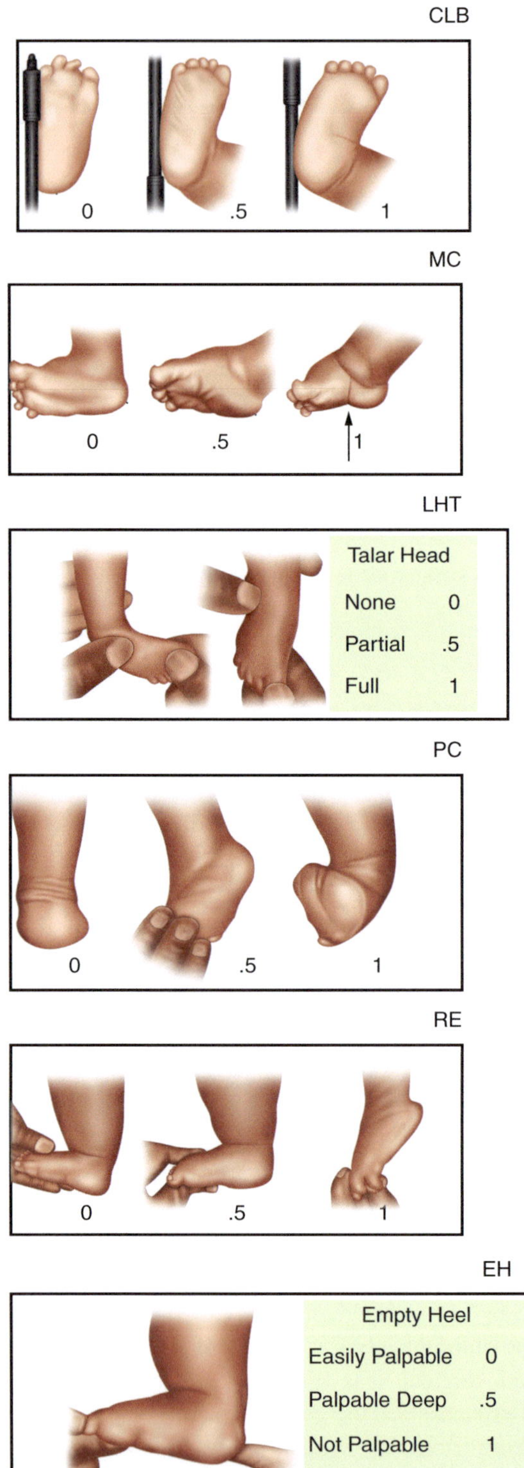

Fig. 12.9 Pirani's schematic classification examples

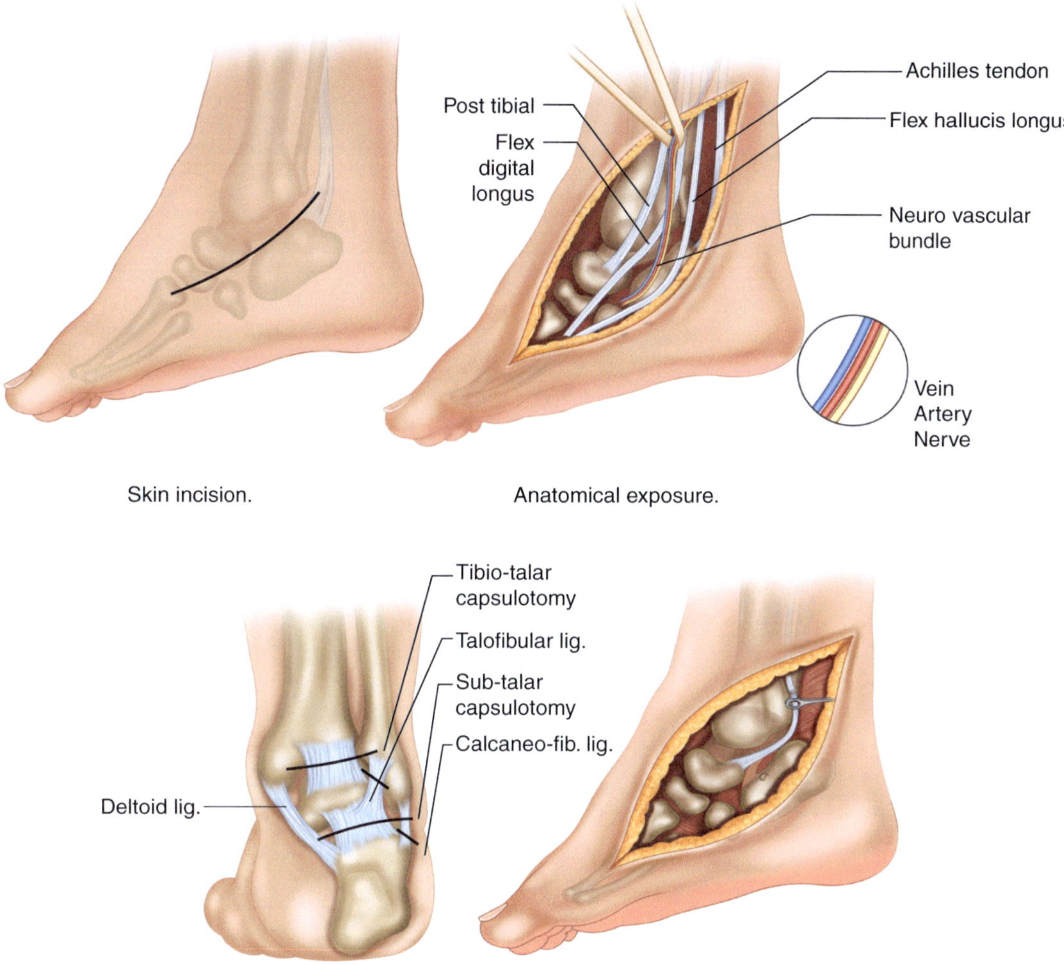

Fig. 12.10 Turco posterior medial approach

for patients with arthrogryposis and spina bifida [75]. Green et al. in 1984 discuss their favorable results of talectomy in children with arthrogryposis multiplex congenita [76]. Chotigavanichaya et al. described primary talectomy in patients with arthrogryposis multiplex congenita [77]. This can be combined with tibial calcaneal fusion and/or calcaneocuboid fusion to help prevent future recurrence of deformities [78]. Shah et al. proposed a treatment algorithm for non-idiopathic clubfeet and suggested that talectomy be considered for the neurogenic and syndromic rigid deformities [79]. El-Sherbini et al. in 2015 reported satisfactory results in 19 feet with severe rigid equinovarus deformities with a minimum of 6.4-year follow-up [80]. Talectomy can be successful for the rigid equinovarus deformity as long as there is complete excision of the talus and the tibial calcaneal axis is optimized by correct alignment (Fig. 12.13).

The French functional method is a form of physiotherapy that was developed in the late 1970s and has been more popular in European countries [81]. The treatment involves daily manipulation and stretching of the medial soft tissues to allow the navicular to move laterally away from the medial malleolus. The manipulation is followed by splintage. The French technique is somewhat labor-intensive, but results of treatment have been favorable [82]. Some authors

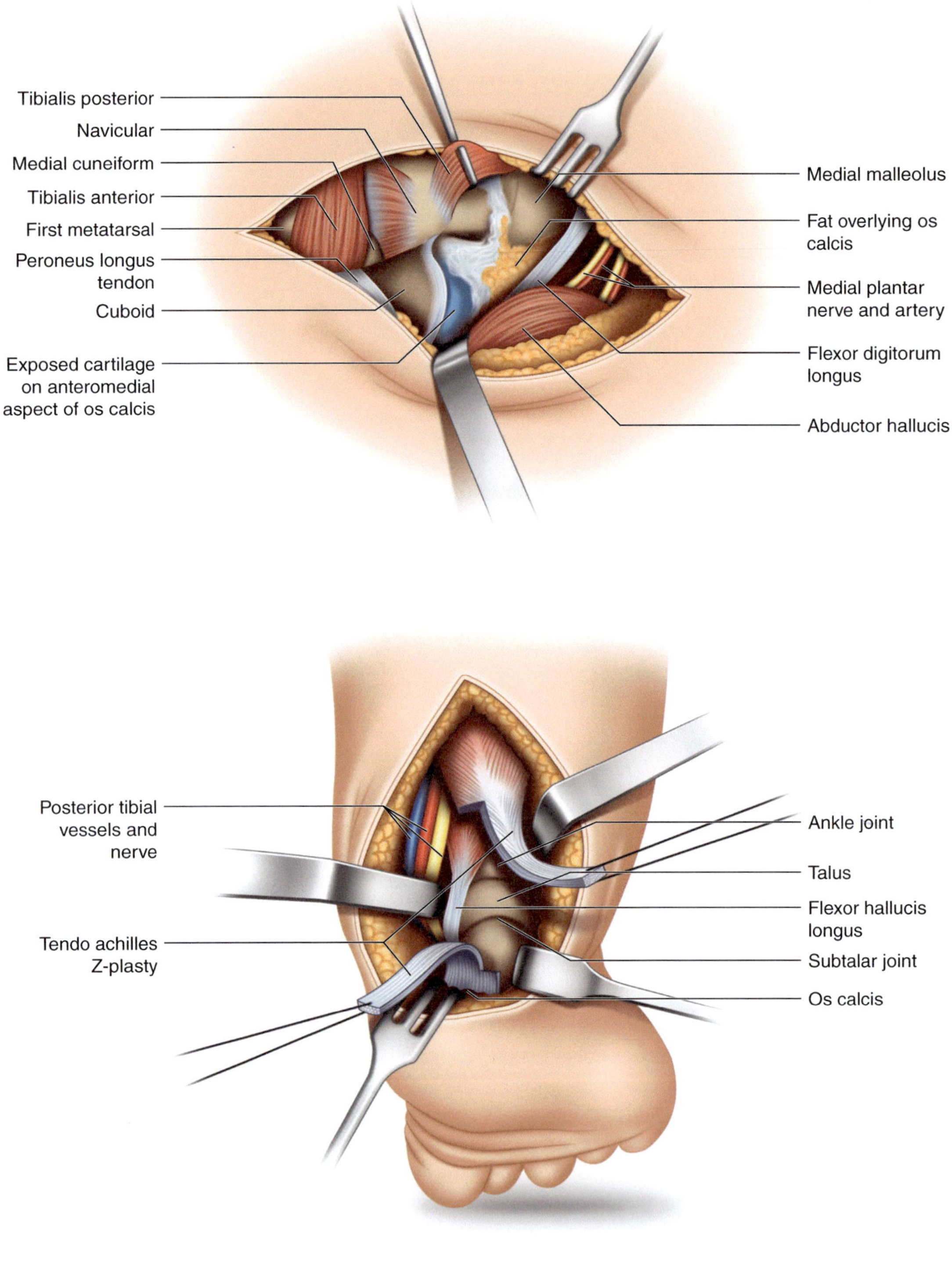

Fig. 12.11 Medial and posterior approaches as advocated by Dr. Carroll

have advocated combing both the French method and Ponseti technique to achieve improved functional motor function [83].

The use of distraction histogenesis (Ilizarov technique) has been reported as being successful in the treatment of pediatric foot deformities [84–86]. The Ilizarov technique has been utilized in the treatment of clubfoot especially in the neglected and recurrent types [87–97]. Ilizarov's principle of "tension stress" demonstrates distracted tissues becoming more metabolically active and regenerative. An alternative form of external fixation for CTEV was reported by Joshi in 1999 [98]. Joshi found his alternative to circular fixation to be easier in application and technique and used non-tensioned K-wires in the

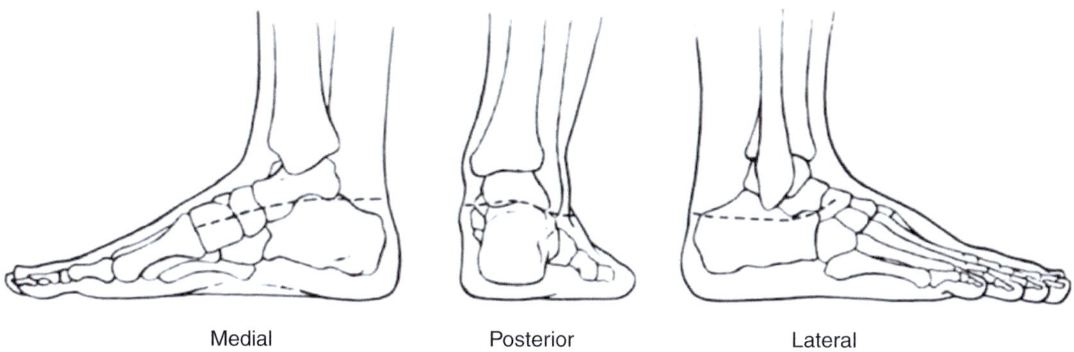

Fig. 12.12 Cincinnati incision

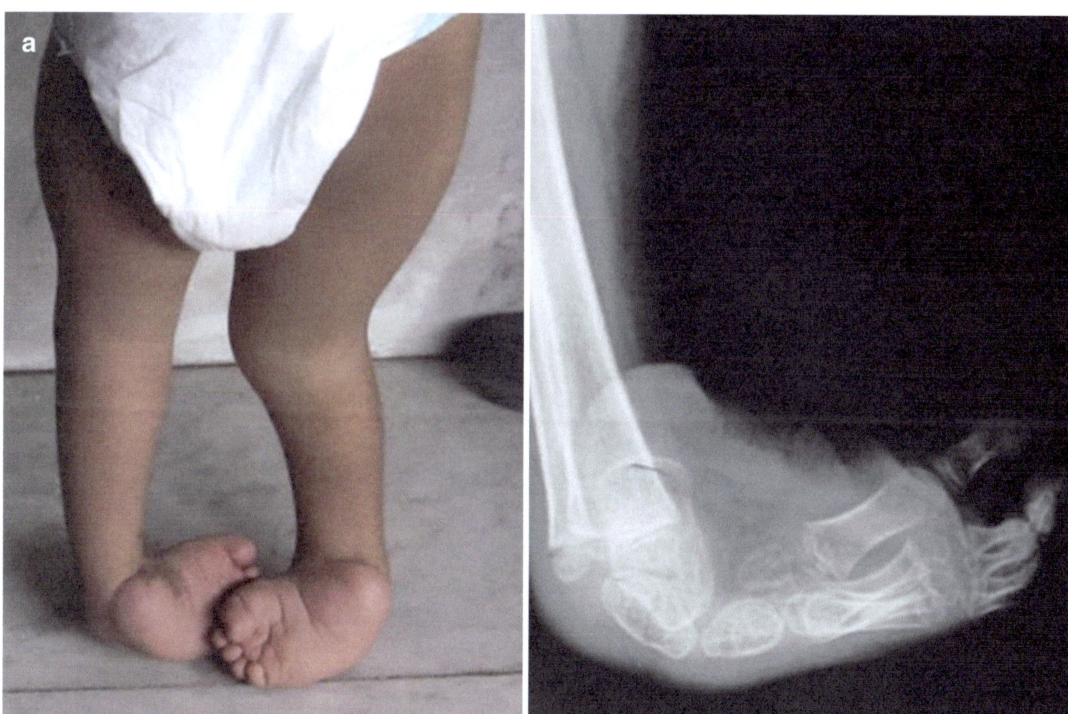

Fig. 12.13 Pre- and post-clinical and radiographic appearance of severe equinovarus foot with talectomy (Reproduced by permission- El- Sherbini). (**a**) Pre-op clinical and radiographic of the right foot. (**b**) Post-operative clinical and radiographic appearance of the right foot

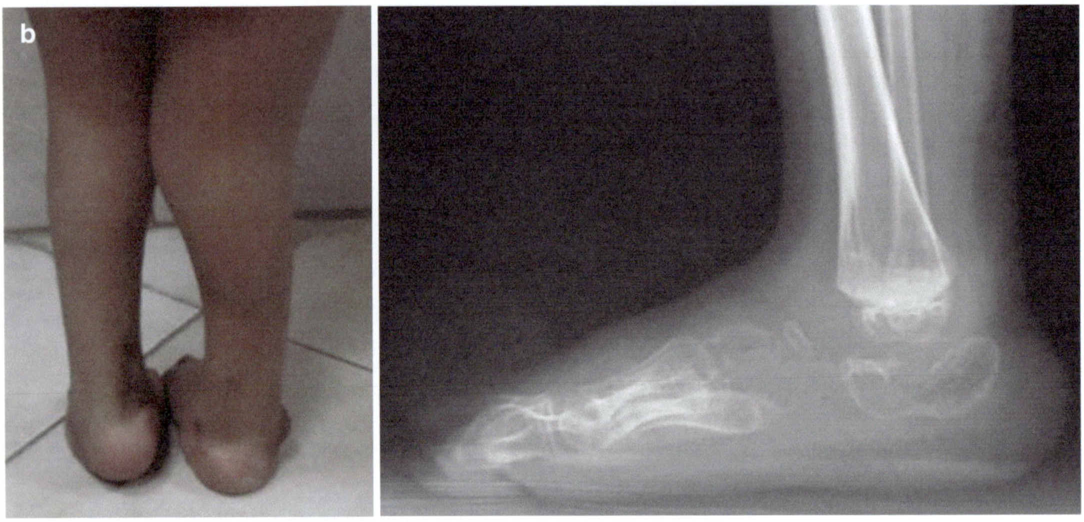

Fig. 12.13 (continued)

tibia, calcaneus, and metatarsals connecting them with rods. Essentially, this created a monolateral form of external fixation for the purpose of distraction and realignment. This technique has favorable results especially when utilized in the recurrent or neglected clubfoot [99–101]. Prem et al. also reported favorable results with Ilizarov distraction in resistant clubfoot [102]. Bradish and Noor, Franke et al., and Barbary et al. reported successful utilization of Ilizarov techniques in adolescent children (approximately 8 years of age) with clubfoot [88, 103, 104]. When the Ilizarov technique is employed, the stabilization of the talus is necessary to prevent external rotation of the talus upon the fibula during correction. Stabilization of the talus is also important as to allow the mechanics of the subtalar joint to facilitate abduction of the anterior process of the calcaneus and subsequent eversion of the heel. This author has successfully employed the use of circular external fixation with both constrained and unconstrained constructs for the treatment of neglected, recurrent, syndromic, and teratologic clubfoot in older children where initial casting was unsuccessful (Fig. 12.14). The method of external fixation used the rotation of the forefoot about the fixed talar pivot point. The use of external distraction histogenesis is an alternative to acute surgical correction techniques as advocated by Dwyer, Evans, and Japas. When these latter methods are performed to offer correction in skeletally immature adolescents, further shortening of the foot, arthrosis, and premature closure of physeal plates are possible outcomes.

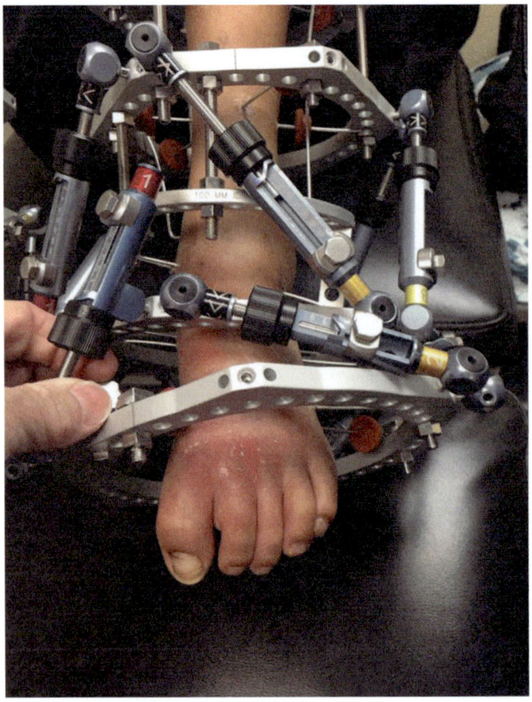

Fig. 12.14 Example of multiplanar frame treatment in neglected 12 y/o male

Delgado reported in 2000 the ability to avoid surgery with the use of botox injections [105]. The use of botulinum toxin has also been reported favorably by Alvarez [106]. This author has used botox in the contracted muscle groups in cases of syndromic and teratologic clubfoot to facilitate manipulation and casting. While this helped facilitate some conditions with castings, those with more rigid contractures went on to be treated with circular external distraction histogenesis.

Ignacio Ponseti (June 03, 1914–October 18, 2009) started his technique of conservative treatment for clubfoot in the 1950s after realizing that surgery left a very scarred and stiff, non-functional foot that often required additional surgeries. He based his concepts on the understanding of foot mechanics initially described by the French anatomist Farabeuf and later by Huson in his dissertation [4, 44]. The main premise of treatment to be understood is that the anterior process of the calcaneus must first abduct before heel eversion can occur. This is accomplished by abducting the forefoot with counterpressure being applied at the lateral aspect of the talar head. Even though Ponseti developed this technique in the 1950s, it did not become popular until the 1990s with the advent of the Internet [107]. Frustrated parents would compare clubfoot treatment results on the Internet yielding a renewed interest in Ponseti technique. Presently, the Ponseti technique is considered the "gold standard" in the treatment of idiopathic clubfoot. There are numerous articles in the current literature that support this technique as the first treatment option for idiopathic clubfoot [108–117]. Ponseti and Smoley reported on their series of 67 patients with 94 clubfeet in 1963 [48]. They had 5–12 years of follow-up and reported 71% good results. Laaveg and Ponseti in 1980 reported on 104 feet in 70 patients yielding good results in 88.7% of the cases [118]. Ponseti in 1992 stated that he had an 89% success rate but a recurrence rate of 50% [119]. At that time he was recommending splinting for only 2 years after his treatment. Later studies would recommend a longer period of splinting (4–5 years) in an attempt to resist the aggressive collagen synthesis up until this age. Recurrence rates would then decrease with improved adherence to the treatment plan and duration of splinting [110]. In 1995 Cooper and Dietz reported on a 30-year follow-up of patients treated with Ponseti technique [120]. They studied 45 patients with 71 clubfeet and found that 78% had good to excellent results. In 2002, Herzenberg reported that his control group of standard serial casting (Kite's method) had 32/34 posterior medial surgical release (PMR) and those treated with Ponseti technique had only 1/34 PMR [121]. In 2006 Dobbs et al. reported on 34 patients who underwent an extensive soft tissue release with a mean follow-up of 30 years. Their results illustrated the poor foot function and decreased quality of life in patients undergoing surgical treatment for the correction of clubfoot [1]. In 2006 at the Pediatric Orthopedic Symposium of North America, Lovell et al. reported on a 50-year follow-up on patients treated for idiopathic clubfoot with Ponseti technique exhibiting satisfactory long-term results and function [122]. Since then there have been many articles in the literature that support the Ponseti technique as the primary method in treating idiopathic clubfoot [61, 72, 115, 123]. Gray et al. in their 2014 Cochrane Review of 14 trials with 607 participants found lower post-treatment Pirani scores in the Ponseti group versus the Kite group [61]. Patients in the Kite group also required more extensive surgery after initial treatment. Additionally, the Ponseti technique is also being utilized in neglected clubfeet in older children [124–128]. With the understanding of foot mechanics and Ponseti's principles, this conservative manipulation technique is being successfully utilized in previously resistant cases such as arthrogryposis [129, 130], in older age groups with neglected clubfoot [124, 127, 128, 131], and even in a reverse Ponseti technique for the treatment of rocker-bottom flatfoot and vertical talus [132].

Treatment Protocols: Ponseti

Ideally the conservative treatment for clubfoot should begin as soon as possible after birth and is best within the first week when the condition is more amenable to manipulation and casting. This also may be due to the practitioner's expertise as some authors advocate treatment after the first 30 days of birth to 3 months [54, 133]. Microscopically, the collagen fibers have a wavy appearance known as crimp. It is the stretching of the collagen and subsequent reappearance of crimp after several days that allow the casting technique to be successful [53]. Additionally, Pirani et al. reported on MRI studies demonstrating that joint adaptation and realignment has occurred after casting [134]. A CT study by Ippolito also confirms realignment [135]. In Ponseti's conservative manipulation treatment protocol, the foot deformities of cavus, adduction, and varus are all treated simultaneously, and the equinus is treated last. The initial cast focuses on the cavus deformity by supinating the forefoot while abducting against counterpressure on the lateral aspect of the talar head (Fig. 12.15). Ponseti identified a common error attempting to get the foot down by pronation. Pronation of the foot is an absolute contraindication that increases the deformity. The forefoot is in varus and any attempt to pronate the forefoot will increase the amount of cavus.

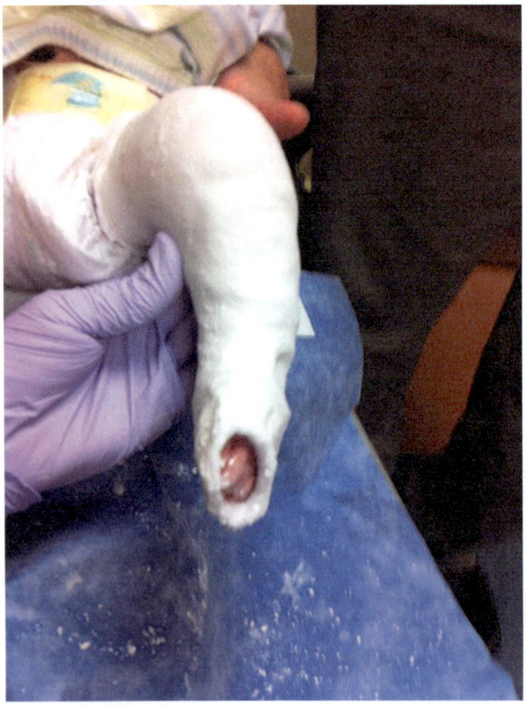

Fig. 12.15 First cast

Subsequent manipulations and casting are continued until the abduction of the foot relative to the leg is approximately 70 degrees. These 70 degrees is a result of motion about the subtalar joint, midtarsal joint, and foot compared to the leg. The average number of treatments to reach this stage is three to six (Figs. 12.16 and 12.17). However, each child is different and manipulations are not stressed or forced to achieve that goal. It sometimes takes more treatment utilizing a gentle stretch to resistance. Gentle manipulations and casting with plaster (Gypsona®) are performed each visit. It is important for the infant to be relaxed and comfortable. Preferably, it is advisable to feed the child during manipulations and casting. It is also desirable to have two people involved in the casting. One person maintains the foot in its corrected position, while the other molds and applies the plaster. The manipulations involve performing Ponseti's maneuver. The thumb of the left hand is against the lateral aspect of the talar head of the baby's right foot and the right hand with full contact along the plantar surface of the foot, abducting the forefoot against the counterpressure of the left thumb (Fig. 12.18). Manipulations and casting are performed to resistance and never forced. Ponseti advocated casting to the groin above the knee in order to be able to abduct the foot around the talus and relative to the lower leg. Additionally, in treating the infant, the long leg cast helps to prevent slippage. Webril® padding is applied from the toes to the knee. Plaster is then applied over the padding while molding the foot and posterior heel. The foot is held in its new position with Ponseti's maneuver while the

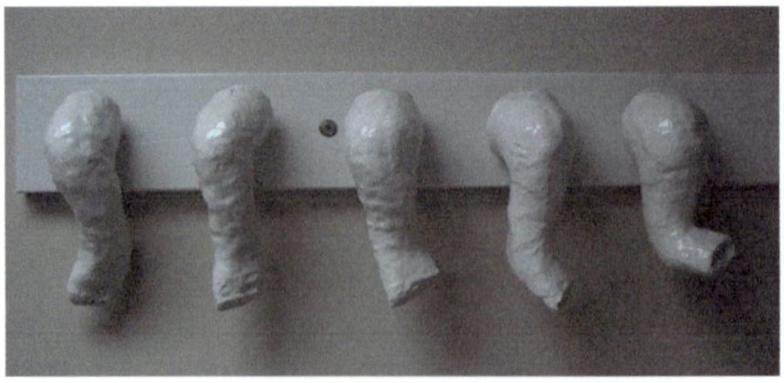

Fig. 12.16 Casting series. Photo by author from Dr. Ponseti's clinic showing typical casting series

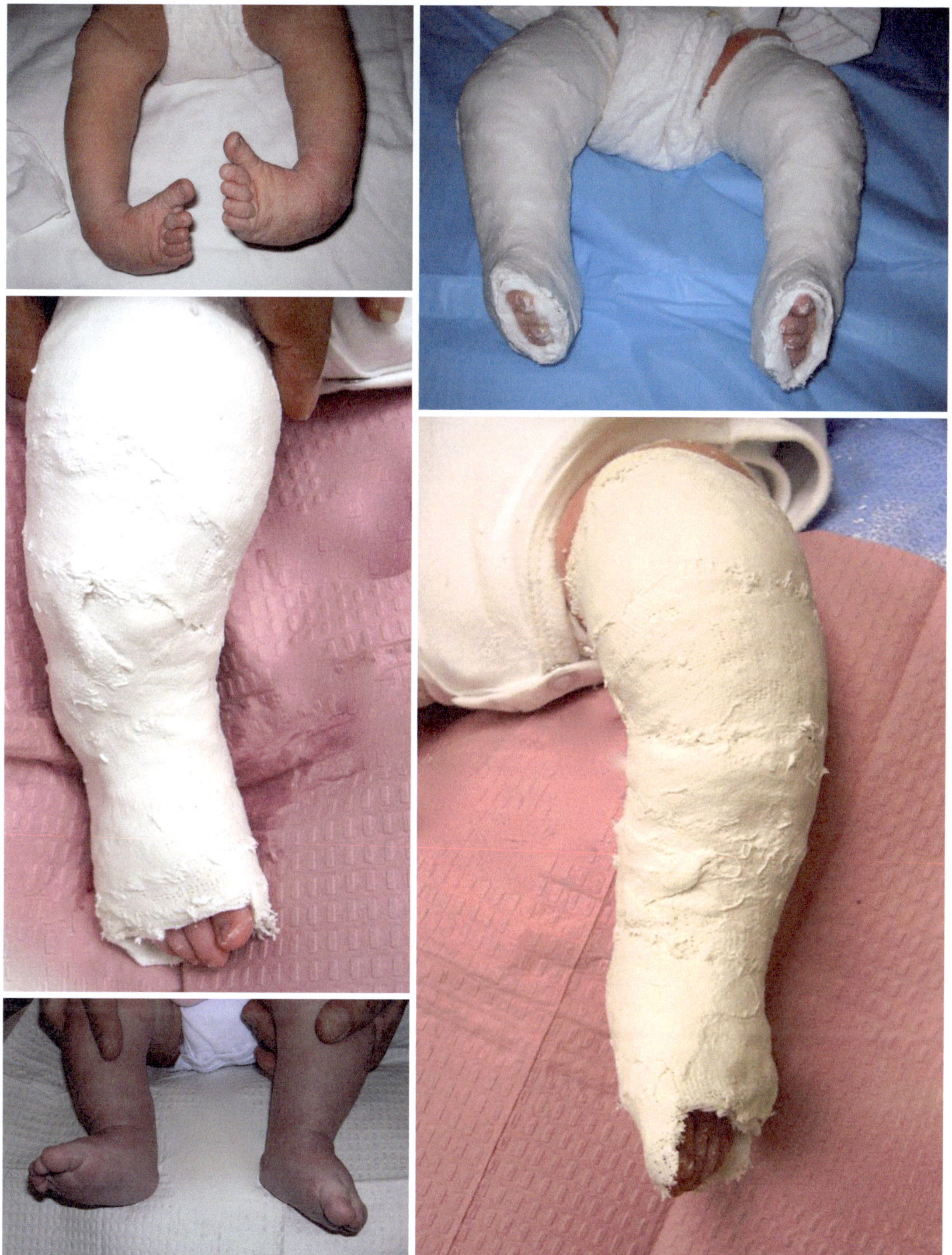

Fig. 12.17 Typical sequence from initial presentation, first cast, and third cast to final presentation

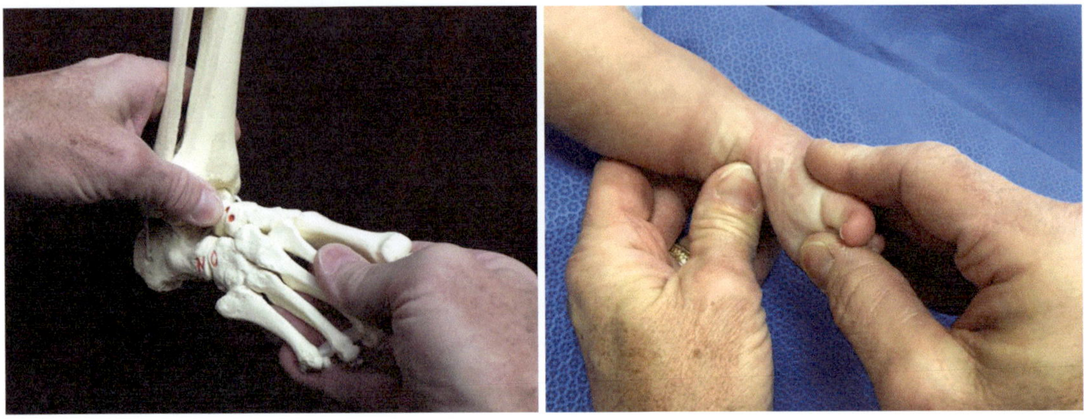

Fig. 12.18 Ponseti's maneuver. Note that the entire plantar surface of the child's foot is in contact with the length of my fingers. I am also supinating the forefoot with abduction against the left thumb pressing against the lateral aspect of the talar head

cast hardens. Care is taken to avoid excessive pressure at the lateral aspect of the talar head that may result in a pressure sore. The plaster is snug on the lower leg and it must be very well molded. Padding is then applied over the proximal portion of the cast to the groin with the knee bent at 90 degrees. The plaster above the knee may be applied with more gentle tension. The toe of the cast is open to visualize vascular status of the digits (Fig. 12.19). An average of six casts are applied with the final ones focusing on the ankle equinus component of the deformity. If resistance is met in correcting the equinus, the decision for a tenotomy of the Achilles tendon is considered. The tenotomy is performed an average of 85–90% of the cases and is a safe procedure for those with the knowledge of the anatomy [136]. It can easily be done in a clinic setting with local anesthetic, thus avoiding a general anesthetic at this age. Grigoriou et al. found that an Achilles tenotomy was as useful as an Achilles tenotomy and posterior capsular release in clubfoot treatment [137]. Therefore, these authors did not recommend a posterior capsular release. Before the procedure a topical anesthetic cream is applied for several hours under occlusion. After a surgical prep, a small subcutaneous wheal of 1% lidocaine plain is created over the Achilles tendon approximately 1 centimeter above the superior aspect of the os calcis. Care is taken to avoid using too much fluid to obscure palpation of the Achilles tendon. Holding the foot in dorsiflexion to create tension on the Achilles tendon, a small stab incision is made with a beaver blade (e.g., #67) adjacent to the tendon. Palpation of the tendon is performed, and it is transected in its entirety such that a noticeable release is felt and heard. After the

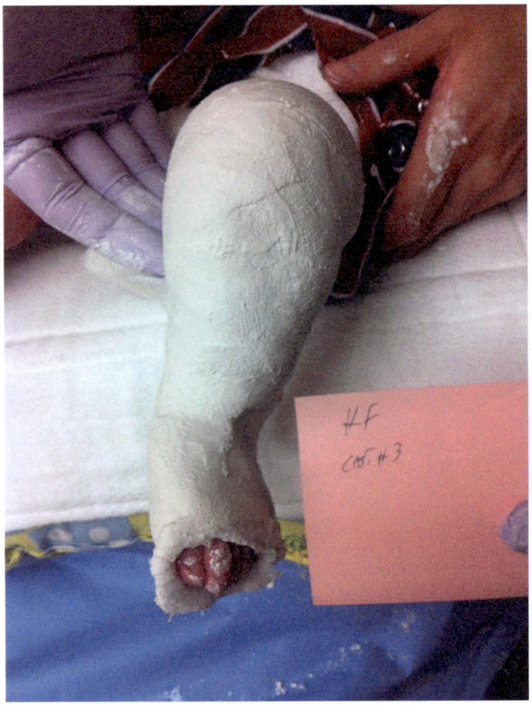

Fig. 12.19 Typical cast appearance

tenotomy, a final cast is applied for 3 weeks. The tendon heals quite readily in this time frame. Ultrasound studies have shown that healing is complete at this time frame [138]. The cast is then removed. And an application of straight lasted shoes on an abduction bar with the amount of abduction set at approximately 70 degrees for the involved foot/feet (Fig. 12.20). Initially, this splint is kept on for 3 months at 23 hours per day. Thereafter, the use of the splint is maintained on for naps and sleeping averaging approximately 16 hours per day. Periodic evaluations every 4 months are made to assess adherence to treatment plan and monitor growth and any chance of recurrence [139]. Later in his career, Ponseti advocated splinting while sleeping until the age of 5 to help reduce the chance of recurrence. Ponseti believed the rapid rate of collagen synthesis beginning at birth contributed to recurrence of the deformity and started to taper down at the age of 5 [4].

Other adjunctive treatment options have been utilized with casting techniques and include the use of the French method, especially after completion of the Ponseti casts, and the use of botulinum toxin as reported by Alvarez.

Relapses

A relapse in the treatment of clubfoot is a partial recurrence of the original deformity usually as a result of premature cessation of treatment [140]. This condition is mostly exhibited by equinus and supination of the foot (Fig. 12.5). Periodic monitoring of the patient after initial treatment (every 3–4 months) is recommended to check for any signs of relapse and proper fit of the shoes and brace. Relapses are infrequent after the age of 5 in part due to the maturity of the collagen fibers. However, it may occur even at the age of 11 as reported by Morcuende [141].

Treatment of a relapsed clubfoot begins with repeat serial casting followed by bracing. If the equinus component is not corrected to 10° dorsiflexion after 4–5 casts in a child less than 4 years of age, then a repeat tenotomy may be necessary [142]. After development of the primary ossification center of the lateral cuneiform and in children over the age of 3, a tibialis anterior tendon transfer may be performed if there is dynamic supination of the foot [143, 144]. The treatment of a recurrent clubfoot by the tibialis anterior tendon transfer is supported by various

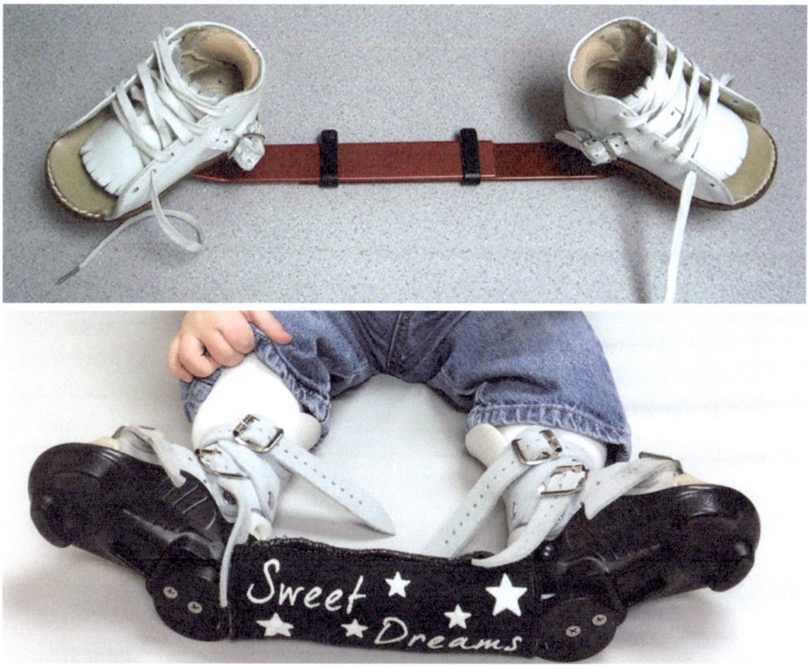

Fig. 12.20 Splinting types

authors [145–147]. Corrective casting is employed initially, in part, to improve the alignment of the foot in order to achieve a better functional transfer of the tibialis anterior due to improved alignment [144]. This technique has been described by Dr. Vincent Mosca in the *Global Health* monograph edited by Dr. Lynn Staheli [53]. The tibialis anterior tendon transfer procedure is performed by a two incisional approach: one is over the insertion of the tendon and the other over the third cuneiform. Incision placement is aided by the use of fluoroscopy. The tendon is carefully freed from its attachment and tagged with 2-0 absorbable suture. It is passed subcutaneously to the lateral incision keeping the superior retinaculum intact (Fig. 12.21). A drill hole is made in the lateral cuneiform, and the tendon is passed through the hole under tension while the foot is held in dorsiflexion. Keith needles are utilized and passed through the bottom of the foot and tied over rolled gauze and sterile button. The above knee cast is applied for 6 weeks to facilitate tenodesis. Usually bracing is not needed afterward.

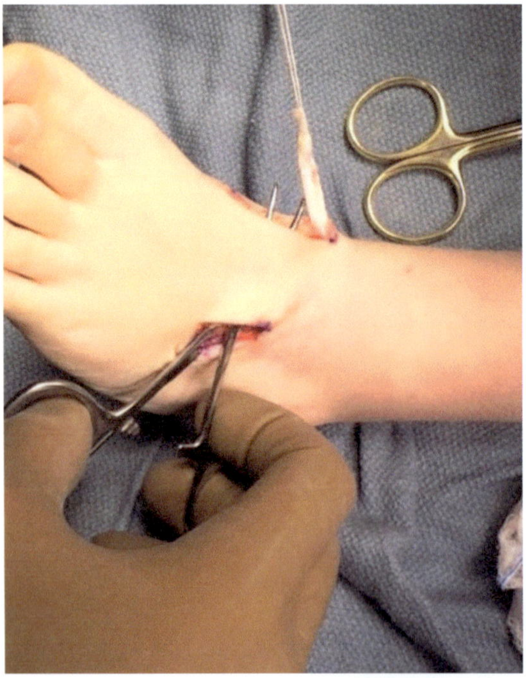

Fig. 12.21 Intra-operative photo of tibialis anterior tendon transfer

Complications

While the Ponseti method is a safe and reliable method for treating idiopathic clubfoot, complications may arise during treatment. Majority of these are usually due to casting errors and include overcorrection, rocker-bottom flatfoot deformity, lateral displacement of the fibula, flattening of the talar dome, and atypical clubfoot [148].

Overcorrection is usually isolated to abduction of the forefoot at Lisfranc's joint. This usually evolves after applying counterpressure along the lateral column of the foot (cuboid) versus the lateral aspect of the talar head.

A rocker-bottom flatfoot (Fig. 12.22) is achieved by early dorsiflexion of the foot relative to the leg before adequate eversion of the heel is achieved. It is also accomplished by dorsiflexing the forefoot alone rather than the entire foot relative to the leg. The example in Fig. 12.22a was treated successfully by a "reverse Ponseti" technique to help realign the talonavicular joint.

Lateral displacement of the fibula occurs when the talus externally rotates within the ankle mortise and usually occurs when the heel is still locked in a varus position. Counterpressure against the lateral aspect of the talar head is important in preventing this complication. A flat talar dome may be seen on a lateral projection radiograph and is usually due to excessive external rotation of the foot to the lower leg.

The atypical clubfoot is an entity that may include clubfoot associated with other conditions that may make it more difficult to treat. These include syndromic, teratologic, and neurogenic conditions. A unique, atypical clubfoot that occurs during the casting process in otherwise normal children is called complex or resistant clubfoot [149]. This foot type is usually increased in girth and has a pronounced equinus component to it both at the ankle and the forefoot. This results in a plantarflexed first ray giving the hallux a shorter appearance. The complex clubfoot is stiffer foot and also presents with a central crease in the arch (Fig. 12.6). The metatarsals are plantarflexed in addition to the heel. Any attempt at reducing heel varus in the usual fashion will lead to hyperabduction of the metatarsals. There are various theories

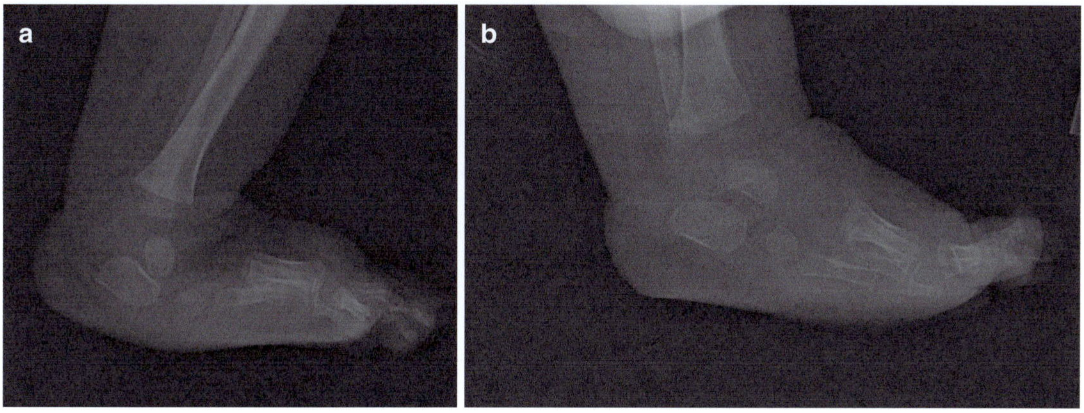

Fig. 12.22 Example of rocker-bottom foot. (**a**) Pre-treatment. (**b**) Post-treatment (reverse Ponseti)

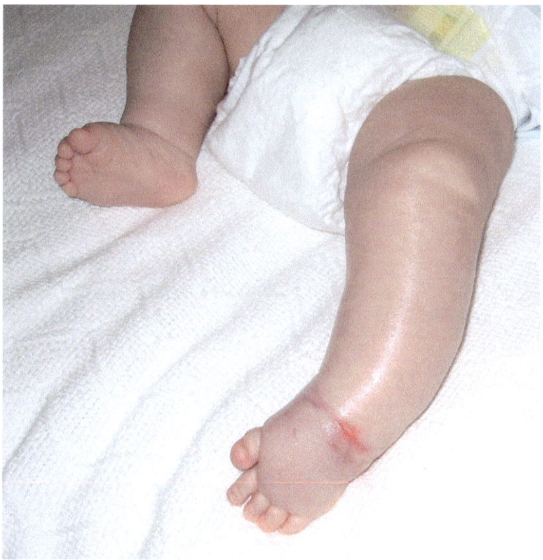

Fig. 12.23 Complex clubfoot appearance. Note increased girth, hyperemia, and taut skin along with short appearing hallux

regarding the etiology of atypical clubfoot ranging from error in treatment to a sympathetic-mediated response during treatment (Fig. 12.23). While chronic regional pain syndromes have been reported in pediatrics, this has not been well documented in infants [150]. The complex clubfoot is a condition that occurs during treatment of clubfoot and not at the onset. An initial sign of concern to the practitioner is when the toes appear to be retracting within the cast (Fig. 12.24). The treatment for complex clubfoot is modified to address the unique nature of the deformity. After applying

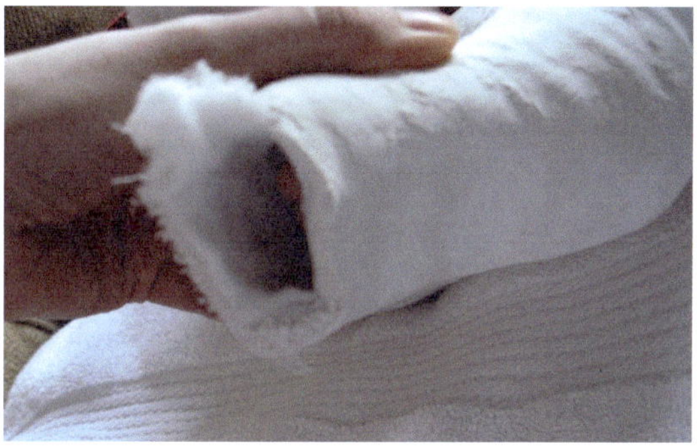

Fig. 12.24 Toes appear retracted in cast

standard Ponseti technique and getting the foot to approximately 30 degrees of external rotation, attention is directed to address the equinus component. The clinician's thumbs are pressed along the first and fifth metatarsals, while the index fingers are on the head of the talus. The cavus and the equinus components are addressed simultaneously . A tenotomy of the Achilles tendon in these cases is most always necessary.

Summary

While the Ponseti technique is presently considered the "gold standard" for the treatment of idiopathic clubfoot, there are still some conditions that may be resistant to this method and may require surgical intervention. Most recently, Wright stated: "The Ponseti protocol has completely changed the treatment of clubfoot with results so obviously superior to extensive surgical release that a randomized controlled trial would not be appropriate." *[72]* Ponseti stated in his book on *Congenital Clubfoot: Fundamentals of Treatment*: "a well conducted orthopedic treatment based upon a sound understanding of the functional anatomy of the foot and on the biologic response of young connective tissue and bone to the changes in direction of mechanical stimuli, can gradually reduce or almost eliminate these deformities in most clubfeet."

References

1. Dobbs MB, Nunley R, Schoenecker PL. Long-term follow up of patients with clubfeet treated with extensive soft tissue release. JBJS. 2006;88-A:986–96.
2. Wynne DR. Family study and the cause of clubfoot. J Bone Joint Surg. 1964;46:445–63.
3. Cartlidge I. Observations on the epidemiology of club foot in Polynesian and Caucasian populations. J Med Genet. 1984;21:290–2.
4. Ponseti IV. Congenital clubfoot: fundamentals of treatment. Oxford: Oxford University Press, USA; 1996.
5. Ponseti I, Staheli LT. Clubfoot: ponseti management. Seattle: Global-HELP; 2005.
6. Burgan HE, Furness ME, Foster BK. Prenatal ultrasound diagnosis of clubfoot. J Pediatr Orthop. 1999;19:11–3.
7. Keret D, Ezra E, Lokiec F, Hayek S, Segev E, Wientroub S. Efficacy of prenatal ultrasonography in confirmed club foot. J Bone Joint Surg Br. 2002;84:1015–9.
8. Aurell Y, Johansson A, Hansson G, Jonsson K. Ultrasound anatomy in the neonatal clubfoot. Eur Radiol. 2002;12:2509–17.
9. Silvani S, DeValentine SJ, Karlin JM, SBL. Moebius syndrome and TEV. JAPA. 1981;71:604–6.
10. Purushothamdas S, Rayan F, Gayner A. Correction of neglected clubfoot deformity in children with Moebius syndrome. J Pediatr Orthop B/Eur Paediatr Orthop Soc N Am. 2009;18:73–5.
11. Böhm M. The embryologic origin of club-foot. J Bone Joint Surg Am. 1929;11:229–59.
12. Irani RN, Sherman MS. The pathological anatomy of club foot. J Bone Joint Surg Am. 1963;45:45–52.
13. Tachdjian MO. The child's foot. Philadelphia: Saunders; 1985.
14. Greider TD, Siff SJ, Gerson P, Donovan MM. Arteriography in club foot. J Bone Joint Surg Am. 1982;64:837–40.
15. Isaacs H, Handelsman JE, Badenhorst M, Pickering A. The muscles in club foot--a histological histochemical and electron microscopic study. J Bone Joint Surg Br. 1977;59-B:465–72.
16. Adams F. The genuine works of Hippocrates. Baltimore: Williams & Wilkins; 1939.
17. Browne D. Congenital deformities of mechanical origin. Br Med J. 1936;1:1182.
18. Dunn PM. Sir Denis Browne (1892–1967) and congenital deformities of mechanical origin. Arch Dis Child Fetal Neonatal Ed. 2005;90:F88–91.
19. Tabor A, Alfirevic Z. Update on procedure-related risks for prenatal diagnosis techniques. Fetal Diagn Ther. 2010;27:1–7.
20. Farrell SA, Summers AM, Dallaire L, Singer J, Johnson J-AM, Wilson RD. Club foot, an adverse outcome of early amniocentesis: disruption or deformation? J Med Genet. 1999;36:843–6.
21. Yazdy MM, Mitchell AA, Louik C, Werler MM. Use of selective serotonin-reuptake inhibitors during pregnancy and the risk of clubfoot. Epidemiology. 2014;25:859–65.
22. Bacino CA, Hecht JT. Etiopathogenesis of equinovarus foot malformations. Eur J Med Genet. 2014;57:473–9.
23. Ippolito E, Ponseti IV. Congenital club foot in the human fetus. A histological study. J Bone Joint Surg Am. 1980;62:8–22.
24. Ponseti IV, Campos J. Observations on pathogenesis and treatment of congenital clubfoot. Clin Orthop Relat Res. 1972;84:50–60.
25. Fukuhara K, Schollmeier G, Uhthoff HK. The pathogenesis of clubfoot. A histomorphometric and immunohistochemical study of fetuses. J Bone Joint Surg Br. 1994;76:450–7.
26. Sano H, Uhthoff HK, Jarvis JG, Mansingh A, Wenckebach GF. Pathogenesis of soft-tissue contracture in club foot. J Bone Joint Surg Br. 1998;80:641–4.
27. Klein D. Genetics of clubfoot. J Genet Hum. 1964;13:385–6.
28. Cowell HRWBK. Current concepts review: genetic aspects of club foot. J Bone Joint Surg. 1980;62-A:1381–4.
29. Chapman C, Stott NS, Port RV, Nicol RO. Genetics of club foot in Maori and Pacific people. J Med Genet. 2000;37:680–3.
30. Wang JH, Palmer RM, Chung CS. The role of major gene in clubfoot. Am J Hum Genet. 1988;42:772–6.
31. Dietz F. The genetics of idiopathic clubfoot. Clin Orthop Relat Res. 2002;401:39–48.
32. Dobbs MB. Clubfoot: etiology and treatment: editorial comment. Clin Orthop Relat Res. 2009;467:1119–20.
33. Idelberger K. Die ergebnisse der zwillingsforschung beim angeborenen klumpfuss. Verh Dtsch Orthop Ges. 1939;33:272.
34. Gurnett CA, Alaee F, Kruse LM, Desruisseau DM, Hecht JT, Wise CA, Bowcock AM, Dobbs MB. Asymmetric lower-limb malformations in individuals with homeobox PITX1 gene mutation. Am J Hum Genet. 2008;83:616–22.
35. Dobbs MB, Gurnett CA. Update on clubfoot: etiology and treatment. Clin Orthop Relat Res. 2009;467:1146–53.

36. Wynne-Davies R, Littlejohn A, Gormley J. Aetiology and interrelationship of some common skeletal deformities. (Talipes equinovarus and calcaneovalgus, metatarsus varus, congenital dislocation of the hip, and infantile idiopathic scoliosis). J Med Genet. 1982;19:321–8.
37. Scarpa A. Memoria chirurgica sui piedi torti congeniti dei fanciulli e sulla maniera di correggere questa deformita, di Antonio Scarpa. G. Comini; 1803.
38. Ippolito E. Update on pathologic anatomy of clubfoot. J Pediatr Orthop B. 1995;4:17–24.
39. Carroll NC. Pathoanatomy of congenital clubfoot. In: Symposium on pediatric clubfoot; 1978. p. 225–32.
40. Herzenberg JE, Carroll NC, Christofersen MR, Lee EH, White S, Munroe R. Clubfoot analysis with three-dimensional computer modeling. J Pediatr Orthop. 1988;8:257.
41. Ponseti IV. Personal communication. 2003.
42. Farabeauf LH. Precis de Manuel Operatoire par L. H. Farabeuf. 4th ed. Paris: Masson; 1893.
43. Huson A. Een Ontleedkundig-functioneel Onderzoek Van de Voetwortel: (An anatomic and functional study of the tarsus). Leiden: Leiden University; 1961.
44. Dobbs MB, Morcuende JA, Gurnett CA, Ponseti IV. Treatment of idiopathic clubfoot: an historical review. Iowa Orthop J. 2000;20:59–64.
45. Manter JT. Movements of the subtalar and transverse tarsal joints. Anat Rec. 1941;80:397–410.
46. Hicks JH. The mechanics of the foot. I. The joints. J Anat. 1953;87:345–57.
47. Sarrafian SK. Biomechanics of the subtalar joint complex. Clin Orthop Relat Res. 1993;(290):17–26.
48. Ponseti IV, Smoley EN. Congenital club Foot: the results of treatment. J Bone Joint Surg. 1963;45:261–344.
49. Irani RN, Sherman MS. The pathological anatomy of idiopathic clubfoot. Clin Orthop Relat Res. 1972;84:14–20.
50. Cosma D, Vasilescu DE. A clinical evaluation of the Pirani and Dimeglio idiopathic clubfoot classifications. J Foot Ankle Surg. 2015;54:582–5.
51. Diméglio A, Bensahel H, Souchet P, Mazeau P, Bonnet F. Classification of clubfoot. J Pediatr Orthop B. 1995;4:129–36.
52. Pirani S, Hodges D, Sekeramayi F. A reliable & valid method of assessing the amount of deformity in the congenital clubfoot deformity. J Bone Joint Surg Br. 2008;90-B:53.
53. Clubfoot SL. Ponseti management. Seattle: Global HELP Organization; 2009.
54. Zionts LE. What's new in idiopathic clubfoot? J Pediatr Orthop. 2015;35:547–50.
55. Lampasi M, Abati CN, Stilli S, Trisolino G. Use of the Pirani score in monitoring progression of correction and in guiding indications for tenotomy in the Ponseti method: are we coming to the same decisions? J Orthop Surg. 2017;25:2309499017713916.
56. Jones R. Discussion on the treatment of club-foot. Br Med J. 1909;2:1065–71.
57. Kite JH. Non-operative treatment of con- genital clubfeet: a review of one hundred cases*. South Med J. 1930;23:337–44.
58. Kite JH. Principles involved in the treatment of congenital club-foot. 1939. Clin Orthop Relat Res. 1972;84:4–8.
59. Sud A, Tiwari A, Sharma D, Kapoor S. Ponseti's vs. Kite's method in the treatment of clubfoot – a prospective randomised study. Int Orthop. 2008;32:409–13.
60. Rijal R, Shrestha B, Singh G, Singh M, Nepal P, Khanal G, Rai P. Comparison of Ponseti and Kite's method of treatment for idiopathic clubfoot. Indian J Orthop. 2010;44:202.
61. Gray K, Pacey V, Gibbons P, Little D, Frost C, Burns J. Interventions for congenital talipes equinovarus (clubfoot). Cochrane Database Syst Rev. 2012;4:CD008602.
62. Codivilla A. Sulla Cura del piede equino varo congenito. Arch Ortop. 1906;23:245–56.
63. Sanzarello I, Nanni M, Faldini C. The clubfoot over the centuries. J Pediatr Orthop B. 2017;26:143–51.
64. Turco VJ. Surgical correction of the resistant club foot. One-stage posteromedial release with internal fixation: a preliminary report. J Bone Joint Surg Am. 1971;53:477–97.
65. Turco VJ. Resistant congenital clubfoot- one stage posteriomedial release with internal fixation. J Bone Joint Surg. 1979;61:805–14.
66. Carroll NC, Gross RH. Operative management of clubfoot. Orthopedics. 1990;13:1285–96.
67. Carroll NC. Surgical technique for talipes equinovarus. Oper Tech Orthop. 1993;3:115–20.
68. Crawford AH, Marxen JL, Osterfeld DL. The Cincinnati incision: a comprehensive approach for surgical procedures of the foot and ankle in childhood. J Bone Joint Surg Am. 1982;64:1355–8.
69. Mahapatra S, Abraham VT. A comparative analysis of the two most common surgical exposures for clubfoot. Int Surg J. 2016;3:1283–6.
70. van Gelder JH, van Ruiten AG, Visser JD, Maathuis PG. Long-term results of the posteromedial release in the treatment of idiopathic clubfoot. J Pediatr Orthop. 2010;30:700–4.
71. Alkar F, Louahem D, Bonnet F, Patte K, Delpont M, Cottalorda J. Long-term results after extensive soft tissue release in very severe congenital clubfeet. J Pediatr Orthop. 2017;37:500–3.
72. Wright JG. Commentary on articles by Kelly A. Jeans, MS, et al.: "Functional outcomes following treatment for clubfoot. Ten-year follow-up," and Bibek Banskota, MRCS, MS, et al.: "Outcomes of the Ponseti method for untreated clubfeet in Nepalese patients seen between the ages of one and five years and followed for at least 10 years.". J Bone Joint Surg Am. 2018;100:e149.
73. Zionts LE, Sangiorgio SN, Ebramzadeh E, Morcuende JA. The current management of idiopathic clubfoot revisited: results of a survey of the POSNA Membership. J Pediatr Orthop. 2012;32:515.

74. Švehlík M, Floh U, Steinwender G, Sperl M, Novak M, Kraus T. Ponseti method is superior to surgical treatment in clubfoot – long-term, randomized, prospective trial. Gait Posture. 2017;58:346–51.
75. Menelaus MB. Talectomy for equinovarus deformity in arthrogryposis and spina bifida. J Bone Joint Surg Br. 1971;53:468–73.
76. Green AD, Fixsen JA, Lloyd-Roberts GC. Talectomy for arthrogryposis multiplex congenita. J Bone Joint Surg Br. 1984;66-B:697–9.
77. Chotigavanichaya C, Ariyawatkul T, Eamsobhana P, Kaewpornsawan K. Results of primary talectomy for clubfoot in infants and toddlers with arthrogryposis multiplex congenita. J Med Assoc Thail. 2015;98:S38–41.
78. Nicomedez FPI, Li YH, Leong JCY. Tibiocalcaneal fusion after talectomy in arthrogrypotic patients. J Pediatr Orthop. 2003;23:654–7.
79. Shah IP, Crawford AH, Tamai J, Parikh SN. Management of non-idiopathic clubfeet. Int J Paediatr Orthop. 2016;2:27–32.
80. El-Sherbini MH, Omran AA. Midterm follow-up of talectomy for severe rigid equinovarus feet. J Foot Ankle Surg. 2015;54:1093–8.
81. Faulks S, Richards BS. Clubfoot treatment: Ponseti and French functional methods are equally effective. Clin Orthop Relat Res. 2009;467:1278–82.
82. Dimeglio A, Canavese F. The French functional physical therapy method for the treatment of congenital clubfoot. J Pediatr Orthop B. 2012;21:28–39.
83. Zapata KA, Karol LA, Jeans KA, Jo C-H. Gross motor function at 10 years of age in children with clubfoot following the French physical therapy method and the Ponseti technique. J Pediatr Orthop. 2018;38:e519–23.
84. Paley D, Foot N, Correction D. Principles of foot deformity correction: Ilizarov technique. In: Gould JS, editor. Operative foot surgery. Philadelphia: WB Saunders; 1994. p. 476–514.
85. Reinker KA, Carpenter CT. Ilizarov applications in the pediatric foot. J Pediatr Orthop. 1997;17:796–802.
86. Lamm BM, Standard SL, Galley IJ, Herzenberg JE, Paley D. External fixation for the foot and ankle in children. Clin Podiatr Med Surg. 2006;23:137–66.
87. Grill F, Franke J. The Ilizarov distractor for the correction of relapsed or neglected clubfoot. J Bone Joint Surg Br. 1987;69:593–7.
88. Franke J, Grill F, Hein G, Simon M. Correction of clubfoot relapse using Ilizarov's apparatus in children 8-15 years old. Arch Orthop Trauma Surg. 1990;110:33–7.
89. de la Huerta F. Correction of the neglected clubfoot by the Ilizarov method. Clin Orthop Relat Res. 1994;(301):89–93.
90. Wallender H, Hansson GTB. Correction of persistent clubfoot deformities with the Ilizarov external fixator. Acta Orthop Scand. 1996;67:283–7.
91. Choi IH, Yang MS, Chung CY, Cho TJ, Sohn YJ. The treatment of recurrent arthrogrypotic club foot in children by the Ilizarov method. A preliminary report. J Bone Joint Surg Br. 2001;83:731–7.
92. Hosny GA. Correction of foot deformities by the Ilizarov method without corrective osteotomies or soft tissue release. J Pediatr Orthop B/Eur Paediatr Orthop Soc Pediatr Orthop Soc N Am. 2002;11:121–8.
93. Utukuri MM, Ramachandran M, Hartley J, Hill RA. Patient-based outcomes after Ilizarov surgery in resistant clubfeet. J Pediatr Orthop B/Eur Paediatr Orthop Soc Pediatr Orthop Soc N Am. 2006;15:278–84.
94. Burns JK, Sullivan R. Correction of severe residual clubfoot deformity in adolescents with the Ilizarov technique. Foot Ankle Clin. 2004;9:571–82.
95. Ferreira RC, Costa MT, Frizzo GG, Santin RAL. Correction of severe recurrent clubfoot using a simplified setting of the Ilizarov device. Foot Ankle Int. 2007;28:557–68.
96. Peterson HA. The Ilizarov method for the treatment of resistant clubfoot: is it an effective solution? Yearbook Orthop. 2007;2007:52–3.
97. Kocaoğlu M, Eralp L, Atalar AC, Bilen FE. Correction of complex foot deformities using the Ilizarov external fixator. J Foot Ankle Surg. 2002;41:30–9.
98. Joshi BB, Laud NS, Warrier S, Kanaji BG. Treatment of CTEV by Joshi's external stabilization system (JESS). Textbook of orthopaedics and trauma. 1st ed. New Delhi: Jaypee Brothers Medical Publishers; 1999.
99. Suresh S, Ahmed A, Sharma VK. Role of Joshi's external stabilisation system fixator in the management of idiopathic clubfoot. J Orthop Surg. 2003;11:194–201.
100. Anwar MH. Short term results of Correction of CTEV with JESS Distractor. J Orthopaedics. 2004;1(1):e3. http://www.jortho.org/2004/1/1/e3&&.
101. Manjappa CN. Joshi's External Stabilization System (JESS) application for correction of resistant clubfoot. Internet J Orthop Surg. 2010;18. https://doi.org/10.5580/1408.
102. Prem H, Zenios M, Farrell R, Day JB. Soft tissue Ilizarov correction of congenital talipes equinovarus--5 to 10 years postsurgery. J Pediatr Orthop. 2007;27:220–4.
103. Bradish CF, Noor S. The Ilizarov method in the management of relapsed club feet. J Bone Joint Surg Br. 2000;82:387–91.
104. El Barbary H, Abdel Ghani H, Hegazy M. Correction of relapsed or neglected clubfoot using a simple Ilizarov frame. Int Orthop. 2004;28:183–6.
105. Delgado MR, Wilson H, Johnston C, Richards S, Karol L. A preliminary report of the use of botulinum toxin type A in infants with clubfoot: four case studies. J Pediatr Orthop. 2000;20:533–8.
106. Alvarez CM, De Vera MA, Chhina H, Williams L, Durlacher K, Kaga S. The use of botulinum type A toxin in the treatment of idiopathic clubfoot: 5-year follow-up. J Pediatr Orthop. 2009;29:570–5.

107. Morcuende JA, Egbert M, Ponseti IV. The effect of the internet in the treatment of congenital idiopathic clubfoot. Iowa Orthop J. 2003;23:83–6.
108. Doherty R. Long term follow up. BMJ Br Med J. 1999;318:233.
109. Colburn M, Williams M. Evaluation of the treatment of idiopathic clubfoot by using the Ponseti method. J Foot Ankle Surg. 2003;42:259–67.
110. Morcuende JA, Dolan LA, Dietz FR, Ponseti IV. Radical reduction in the rate of extensive corrective surgery for clubfoot using the Ponseti method. Pediatrics. 2004;113:376–80.
111. Zwick EB, Kraus T, Maizen C, Steinwender G, Linhart WE. Comparison of Ponseti versus surgical treatment for idiopathic clubfoot: a short-term preliminary report. Clin Orthop Relat Res. 2009;467:2668–76.
112. Clarke NMP, Uglow MG, Valentine KM. Comparison of Ponseti versus surgical treatment in congenital talipes equinovarus. J Foot Ankle Surg. 2011;50:529–34.
113. Zionts LE, Zhao G, Hitchcock K, Maewal J, Ebramzadeh E. Has the rate of extensive surgery to treat idiopathic clubfoot declined in the United States? J Bone Joint Surg Am. 2010;92:882. https://doi.org/10.2106/JBJS.I.00819.
114. Halanski MA, Davison JE, Huang J-C, Walker CG, Walsh SJ, Crawford HA. Ponseti method compared with surgical treatment of clubfoot: a prospective comparison. J Bone Joint Surg Am. 2010;92:270–8.
115. Lykissas MG, Crawford AH, Eismann EA, Tamai J. Ponseti method compared with soft-tissue release for the management of clubfoot: a meta-analysis study. World J Orthop. 2013;4:144–53.
116. Mayne AIW, Bidwai AS, Beirne P, Garg NK, Bruce CE. The effect of a dedicated Ponseti service on the outcome of idiopathic clubfoot treatment. Bone Joint J. 2014;96:1424–6.
117. Ganesan B, Luximon A, Al-Jumaily A, Balasankar SK, Naik GR. Ponseti method in the management of clubfoot under 2 years of age: a systematic review. PLoS One. 2017;12:e0178299.
118. Laaveg SJ, Ponseti IV. Long-term results of treatment of congenital club foot. J Bone Joint Surg Am. 1980;62:23–31.
119. Ponseti IV. Treatment of congenital club foot. J Bone Joint Surg Am. 1992;74:448–54.
120. Cooper DM, Dietz FR. Treatment of idiopathic clubfoot. A thirty-year follow-up note. J Bone Joint Surg Am. 1995;77:1477–89.
121. Herzenberg JE, Radler C, Bor N. Ponseti versus traditional methods of casting for idiopathic clubfoot. J Pediatr Orthop. 2002;22:517–21.
122. Lovell ME, Oji DE, Dolan LA, Ponseti IV. Others Health and function of patients with treated idiopathic clubfeet: 50 year follow-up study. Annual meeting of the Pediatric Orthopedic Society of North America. San Diego: 2006.
123. Jowett CR, Morcuende JA, Ramachandran M. Management of congenital talipes equinovarus using the Ponseti method: a systematic review. J Bone Joint Surg Br. 2011;93B:1160–4.
124. Banskota B, Banskota AK, Regmi R, Rajbhandary T, Shrestha OP, Spiegel DA. The Ponseti method in the treatment of children with idiopathic clubfoot presenting between five and ten years of age. Bone Joint J. 2013;95-B:1721–5.
125. Aroojis A, Pirani S, Banskota B, Banskota AK, Spiegel DA. Clubfoot etiology, pathoanatomy, basic Ponseti technique, and Ponseti in older patients. In: Global orthopedics. New York: Springer Science+Business Media; 2014. p. 357–68.
126. Faizan M, Jilani LZ, Abbas M, Zahid M, Asif N. Management of idiopathic clubfoot by Ponseti technique in children presenting after one year of age. J Foot Ankle Surg. 2015;54:967–72.
127. Digge V, Desai J, Das S. Expanded age indication for Ponseti method for correction of congenital idiopathic talipes equinovarus: a systematic review. J Foot Ankle Surg. 2018;57:155–8.
128. van Praag VM, Lysenko M, Harvey B, Yankanah R, Wright JG. Casting is effective for recurrence following Ponseti treatment of clubfoot. J Bone Joint Surg Am. 2018;100:1001–8.
129. Morcuende JA, Dobbs MB, Frick SL. Results of the Ponseti method in patients with clubfoot associated with arthrogryposis. Iowa Orthop J. 2008;28:22–6.
130. Kowalczyk B, Felus J. Ponseti casting and Achilles release versus classic casting and soft tissue releases for the initial treatment of arthrogrypotic clubfeet. Foot Ankle Int. 2015;36:1072–7.
131. Lourenço AF, Morcuende JA. Correction of neglected idiopathic club foot by the Ponseti method. J Bone Joint Surg Br. 2007;89:378–81.
132. Dobbs MB, Purcell DB, Nunley R, Morcuende JA. Early results of a new method of treatment for idiopathic congenital vertical talus. J Bone Joint Surg Am. 2006;88:1192–200.
133. Liu Y-B, Li S-J, Zhao L, Yu B, Zhao D-H. Timing for Ponseti clubfoot management: does the age matter? 90 children (131 feet) with a mean follow-up of 5 years. Acta Orthop. 2018;89:662–7.
134. Pirani S, Zeznik L, Hodges D. Magnetic resonance imaging study of the congenital clubfoot treated with the Ponseti method. J Pediatr Orthop. 2001;21:719.
135. Ippolito E, Fraracci L, Farsetti P, Di Mario M, Caterini R. The influence of treatment on the pathology of club foot. CT study at maturity. J Bone Joint Surg Br. 2004;86:574–80.
136. Dobbs MB, Gordon JE, Walton T, Schoenecker PL. Bleeding complications following percutaneous Tendoachilles Tenotomy in the treatment of clubfoot deformity. J Pediatr Orthop. 2004;24:353.
137. Grigoriou E, Abol Oyoun N, Kushare I, Baldwin KD, Horn BD, Davidson RS. Comparative results of percutaneous Achilles tenotomy to combined open Achilles tenotomy with posterior capsulotomy in the correction of equinus deformity in congenital talipes equinovarus. Int Orthop. 2015;39:721–5.

138. Niki H, Nakajima H, Hirano T, Okada H, Beppu M. Ultrasonographic observation of the healing process in the gap after a Ponseti-type Achilles tenotomy for idiopathic congenital clubfoot at two-year follow-up. J Orthop Sci. 2013;18: 70–5.
139. Shabtai L, Segev E, Yavor A, Wientroub S, Hemo Y. Prolonged use of foot abduction brace reduces the rate of surgery in Ponseti-treated idiopathic club feet. J Child Orthop. 2015;9:177–82.
140. Dobbs MB, Rudzki JR, Purcell DB, Walton T, Porter KR, Gurnett CaBeck RW. Factors predictive of outcome after use of the Ponseti Method for the treatment of idiopathic clubfeet. JBJS. 2004;86-A:22–7.
141. McKay SD, Dolan LA, Morcuende JA. Treatment results of late-relapsing idiopathic clubfoot previously treated with the Ponseti method. J Pediatr Orthop. 2012;32:406–11.
142. Dietz FR. Treatment of a recurrent clubfoot deformity after initial correction with the Ponseti technique. Instr Course Lect. 2006;55:625–9.
143. Alonso J, Davis N, Harris R. Surgical relevance of delayed ossification of lateral cuneiform in children with clubfoot. J Bone Joint Surg Br. 2009;91-B: 56–7.
144. Holt JB, Oji DE, Yack HJ, Morcuende JA. Long-term results of tibialis anterior tendon transfer for relapsed idiopathic clubfoot treated with the Ponseti method. J Bone Joint Surg. 2015;97:47–55.
145. Garceau GJ, Manning KR. Transposition of the anterior tibial tendon in the treatment of recurrent congenital club-foot. J Bone Joint Surg Am. 1947;29:1044–8.
146. Kuo KN, Hennigan SP, Hastings ME. Anterior tibial tendon transfer in residual dynamic clubfoot deformity. J Pediatr Orthop. 2001;21:35–41.
147. Holt JB, Oji DE, Yack HJ, Morcuende JA. Long-term results of tibialis anterior tendon transfer for relapsed idiopathic clubfoot treated with the Ponseti method: a follow-up of thirty-seven to fifty-five years. J Bone Joint Surg Am. 2015;97:47–55.
148. Ponseti IV. Common errors in the treatment of congenital clubfoot. Int Orthop. 1997;21:137–41.
149. Ponseti IV, Zhivkov M, Davis N, Sinclair M, Dobbs MB, Morcuende JA. Treatment of the complex idiopathic clubfoot. Clin Orthop Relat Res. 2006;451:171–6.
150. Low AK, Ward K, Wines AP. Pediatric complex regional pain syndrome. J Pediatr Orthop. 2007;27:567–72.

Sports Medicine of the Pediatric Foot and Ankle

13

Robert Duggan

With recreational adolescent sports participants' number at over 35 million and growing in the United States, the numbers of associated sports-related injuries are increasing with lower extremity injuries presenting more frequently for care than upper extremity injuries [1]. This chapter will touch on a number of these factors and identify some of the injury patterns that can assist the sports medicine physician with assessment, diagnosis, and treatment of the athlete child.

It is well established that exercise and wellness go hand in hand. Many of our young children will participate in competitive sports that they were first exposed to as recreational activities either in community programs or through school activities. Levels of exercise in young children correlate with fitness, and the lack of exercise is seen in the obese child [2].

Since the later part of the twentieth century, children's free time has decreased. The trend for less physical activity during the normal school day and the decrease in school-related opportunities for physical activity have contributed to an overall negative effect on the levels of fitness in children. The rise in organized sports has, in many areas, replaced the "free" playtime for many American children. With this information the American Academy of Pediatrics made its recommendation that organized sports should not replace play activities and physical activity, but should augment it [3].

In the child athlete, both insufficient and excessive levels of activity can contribute to injury in recreational and competitive sports. One of the challenges of the sports medical professional is to find the levels of physical activity that enhance wellness and sports enjoyment for the child and at the same time prevent or at least limit the number and frequency of sports-related injuries.

Several epidemiologic studies have identified the number of injuries in a variety of sports and their rate of occurrence. Overuse-type injuries have been identified as half of these injuries [4]. Herring and Nilson have defined overuse injuries as "repetitive application of submaximal stress to otherwise normal tissue, overwhelming the normal repair process" [5]. A significant number of these sports-related injuries are associated with the lower leg, ankle, and foot [6]. In a retrospective study, Stracciolini looked at 2133 charts at Boston Children's Hospital and found that female athletes had more overuse injuries (62.5%) than males (41.9%). The remaining percentages were listed as traumatic injuries. The lower extremity accounted for 60.2% of all injuries in the samples

R. Duggan (✉)
Caldwell Foot and Ankle, Caldwell UNC Health Care, University of North Carolina Healthcare, Lenoir, NC, USA

University of Central Florida College of Medicine, Orlando, FL, USA
e-mail: RDuggan@paof.com

M. L. Butterworth, J. T. Marcoux (eds.), *The Pediatric Foot and Ankle*,
https://doi.org/10.1007/978-3-030-29788-6_13

Table 13.1 Risk factors for overuse injuries in children

Intrinsic risk factors	Extrinsic risk factors
Growth-related factors	Training workload (intensity, time)
Previous injuries	Training and competition schedule
Previous level of conditioning	Equipment/footwear
Anatomic factors	Environmental
Psychological and development factors	Sport technique
Athlete specific	Psychological factors
	Adult and peer influences

Adapted from DiFiori [10]

Table 13.2 Recommendations regarding intensive training and sports specialization

Participate in activities at the child's skill level
Ensure coaches are knowledgeable and trained in physical, technical, and psychological aspects of coaching children as well as knowledge of equipment and competition
Early and adequate recognition of injury especially overuse-type injuries
Recognize signs and symptoms of overtraining
Ongoing nutritional assessment with attention to calories and vitamin intake
Educate all those involved including parents in heat-related conditions and prevention

Pediatrics [13]

reviewed [7]. Track-related injuries in children and adolescents treated in emergency departments have increased from the early 1990s. High school track athletes have a lower extremity injury rate of 58.2%, with foot and ankle injuries comprising a total of 30.2% [8].

There are several intrinsic, as well as extrinsic, factors that are associated with sports-related injuries in the child [9].

Table 13.1 lists some of the risk factors that can influence the occurrence and rate of overuse injuries. Intrinsic factors are those things specific to the individual. Extrinsic factors are independent to the individual child. It is reasonable to also include current illness and/or injuries.

In recent years, the practice of early single-sport specialization has come into question. Not only have athletes chosen a single year-round sport at earlier ages, but the intensity of exercise and activity has increased. There is little data to show that early single-sport specialization improves long-term or future athletic performance. There is, however, significant evidence that shows increased hours of participation in training and intensity correlate directly with overuse-type injuries [11].

It has also been questioned whether early single-sport specialization has a long-term overall permanent health benefit for the child, despite some athletes having significant early sport skill development. With increased sport specialization in our young athletes, training intensity increases. Coaching time is increased and skill levels are trained to higher expectations. The American Academy of Pediatrics has made specific recommendations in 2000 regarding intensive training and sports specialization in young athletes. Table 13.2 describes these recommendations [12].

Cuff et al. found that student athletes that played all year had 42% more overuse injuries than those that played fewer seasons [14]. There is also evidence that injury increases as the ratio of time in organized sports to the time spent in free play increases. A ratio of greater than 2:1 time spent increases injuries. The overwhelming type of injury was found to be overuse type at 67.4% and acute injury at 32.6% [15].

It is reasonable given the current information available that early single-sport specialization can increase the risk for injuries in our young athletes. The pressure for early success and efforts to improve performance may not be in the best interest in the young athletes' health. Decisions regarding treatment of injuries in young athletes and the eventual return to athletics have significant roles for the sports medicine professional. Several factors must be taken into consideration when advising a young athlete on sports injury and their return to play. Those treating the athlete should not only have expertise in foot and ankle treatment, but they must also have significant knowledge of the individual's sport and the athlete's role in that sport. The sports medicine practitioner must have a working knowledge of the athlete's needs and the total demands of each sport. Healing of an injury must be evaluated and compared to the ability of the athlete and the injured part to withstand the demands of the sport upon return to all or part of the sport. Consideration of the impact on family, school, and the young athlete especially must be reassessed often as the healing process progresses.

Not only is the physical injury a concern in our young athletes, but psychological and social concerns exist as well. Our young athletes place significant value in their ability to play sport and often have identity as team members. Adolescent athletes with self-reported injuries had lower quality of life scores than uninjured adolescents. Not only were these scores related to physical functioning, but the injured athletes had lower scores in social and global functioning [16]. This means that a segment of injured young athletes may be unable to manage the complexities of the athletic injury without help. Again, early recognition of these situations is critical to full recovery and return to activity and competition. Every effort should be made to assure the total return of the young athlete's pre-injury life activities, including social and academic function. Failure to heal the whole patient will compromise the return of wellness.

Strength Training in the Young Athlete

An additional feature of early sports specialization in young athletes is the additional concentration on resistive strength training. As young athletes become more focused on a single sport, the culture of competition often will add to the training of the young athlete. One of the areas included is strength training, not to be confused with weight lifting, which is usually a competition aimed at highest weight totals lifted. Resistive weight training is designed to strengthen the total athlete in an effort to both increase protective muscular strength and increase physical performance. The acceptance of strength training by the medical community has not always been generally the case. As recent as 1983, the American Academy of Pediatrics discouraged strength training in the prepubescent and skeletally immature athlete [17]. Early references to children and adolescents incorporating resistance training discussed the potential for muscles to increase in strength without the associated muscular hypertrophy. The resulting increase in strength was associated with neuromuscular activation and coordination rather than hypertrophy [18].

More recent recommendations have noted significant benefits to the young athlete that incorporates a well-designed, supervised strength training program [19]. These programs highlight the overall strength development and musculoskeletal function of the young athlete. When done with appropriate supervision and care, these strength development programs augment normal growth and development.

Restive strength training has also been found to be beneficial in a growing population of adolescents with comorbidities associated with obesity, insulin-dependent diabetes, and cardiovascular disease [20]. Exercise protocols in these patient populations require coordination with all those involved with the athletes' care so that the physical limitations and physiologic requirements can be optimized for each individual athlete. Quantity and intensity of exercise will be a challenge throughout the conditioning process.

Resistive training is a component of a complete training program that includes cardiovascular training, flexibility, balance, agility, reaction time, as well as other components as demanded by the sport or activity. Daily physical maintenance is required of every athlete but is learned as a young child. Rest and sleep are vital for growth and repair. Hydration and nutrition should be focused on food types and their quantities and timing of meals.

Team, coach, parents, and medical personal all must give the young athlete guidance as the healing process progresses. Often, external pressure is felt by the athlete to return to activity, especially when competition looms. It is important to stress to the athlete and all those involved that the child's health is paramount in all decisions with regard to return to play.

Cardiovascular Training in the Pediatric Athlete

Often used as the main method of cardiovascular fitness development in the school setting, running is often a major form of conditioning in the child, as well as a cause of injury. As with all forms of exercise, running should be thought of as a stressor of the young body having a wide range of effects. The continuum of running effects is related to both intensity and duration. The running environment will affect the individual child's response as well. At the very least, the dose-related individual child response to running must be tracked to ensure positive outcome and track the desired conditioning effect.

At levels of exercise, in this case running, that create injury, the individual response to running may move toward the overuse or injury spectrum. This can interfere with the child's growth and development at least temporarily. Injury creates tissue disruption and limits activity levels in the otherwise healthy child. Time lose to injury is also time lose to normal activity and potentially normal development depending on severity of injury and tissues involved.

Positive levels of running or any cardiovascular exercise can be identified through a graduated program that allows for exercise response and recuperation over time. Cross training, using several forms of exercise appropriately coached, is recommended in early childhood, in an effort to discourage early single-sport commitment. Studies have identified the injuries seen with running and the child athlete. In the adolescent athlete, the running response is similar in both male and female athletes. As the young athletes grow, a shift is seen toward male to female injury ratio changes with the female athletes having a higher risk for overuse types of injury. There is evidence that a modest decrease in running mileage can reduce injury rate [21].

The History and Physical

The young athlete should have a preparticipation physical evaluation. Screening for cardiac issues may include special testing if risk factors are present. Concussion protocols are now more commonly included in preseason or baseline evaluations. Standardly, a complete musculoskeletal evaluation is also included [22].

A sports medicine trained physician is the best choice to perform preseason, the preparticipation history and physical is a sports medicine physician. The pediatrician with sports medicine background, which has cared for the athlete and knows his or her medical history and the family dynamics, is an excellent choice for the athlete. This same physician can give valuable insights on pre-injury status as well, should there be an injury that needs treatment. A discussion with the athlete's primary care physician can be very valuable. The need for additional testing or baseline studies can be determined prior to increases in physical activity. This information can be very valuable when assessing post-injury status. The addition of balance and specific strength testing can also be very helpful.

Comprehensive Training and Conditioning Programs

Every sport will require some training and conditioning. Preseason, in-season, post-, or out-of-season training should be coordinated on an individual basis and incorporated with the athlete's year-round activities to avoid overtraining and injuries. Significant attention should be given to rest and the athlete educated on progression of each component of conditioning.

The American College of Sports Medicine published its first set of guidelines for physical activity. At that time the recommendation was for 20–30 minutes of vigorous exercise daily [23]. Following those recommendations, guidelines have evolved from several groups, and many groups will suggest up to 60 minutes per day of moderate activity.

Growth and development is a hallmark of the growing, young athlete. This growth affects the training and performance of the child. Growth does not occur at a steady rate and is not the same from child to child. The child's musculoskeletal and neural development has unique stages of maturation that will affect training as well as skill development [24].

Many organizations have suggested that children participate in a variety of different activities. The young athlete has many opportunities for varied activities, and an effort should be made to incorporate these in the growing athlete. It is prudent to suggest to the young athlete to vary participation in sport and play activities.

Exercise Intensity and the Young Athlete

Any physical activity taken beyond the conditioning level or having a duration or intensity that goes beyond the physical maximum of the tissues involved, without sufficient rest or recuperation, will approach the level of tissue breakdown and eventual injury. Every effort should be made to gradually increase exercise intensity, so the child can tolerate the increase without injury. Some of the physical effects of conditioning will be fatigue, muscle soreness, and some general discomfort after maximum effort. These effects normally should resolve by the next exercise bout or training episode. It is reasonable to conclude that cardiovascular and musculoskeletal conditioning not performed properly or developed gradually can cause injury. It is also reasonable to conclude that the absence of proper graduated types of conditioning in young athletes may lead to fatigue, skill deterioration, and possibly injury. The goal of conditioning is to prepare the young athlete for the rigors of the sport and to protect them from injury. Training errors, such as too much activity or conditioning, as well as nonexistent or too little conditioning, are often the source of early season injuries. Training and conditioning errors that go unnoticed can lead to injuries at any point in the sport season. Athletes should be examined for training error injuries or previous injuries that may be exacerbated any time the athlete's progress fails to respond.

Sport Selection

Many factors can limit the athlete's exposure to a number of organized sports. Geographic and cultural influences may limit the type of sport played in neighborhoods or regions. Economics may play a role where there is limited access to sports that require financial investment in equipment, instruction, and often rental fees for court or playing venue time. Transportation to and from practice and competitions can also be burdensome for some young athletes. These factors, along with the ever-increasing sport skill levels in our children, contribute to more and more single-sport selection by a greater number of young athletes. The hope for college scholarships and eventual positions in professional sports is often a dream of many young athletes and their parents, even though the statistics are against that happening. With nearly eight [8] million high school student athletes and a NCAA total of 480,000 college athletes, the chance of participating in sports after high school is about 6%. The chance of receiving a scholarship of any amount is about 2%. The average college scholarship is approximately $11,000 per year. Therefore, the young high school athlete must realize that sport enjoyment must be paramount and that health and wellness are the long-term goals of any successful sports program.

Coaching plays an important role in the safety and enjoyment in sports. Experienced coaches with sport-specific training have lower injury rates [25]. Parents are often the major supporters for the young athlete. Both financial and psychological supports are essential for success and enjoyment. The balance of support and drive for success in sport is often difficult for those close to the young athlete. Every effort should be made to allow the young athlete to direct the progress and participation in sport. Athletics in the high school athlete is an excellent time to develop personal commitment and team responsibilities. The athletes that "own" their sport are always the happiest.

Growth and Development and a Pediatric Athlete

Many of the recent research on young athletes are aimed at the potential risk vs children benefit from strength training and growth and development. Children and adolescence should be encouraged to participate in a variety of sports and recreational activities to enhance their physical and psychosocial development and establish good health habits at an early age. Along with other types of physical activity, youth strength training has been shown to have a positive influence on several measurable indices of health, including cardiorespiratory fitness, body composition, bone mineral density, blood lipids, and selected psychosocial measures [26]. With review of current information, it appears that strength training does enhance growth and development if done with trained coaches and in programs specific to each child. Running and cardiovascular conditioning can be beneficial to most young athletes. As with every activity, gradual conditioning and proper, well-coached training are essential. Medical supervision and avoidance of adult training programs are recommended.

Sport-Specific Injuries

In 2002, Luckstead and colleagues reported injury rates in American youth sports. Sports with both overuse injuries and traumatic injuries were examined. The largest numbers of injuries were in cross country with 61.4% chance of injury, followed by football with 58.8%. Golf, tennis, and swimming showed the lowest risk. The sports that had both male and female team participation had greater injuries in the female teams were cross country and track specifically (61.4% vs 43.7%) and (24.8% vs 17.3%). Training, strength, biomechanics, and other causes have all been implicated in possible reasons for this difference [27].

Often pain is the presenting finding in the sports injuries, and many of the young athletes are not familiar or unable to differentiate conditioning discomfort with injury pain. Dalton staged mechanical pain with overuse-type injuries.

- Stage I Pain after physical activity
- Stage II Pain during physical activity with no impact on function (can continue participating in activities)
- Stage III Pain during physical activity that lasts all day and has no impact on function (need to decrease or even stop the activities)
- Stage IV Pain during all physical activities, even basic musculoskeletal functions [28]

The Foot- and Ankle-Specific Injuries and Injury Patterns

The cavus foot is a poor accommodator to terrain changes and can be associated with many injuries. Metatarsalgia, stress fractures, recurrent inversion ankle sprains, as well as plantar fasciitis and cuboid injuries are all seen in this foot type. Peroneal tendon injuries are seen often (Fig. 13.1). Many chronic peroneal injuries are seen because of the mechanical position of the peroneal tendons. The peroneus brevis can develop stenosing tenosynovitis because of the "sawing "action of the peroneus longus rubbing against the brevis. This is exacerbated in the cavus foot when the mechanical advantage of the longus is increased at the level of the cuboid. This mechanical advantage is less in the flat foot as the angle at the cuboid groove is less acute [29].

Os peroneum friction syndrome has been reported as well. The lateral plantar foot is frequently painful at the region where the peroneus longus and peroneus brevis intersect. The presence of an os perineum bone can be seen in

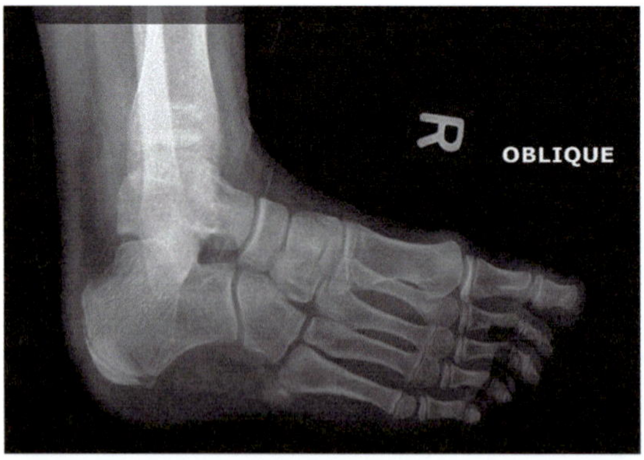

Fig. 13.1 Ten-year-old male athlete with pain at the fifth metatarsal base at the peroneus brevis tendon insertion site. This is a normal appearance of the growth plate

approximately 5–14% of asymptomatic individuals. The radiographic presence is 5% [30].

Chronic irritation in this area and mechanical stress can injure the os peroneum to the point of fracture (Fig. 13.2). Often the athletes can be rested, braced, and returned to activity, but may present with chronic pain that fails conservative care. Excision of the fractured os peroneum is often necessary. Surgical excision and repair as needed of the peroneal complex has shown good results. The athletes often return to full activity without compromise to function and mobility [31].

Often seen on standard radiographs of the foot and ankle, accessory ossicles and sesamoid bones are frequent findings. The os trigonum is one of the largest and most common ossicles found in the foot seen in approximately 1–25% of the population. It is located in the posterior talar region and is connected to the talus by fibrocartilaginous structures forming a synchondrosis. In those athletes where the os trigonum is present from a previous fracture (called a shepherd's fracture), the area can be chronically painful and irritated secondary to impingement of the os trigonum with tissue associated with the flexor hallucis longus tendon. Conservative treatment is often successful, but with continued pain and inability to perform, resection of the os trigonum is often needed to return the athlete to full function.

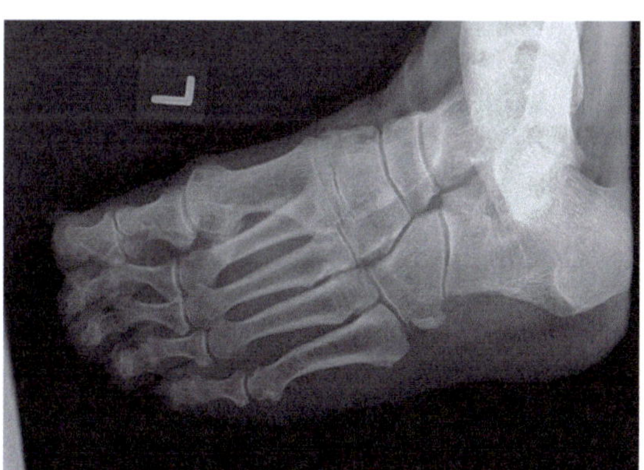

Fig. 13.2 The location where the peroneus brevis and peroneus longus tendons intersect is a very common place for pain in the young athlete. An os peroneum is present and has actually fractured secondary to continued stress on the area

Accessory Navicular

The accessory navicular bone is present in approximately 1.7–7.7% of patients. First described by Bauhin in 1605, the structure is identified as a bony prominence medial posterior to the tarsal navicular. The type II accessory navicular, which is a persistent accessory ossification center of the navicular itself, is often an injury pattern associated with the synchondrosis between the ossicles in the body of the navicular. Athletes will complain of pain swelling and inability to function at this level. This entity is often associated with a pes planus foot type and decreased propulsion complaints by the athlete. Initial treatment consists of bracing, icing, and rest. The athlete may also benefit from orthotic therapy to decrease the stress on the tendon insertion of the tibialis posterior. Those athletes that fail conservative treatment may progress on to surgical resection of the bone with repair of the tibialis posterior and its tendinous insertion on the navicular. MRI is often used not only to identify navicular body changes but also to monitor the progress of healing [32].

Navicular Stress Fracture

Stress fracture to the navicular in our young athletes is not common. Overall track athletes will show a 20% incidence of stress fracture [33]. Often pain, swelling, and point tenderness to the navicular can be diagnostic for this condition when it is associated with an increase in exercise intensity and/or duration. Keys to treatment include rest, decreased weight-bearing, and a slow return back to activity. Return to activity too soon will exacerbate the condition. Frequent monitoring and sequential radiographs can be of some value in a more difficult condition. In our younger athletes, care must be taken to prevent vascular compromise to the navicular and progression of the deformity.

Cuboid Injuries

The cuboid is injured secondary to stress applied often as the lateral side of the foot abducts, compressing the bone against the calcaneus. Cuboid stress injuries are often seen in athletes with increase in training intensity and/or duration. Injuries to the cuboid are difficult to initially diagnose because of nonspecific findings of pain. Limited swelling to the lateral foot is often seen, and standard foot radiographs are often within normal limits. Persistent pain with compression of the cuboid on physical exam, and information obtained from special studies such as MRI or bone scan, can confirm the diagnosis of cuboid injury. Findings are often nonspecific swelling that can progress to a stress fracture diagnosis. Treatment includes rest, ice, and decreasing abductory forces to the foot.

Exercise-Induced Compartment Syndrome

Lower leg injuries in the child athlete can often be seen as a continuum of stress. The compartments of the lower leg function routinely without insult in most children. In some cases, the secondary effect of conditioning or running, with or without a specific history of injury, can cause chronic exertional compartment syndrome (CECS). This condition presents with pain with running. The pain is reproduced at consistent levels of exercise or distance of running. The pain is limited to one or more fascial compartments of the lower leg. The pain of CECS is often associated with a complaint of numbness or other neuritic complaints because of the intercompartmental pressure placed on the neurovascular structures that are compressed in the associated compartment. The condition is considered a diagnosis of exclusion because of its infrequent diagnosis. MRI and nerve conduction studies are recommended to rule out structural and functional changes to the neuromuscular structures. Intercompartmental pressures can be measured both at rest and after exercise to confirm the diagnosis of CECS. A noninvasive test that can be done in an office setting is perceived pain indexing of the compartments of the lower leg using a sphygmomanometer. The cuff is inflated on each leg, and the patient is asked to notify the test or when the area is painful. The patient is then exercised, and the sphygmomanometer cuff is inflated again with the patient identifying the point of pain once again. Patients with CECS will oftentimes have a post-exercise sphygmomanometer reading of approximately 50% of the pre-exercise reading. This test can indicate the existence of CECS but is not specific to the compartment involved. Physical therapy, anti-inflammatory medicine, and rest are all included in the treatment plan for these patients. Patients would have to fail conservative care before surgical release of the involved compartment is considered.

Osteochondritis

Freiberg's Infarct

The most common location of a Freiberg-type injury is the second metatarsal. Freiberg's disease has a 5:1 female predilection [34]. The injury is first seen as a painful swollen joint of the metatarsal-phalangeal articulation. The evidence is not definite on the mechanism of injury. There is an injury, either contusion or stress related, that causes injury to the region of the subchondral metatarsal head. This may have primary and/or secondary vascular compromise that causes collapse of the subchondral bone. Over time, the metatarsal head presents flattened and does not allow normal metatarsophalangeal joint motion. The patient may not present for care until an additional injury is sustained or the area is noted on a subsequent radiograph.

Koehler's Disease

Osteochondritis of the tarsal navicular is thought to also be a pathology that may be related to vascular injury to the bone with or without compression force injury. The architectural change is seen in the disc appearance of the bone often referred to as "silver dollar" navicular. Treatment is based on off-loading the bone as well as immobilization to allow revascularization of the injured bone. This condition stresses the need for strict monitoring of the athlete's condition to ensure architectural changes do not present in conditions of stress and inflammation of the navicular.

Sever's Disease and Calcaneal Stress Fracture

Another injury more commonly identified is a calcaneal stress fracture. The most common sports resulting in this injury are gymnastics and jumping sports (Fig. 13.3). The gymnast's foot that has an open calcaneal growth plates can develop an inflammatory condition because of chronic traction and compression of the enthesis of the Achilles tendon. This area develops a level of inflammatory conditions that is called Sever's disease. A growing number of injuries to the calcaneus are being seen in female gymnasts. The intensity of training and the numbers of landings that contuse the heel in conjunction with errors in technique create a situation at the posterior heel where the ground reactive stress to the inferior calcaneus is opposed to the pull of the Achilles tendon. This, in addition to a contusion mechanism of the calcaneus, has led to an increase in calcaneal stress fractures involving the calcaneus apophysis.

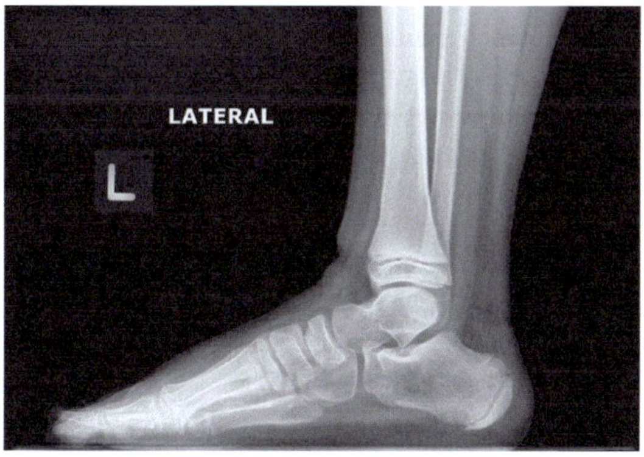

Fig. 13.3 Notice the calcaneal stress fracture in this young female gymnast. This is common secondary to the repetitive impact and stress on the heel in these athletes

Talar Stress Fracture

The talus in young athletes has more recently been implicated in more injury patterns. Stress fractures to the talar body are more and more common in elite female gymnasts. Gymnastics and dance activities have a greater number of confirmed talar stress fractures. The studies on talar body stress fractures, in females aged 15–17, have all reported early normal radiographs [35].

Events of floor exercise and vault require a landing of the athlete that often hits the heel on the ground with significant frequency. As the athlete progresses in skill and strength, the force on landing increases. As the frequency of landings increases, due to the requirements to develop skill, the talus accepts a substantial force. Talar stress fractures are becoming more common in the higher-level gymnasts. The athlete presents with anterior ankle pain with mild to moderate swelling. The clinical hallmark of this injury is pain on palpation of the talar neck. Often, only high-definition MRI will show definitive evidence of a talar stress fracture. Removing the repetitive impact is the treatment of choice. Often, immobilization is not necessary. Four to 6 weeks is not an unusual time frame for healing, with gradual return to activity being the recommendation.

Sesamoid Apparatus Dysfunction

The author has grouped injuries to the sesamoids, first metatarsophalangeal joint capsule, and extensor hallucis longus tendon under one collective group called sesamoid apparatus dysfunction. This group of structures is rarely injured alone. Often a turf toe-type injury is sustained, and the associated first metatarsal phalangeal joint capsule swells secondary to frank tissue damage or associated with compensatory change in gate. As movement of the sesamoids is limited, the extensor hallucis longus tendon is strained in its effort to dorsiflex the joint. This creates more swelling and sesamoid movement decreases. The sesamoids have approximately 12–14 mm of movement on the head of the first metatarsal, and with injury, this normal movement is limited. The sesamoids are then more prone to further injury without their normal movement pattern. As with any injury, the acute inflammation must decrease and the movement pattern of the sesamoids returned. Both metatarsophalangeal joint and sesamoid movement must be restored for full return to activity, or the joint is destined for reinjury. Metatarsophalangeal joint distraction, metatarsophalangeal joint glides, and sesamoid rocking are all techniques that can be used to reestablish normal sesamoid apparatus function.

Tendon Injuries in the Pediatric Athlete

Tibialis Posterior Tendon Injuries

When tibialis posterior tendon injuries are seen in a child, they typically have a more pronatory and abducted foot position. The most common area of tenderness and inflammation is the area of maximum angular change in the tendons course. This is just posterior and inferior to the distal tibia and is also the most common area of tearing.

Treatment consists of efforts to decrease swelling and inflammation. Ice, rest, or bracing is useful. Orthotic management of contributory mechanics is useful in those cases. Identifying the apex of the pathology is critical. The tendon-bone interface at the navicular can represent an area of intense pain. This area can also have associated with it a navicular tuberosity fracture or accessory navicular that can influence the healing process. Surgical repair of the tibialis posterior tendon is reserved for those injuries that fail conservative care.

Tendon-Bone Interface or Enthesis Injury

Accessory ossicles have also been implicated in athletic injuries. Children can develop tendon/accessory bone pain as they grow. As body weight and level of activity increase, the potential for injury to the tendons of the foot can occur. The Achilles tendon is often implicated in Sever's disease, as well as in conditions that are associated with progressive or long-standing ankle joint loss of motion. The equinus-type position creates stress to the tendon that increases at the propulsive phase of gait. This condition is often bilateral and may or may not be associated with a specific injury event. The treatment is directed to increase ankle range of motion both with the knee straight as well as with the knee bent. Subtalar joint mobilization and strength balancing of the lower leg are indicated.

The tibialis posterior tendon has also been associated with painful foot complaints. The association with a mild to moderate flatfoot structure can be an aggravation to the young athlete. Pain associated with the tendon as it passes the medial malleolus as well as pain at the level of tendon insertion at the navicular bone is seen and slips to adjacent bone. A significant accessory bone is often the most difficult pathology to resolve in young athletes. The navicular can have a hypertrophic tuberosity or sustain a fracture. Posterior tibial tendon dysfunction is a chronic condition that has its etiology with conditions often seen in the growing child. The clinician must differentiate the apex of the deformity and the tissue planes involved. As with all injuries, this differentiation is the crucial part of deciding a treatment plan. If the accessory navicular component cannot be relieved using a resting brace and physical therapy, the bone is removed in those that fail the conservative treatment. The tendon is repaired as necessary and the insertion assured its position on the navicular.

Lateral Ankle Sprain

The young athlete is at risk for ankle sprains. The most common athletic injury seen is the lateral ankle sprain. They also have the highest recurrence rate [36]. Recurrence of the lateral ankle sprain is likely in one of three high school athletes. Many may have ongoing issues with the ankle [37].

Young athletes sustaining lateral ankle sprains begin by following a common course of treatment. The apex of the injury of the lateral ankle is, in many cases, the focus of the treatment plan. Early immobilization of the injured structure is necessary to decrease pain and swelling. Once the athlete is able to weight-bear, aggressive physical therapy modalities are used to decrease swelling, as well as to decrease disuse changes to the rest of the foot and ankle. Range of motion, exercise strengthening, proprioception, and balance are incorporated early in the rehabilitation program. A comprehensive examination of the lower limb is needed to rule out osteochondral damage of the distal tibia or talus, as well as associated injuries to the peroneal tendon complex and syndesmotic ligaments of the lower leg. Dynamic bracing of the ankle, allowing for normal joint motion and limiting extreme inversion, has been useful. Follow-up examinations of the young athlete are important to ensure complete rehabilitation of the sprained ankle.

Controversy exists regarding the use of lace-up ankle brace in ankle sprain patients. Recent studies of athletes using ankle sprain bracing show a decrease in recurrent ankle sprains, as well as no difference in the indices of acute knee or other lower extremity injuries [38]. To this point, it appears reasonable to protect post-ankle sprain youth athletes with a dynamic lace-up ankle brace and to follow them for any secondary changes or for any signs of an incomplete rehabilitation (Fig. 13.4).

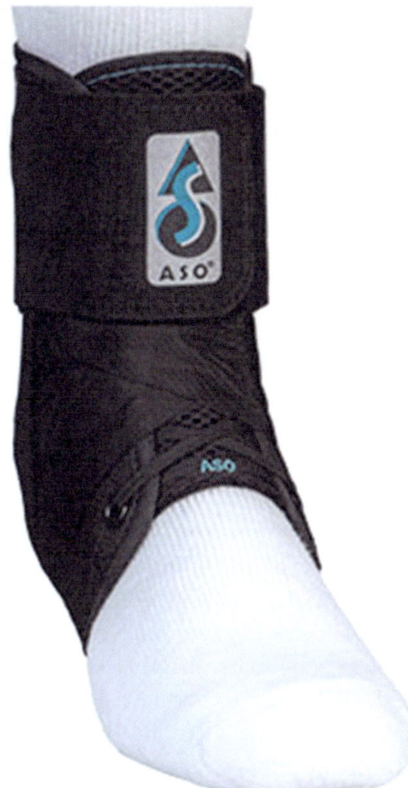

Fig. 13.4 An ankle brace utilized post lateral ankle sprain

Bare Foot Running

Recent studies have listed several running injury patterns that are decreased in the unshod or minimal shoe gear runners. The injury pattern of the Achilles tendon is lessened with the change in position of foot strike force. It has been reported that barefoot running or athletes using minimal shoe gear have decreased complaints of knee pain. There are also reports of decreased impact stress to the single limb with running because of a movement of foot strike farther toward the forefoot. Additionally, stride length is shorter in unshod runners. Recently, studies have shown that there is no mechanical or physiologic benefit with running wearing minimal shoes as opposed to traditional shoes [39].

It is becoming clearer that unshod running demands training and conditioning that is similar but slightly different than traditional shoe running. Intrinsic muscle strength of the foot must be trained. Fatigue injuries to interossei and lumbrical muscles have been identified in young runners moving quickly from shod to unshod running. It is also beneficial in these runners to begin training on soft, uneven surfaces and progress slowly to surfaces that are less forgiving. Further investigation is needed, and recommendations for young athletes must be individualized.

High school runners in both shod and unshod groups had increased risk for medial tibial stress syndrome or tibial stress fracture as both intensity and duration of running increased. A significant relationship was found between body mass index, internal rotation angle, and medial tibial stress syndrome in female high school athletes that were runners. Also, a significant relationship was found between limited straight leg raise stress fractures in male high school runners [40]. This information gives the clinician reason for preseason evaluation of range of motion and strength, not only in the lower extremity but in the whole leg. One should also use caution with intensity and duration for running in high school athletes with increased body mass index.

Female Athlete

Male and female youth athletes have similar performance capabilities up until age 10–12. At that age female athletes begin to have more body fat and less lean body mass than males. This can be attributed to changes in hormone levels in both the male and female. Additional differences include decreased upper body strength in females, even with strength training. Lower extremity strength is much more similar between males and females. Even with these differences, there is very similar work capacity with physiologic training for males and females. Mechanically, the female is more likely to have an increased Q angle of the knee, be more flexible, and have a compensatory pes planus foot with forefoot pronation [41].

Training and conditioning in the female athlete should be monitored for any secondary physiological changes to maximize both conditioning and competitive events. Exercise and running have been shown to lower body fat in runners, and recent studies have shown no detrimental effects in bone mass in female runners. Close communication with the female athlete's primary care physician improved both overall and physical training outcomes [42].

Overtraining and Burnout

Overtraining in children's athletics is a common etiologic factor leading to injury. In many cases, signs of burnout are not recognized. Coaches, teachers, parents, and the athlete themselves all should play a role in early identification of burnout syndrome. Overtraining syndrome can be defined as a series of psychological, physiological, and hormonal changes that result in decreased sports performance [43].

References

1. Davis KW. Imaging pediatric sports injuries: lower extremity. Radiol Clin North Am. 2010;48:1213–35.
2. Richmond SA, Kang J, Emery CA. Is body mass index a risk for sports injuries in adolescence? J Sci Med Sport. 2013;16(5):401–5.
3. Young WK, Metzi JD. Policy statement organized sports for children and adolescents. Pediatr. 2001;107:1459.
4. Soprano JV. Musculoskeletal injuries in the pediatric and adolescent athlete. Curr Sports Med Rep. 2005;4(6):329–34.
5. Herring SA, Nilson KL. Introduction to overuse injuries. Clin Sports Med. 1987;6:225–39.
6. Stracciolini A, Casciano R, Levey Friedman H, Meehan WP 3rd, Micheli LJ. Pediatric sports injuries an age comparison of children versus adolescence. Am J Sports Med. 2013;41(8):1922–9.
7. Stracciolini A, et al. Pediatric sports injuries: a comparison of male versus female. Am J Sports Med. 2014;42:965–72.
8. Reid JP, Nelson NG, Roberts KJ, LB MK. Track related injuries in children and adolescents treated in US emergency departments from 1991 through 2008. Phys Sports Med. 2012;40(2).
9. Caine D, Maffulli N, Caine C. Epidemiology of injury and child and adolescent sports: injury rates, risk factors, and prevention. Clin Sports Med. 2008; 27:19–50.
10. DiFiori JP. Evaluation of overuse injuries in children and adolescents. Curr Sports Med Rep. 2010;9(6):372–8.
11. Smucny M, et al. Consequences of single sport specialization in the pediatric and adolescent athlete. Orthop Clin N Am. 2015;46:249–58.
12. Committee on Sports Medicine and Fitness. Intensive training and sport specialization in the young athletes. Pediatr. 2000;106:154.
13. Pediatrics. 2000;106(1).
14. Cuff, et al. Clin Pediatr. 49(8):731–6.
15. Jayanthi N, LaBella C, Fisher D, Pasulka J, Dugas L. Am J Sports Med. 2015;43:794.
16. Valovich MT. J Athl Train. 2009;44(6):603–10.
17. American Academy of Pediatrics. Phys Sports Med. 1983;11(3): 157–161.
18. Guy J, Micheli L. J Am Acad Orthop Surg. 2001;9(1):29–36.
19. Miller M, Cheatham C, Patel N. Pediatr Clin N Am. 2010;57(3):671–82.
20. Young W, Metzl J. Pediatr Ann. 2010;39:295.

21. Fredericson M, Tenforde A, et al. Phys Med Rehabil. 2016;27.
22. Heinke B. Common issues encountered in adolescent's sports medicine. Primary Care Clin. 2014;41:539–55.
23. American College of Sports Medicine. Position Stand. Physical activity, physical fitness, and hypertension. Med Sci Sport Exerc. 1993;25(10):i–x.
24. American Academy of Pediatrics. Weight training and weight lifting: information for the pediatrician. Phys Sports Med. 1983;11(3):157–61.
25. Caine D, et al. Ethics and sports medicine. Clin Sports Med. 2008;27:19–50.
26. Faigenbaum AD. Pediatric and adolescent sports injuries. Clin Sports Med. 2000;19(4).
27. Luckstead EF, et al. Sports injury profiles, training and rehabilitation issues in American sports. Pediatr Clin N Am. 2002;49:753–67.
28. Dalton SE. Overuse injuries in adolescent athletes. Sports Med. 1992;13:58–70.
29. Munk RL, Davis PH. Longitudinal rupture of the peroneus brevis tendon. J Trauma. 1976;16(10):803–6.
30. Takahashi M, et al. Magnetic resonance imaging and adolescent symptomatic navicular tuberosity fractures. J Med Investig. 2014;61:22–7.
31. Bashir WA, et al. Os peroneum friction syndrome complicated by sesamoid fatigue fracture: a new radiological diagnosis? Case report and literature review. Skelet Radiol. 2009;38:181–6.
32. Carmont MR, et al. Current concepts review: Freiberg's disease. Foot Ankle Int. 2009;30:167–76.
33. Bennell KL, Malcolm SA, Thomas SA, Reid SJ, Brukner PD, Edeling PR, Wark JD. Risk factors for stress fractures in track and field athletes: a 12-month process of active study. Am J Sports Med. 1996;24(6):810–8.
34. Carmont MR, et al. Current concepts review: Freiberg's disease. Foot Ankle Int. 2009;30:167–76.
35. Rossi F, Dragoni S. Talar body fatigue stress fractures: 3 cases observed in a lead female gymnast. Skelet Radiol. 2005;34(7):389–94.
36. Swanson DM, et al. Patterns of recurrent injuries among US high school athletes, 2005–2008. Am J Sports Med. 2009;37(8):1586–93.
37. Gerber JP, et al. Persistent disability associated with ankle sprains: a perspective examination of an athletic population. Foot Ankle Int. 1989;19(10):653–60.
38. McGuine, et al. The effect of lace up ankle braces on injury rates in high school football players. Am J Sports Med. 2012;40(1):49–57.
39. Kahle A, Brown GA, Shaw I, Shaw BS. Mechanical and physiological analysis of minimalist versus traditionally shot running. J Sports Med Phys Fitness. 2016;56(9):974–9.
40. Yagi S, Muneta T, Sekiya I. Knee surgery sports traumatology and. Arthroscopy. 2013;21(3):556–63.
41. Ireland ML, Ott S. Special concerns of the female athlete. Clin Sports Med. 2004;23:291–8.
42. Lucas J, Lucas P, Vogel S, Gamble G, Evans M, Reid I. Effects of sub-elite competitive running on bone density, body composition and sexual maturity of adolescent females. Osteoporos Int. 2003;14:848–56.
43. Small E. Chronic musculoskeletal pain in young athletes. Pediatr Clin N Am. 2002;49:655–62.

Fractures of the Pediatric Foot and Ankle

14

Brian B. Carpenter and Mitzi L. Williams

Pediatric Fractures

Physiology and Anatomy of Pediatric Fractures

Proper management of fractures through the physis in the immature skeleton is extremely important because these injuries are common and have a high rate of complications. There are many factors that contribute to this high rate of complication that include nature and force of the injury, displacement of the fracture, reduction of the fracture, atraumatic operative techniques, and vascular injury at the fracture site both from the injury and from the surgical repair. Complications can be severe and life changing. Some of these complications are premature closure of the physis and premature closure of part of the physis which can result in a limb length deformity, joint incongruency, and angular growth. Trauma to the immature ankle skeleton results in unique fracture patterns that transform over time as the physis closes at different levels of skeletal maturity. Albeit the mechanism of the injury or force generated may be the same for both adult and pediatric patients, the chronobiologic nature of the pediatric skeleton will produce various fracture patterns depending on the temporal biologic physeal development. The fracture morphology in the immature skeleton is dependent not only on the time point of its development but also on the location of the fracture within the growth plate. The immature skeleton is made up of a cartilage model that with maturation is replaced by endochondral ossification of the bone [1]. In the foot and ankle, long bone fractures can occur in the epiphysis, physis, metaphysis, and diaphysis. The epiphysis as it matures will create a subchondral plate parallel and adjacent to the physis. The subchondral surface is osseous and more rigid as compared to the softer and more flexible supra physeal surface. The perichondrium is a layer of connective tissue that envelops the epiphysis and blends with the periosteum. It consists of two separate layers: an outer fibrous layer and inner chondrogenic layer which form the growth plate, which encircles the bone. The fibrous layer contains fibroblasts, which produce collagenous fibers. The chondrogenic layer remains undifferentiated and can form chondroblasts or chondrocytes. The juncture of the two circumferential exterior structures provides

B. B. Carpenter (✉)
Department of Orthopaedics, The University of North Texas Health Science Center, Fort Worth, TX, USA

M. L. Williams
Kaiser San Francisco Bay Area Foot and Ankle Residency Program, Department of Orthopedics and Podiatric Surgery, Kaiser Permanente, Oakland, CA, USA

Pediatry Institute Faculty Member, American Academy of Foot and Ankle, Osteosynthesis, Oakland, CA, USA

M. L. Butterworth, J. T. Marcoux (eds.), *The Pediatric Foot and Ankle*,
https://doi.org/10.1007/978-3-030-29788-6_14

biomechanical strength and stability for the physis at the zone of Ranvier [2, 3]. The physis or "growth plate" allows for skeletal growth via endochondral ossification. The natural epiphysiodesis that occurs within the distal tibia and fibula is asymmetric. The tibial physis initially ossifies centrally and then is directed medially and posteriorly. The anterolateral aspect of the distal tibia is the last anatomical region to ossify. The fibular physis normally will ossify 1–2 years after the distal tibia. The continued development of a physis is dependent on the ability of the epiphyseal vasculature to transverse the subchondral plate that parallels the physis. Damage to the epiphyseal subchondral plate can lead to vascular arrest in various areas of the physis resulting in premature arrest and progressive deformity. This is a well-established surgical treatment in the management of leg length discrepancy, but even in controlled surgical environment, complications occur [4]. Trauma to the physis heals via endochondral bone and cartilage formation. Three types of physeal healing can occur. The first reparative process is via cellular columns. This creates a temporary widening of the physis. The epiphyseal and metaphyseal vasculature become hyperemic producing increased cellular proliferation at the zone of Ranvier. This process can take 3–4 weeks until normal anatomy has been restored. The second method of repair occurs when there is increased hemorrhagic and fibrous tissue within the physis creating increased physeal displacement. In this situation, the metaphyseal vasculature has a more difficult means of crossing the physis to the epiphysis for repair because of the cartilaginous callus and increased damage to the cellular columns. The chondroprogenitor cells within the perichondrium (zone of Ranvier) respond to injury and contribute to articular cartilage healing [5]. The length of time that is required for the metaphyseal vascular to reestablish anastomosis with the epiphyseal vascular varies and is dependent on physeal displacement and periosteal damage and/or imbrication. This process can take 3–6 weeks, but final remodeling to a more normal anatomy can take several months to a year. The third method of physeal repair occurs when a significant amount of physeal separation is filled with fibrous tissue. It is critical in these scenarios that anatomic reduction occurs to minimize the increased physeal displacement. Failure to achieve anatomic reduction or iatrogenic damage to physis from an open reduction procedure can result in metaphyseal epiphyseal bony bridge resulting in premature growth arrest and deformity [6].

The metaphysis is highly osteobiologic and is composed of cortical fenestrations as it is maturing. The porous cortical bone allows for endosteal nutrient channeling between the metaphyseal marrow and subperiosteum. The anatomical nature of the metaphysis with trabecular fenestration is what precludes a higher incidence of torus-type fractures rather than complete fracture patterns. As the metaphysis matures, the underlying woven bone changes to lamellar bone. This impart contributes to the cortical thickening in adults which is fundamentally why torus fractures are not seen in adults without osteopenic disorders. The trabecular bone in the immature skeleton is what also can cause Harris or Park growth arrest lines. The sclerotic line, which runs parallel to the physis, is a result from disuse after trauma and infection. If longitudinal development is delayed for this reason, then the spongy trabeculations become horizontal rather than vertically oriented. This will autocorrect as normal growth and metaphyseal remodeling resumes. The transverse visible sclerotic line will normally disappear as they embark into the diaphysis. The periosteum in children possesses greater osteogenic potential than in adults and is tightly adhered to the zone of Ranvier. The thick pediatric periosteum provides for physeal displacement with trauma but can also interfere with reduction if the integrity has been compromised.

Imaging

When evaluating these fractures, it is essential to obtain the appropriate imaging. Standard radiographs are usually adequate for determining the management of physeal injuries. However, numerous reports have advocated the use of CT scans for assessing transitional fractures. They are useful in determining surgical indications.

Furthermore, if conservative management is going to be employed after a closed reduction, the CT scan should be obtained post-reduction. It is also strongly recommended for determining the fracture fragments in triplane fractures. The CT scan along with three-dimensional reconstruction is a useful tool in planning incisions, placement of reduction clamps, and orientation of screws. It also makes surgical management amenable to minimally invasive approaches.

Closed Management of Physeal Fractures

Most fractures in the immature skeleton that demonstrate greater than 2 mm of articular incongruency and/or physeal displacement should undergo an attempt of closed reduction with either conscious sedation or local anesthesia. Determining which fractures are best suited for closed reduction and with which type of anesthesia has not been well elucidated in the literature.

Surgical Management

Many differences exist in fracture healing and management between the pediatric and adult population. The pediatric patient has a thicker and more active periosteum, which provides greater fracture stability and leads to more rapid and reliable fracture healing. This physiologic advantage, along with the ability to recover soft tissue loss, can influence the surgeon's urgency for surgical management of open pediatric fractures. Overall, the infection rate is relatively low (3%), but has been shown to increase with higher-grade trauma.

Open Fractures

Although a modification of the Gustilo-Anderson grading system to better suit the pediatric population has been proposed, clinical validation is still pending. The reality is that there are no clear guidelines or algorithms for the management of pediatric open fractures, and care varies among training institutions [7]. Open fractures in the pediatric population involving the foot most commonly occur from lawnmower injuries and are very destructive. This occurs when small children are riding on a mower with a parent or chasing the parent on a mower and are unseen. Open fractures are seen in motor vehicular accidents and fall from heights, usually involving the tibia and forearm. Accordingly, the majority of studies review open tibia and forearm fractures but very few other pediatric open fractures. Very limited information is available for the management of the open foot and ankle fractures. Fortunately, only 6.6% of all pediatric open fractures involve the foot and ankle.

Pediatric Ankle Fractures

Epidemiology

Children have unique ankle fracture patterns, which in return can lead to various complications. Children's ankle fractures are the second most common growth plate fractures in humans [8]. Our goal when treating any pediatric fracture is to restore alignment and promote normal function with ongoing growth. Unfortunately, increased osseous and cartilaginous damage at the time of injury is associated with poorer outcomes such as growth disturbance, angular deformities, and posttraumatic arthritis. This in turn may lead to pain and functional deficits into adulthood. While children may remain asymptomatic with angulation of 5 degrees in the coronal plane or 10 degrees in the sagittal plane, they have shown to develop pain and degenerative changes into adulthood [9]. Hence, anatomic alignment should be the goal.

Ankle fractures represent about 5% of all fractures and remain the most common physeal injury in the lower extremity [10–13]. While all children are at risk of physeal injuries, the adolescent population is specifically at risk of transitional ankle fracture patterns given the nature of both the closing physis and the manner in which it closes. Quite often the process for physis closure takes 18 months. Displacement and angulation guide the surgeon toward treatment pathways. Some studies indicate that the incidence of ankle fractures is higher in children with greater body mass index [14, 15]. Thus, this may add increased challenges to the existing complexity of these fractures.

Pediatric Ankle Anatomy

The distal tibial physis closes over an 18-month period of time for most children. The transitional fracture patterns exist due to the anatomy of the ankle as well as the manner in which the distal tibial growth plate closes. In an asymmetric pattern, the distal tibia's physis closes from middle, to medial, and finally lateral. Hence, this is the reason for transitional triplane and Tillaux ankle fracture patterns. As for the younger child, one may present with Salter-Harris I injuries, as the growth plate tends to be weaker than the robust ligaments. With any fracture, the displacement tends to be minimized by the thick periosteum as compared to the adult population.

The degree of injury, displacement, fragmentation, and cartilaginous injury increases the child's risks for degeneration over time. It is important to educate the patient, parents, and/or respective guardians on this issue. Once articular cartilage is damaged by injury, overload, or wasting over age, the defect site does not usually regain original structure and function and may undergo degeneration [5]. There is limited regenerative capacity of articular cartilage which is likely due to low metabolic activity of articular chondrocytes and scarcity of resident mesenchymal progenitors [5]. While research continues to improve with respect to cartilage regeneration, it remains essential to obtain anatomic reduction of the ankle joint to minimize progressive degeneration that may occur from any residual deformity. There is a certain degree of degeneration that may take place due to the traumatic joint injury and cartilage injury at the time of fracture despite anatomic reduction.

When examining patients, it is important at times to obtain contralateral x-rays as subtle differences may be noted. These images are often supplemented with CT scans for review of accuracy of reduction, gap distance of fragments, and displacement. As transitional fractures occur near physis closure, it is generally not the culprit for growth arrest. Historically, x-rays have underrepresented these fracture patterns.

Radiographs

Plain film x-rays including anteroposterior (AP), Mortise, and lateral views are important for initial evaluation of alignment and fragmentation. These images can underestimate true displacement [16]. X-rays significant for displacement should lead to closed reduction of ankle fractures and splinting to maintain reduction. The AP x-ray shows a distal tibia Salter-Harris III fracture, while the lateral x-ray shows a Salter-Harris II or IV fracture. Multiple attempts at closed reduction or inappropriate maneuvers toward reduction have been associated with further joint damage. A CT scan is advised for true evaluation of transitional ankle fractures following closed reduction.

CT Scans

Anatomic reduction of the epiphysis and joint itself is important to minimize impending deformities and degeneration. After closed reduction is performed, a CT scan is utilized to evaluate any further step-off or gapping greater than 2 mm in any plane. Displacement of greater than 2 mm in any plane is an indication for surgery for both Tillaux and triplane fractures [17]. Eismann et al. noted an increase in operative treatment, with 26% of cases originally assigned nonoperative treatment when using radiographs being changed to operative treatment after review of CT scan [18]. As most surgical approaches are completed via a percutaneous technique and/or arthroscopy, a CT scan is essential in reviewing all fragments and location of fragments requiring fixation.

After review of CT scans by Eismann et al. [18], 39% of triplane fractures classified as ≤2 mm displaced by radiographs were changed to >2 mm displaced, which may have warranted a change in treatment on the basis of guidelines recommending surgery [8, 17, 19]. There can be variation of fragments especially among triplane fractures. Axial fracture lines determine optimal screw trajectories for fixation [20]. Triplane fractures have historically been characterized by the number of fracture fragments.

Cooperman et al. [21] described the two-part triplane fracture characterized by displacement of the posterior metaphysis, posterior epiphysis, and lateral epiphysis as a single bone fragment with attachment of the remaining anteromedial epiphysis to the tibial shaft. Marmor recognized the three-part fracture [22]. An anterolateral epiphyseal fragment and posterior metaphyseal fragment attached to the remaining epiphysis and tibial shaft were noted with three-part triplane fractures. Finally, Kärrhom et al. [14] described the four-part triplane fracture. The four fragments of the distal tibia included an anterolateral epiphyseal fragment, an anteromedial epiphyseal fragment, the remaining posterior epiphyseal fragment attached to the posterior metaphyseal fragment, and the tibial shaft.

There are now variants described with respect to triplane fractures, hence the importance of CT scans for assistance with hardware placement. A medial two-part fracture, two variants of the three-part fracture, and at least three variants of the four-part fracture have been described [15–29]. As these fracture lines may be difficult to appreciate intraoperatively, it is important to review the CT scan and have the knowledge of these fracture patterns.

Classification

Fracture mapping of triplane fractures has elucidated class-independent and class-dependent fracture patterns [20]. Hadad et al. noted that metaphyseal fractures are consistent across all triplane fractures and manifest most commonly as a medial-lateral fracture in the posterior metaphysis. Epiphyseal fractures have a common anterior fracture component and class-dependent posterior fracture patterns [20].

Salter-Harris classification 1963 [30]

Salter-Harris	Pattern	Characteristics
I	Separation through physis	May not be visible on x-ray
II	Metaphyseal fragment, above physis	Most common, Thurston-Holland fragment
III	Articulation, enters physis and exits epiphysis	Tillaux, intra-articular
IV	Complete, epiphysis then through physis and exits metaphysis	Risk of physeal arrest
V	Crushing/compression	Injury to physis, appositional growth disturbance risk
VI (Rang)	Injury to perichondral structures	Direct open injury

The Salter-Harris classification [30] of physeal fractures has been expanded to six types. Ogden from a series of 443 physeal fractures has added 3 further subsets [31]:
Ogden VII: Epiphyseal fractures not involving physis
Ogden VIII: Metaphyseal fractures affecting later growth
Ogden IX: Periosteal damage affecting later growth

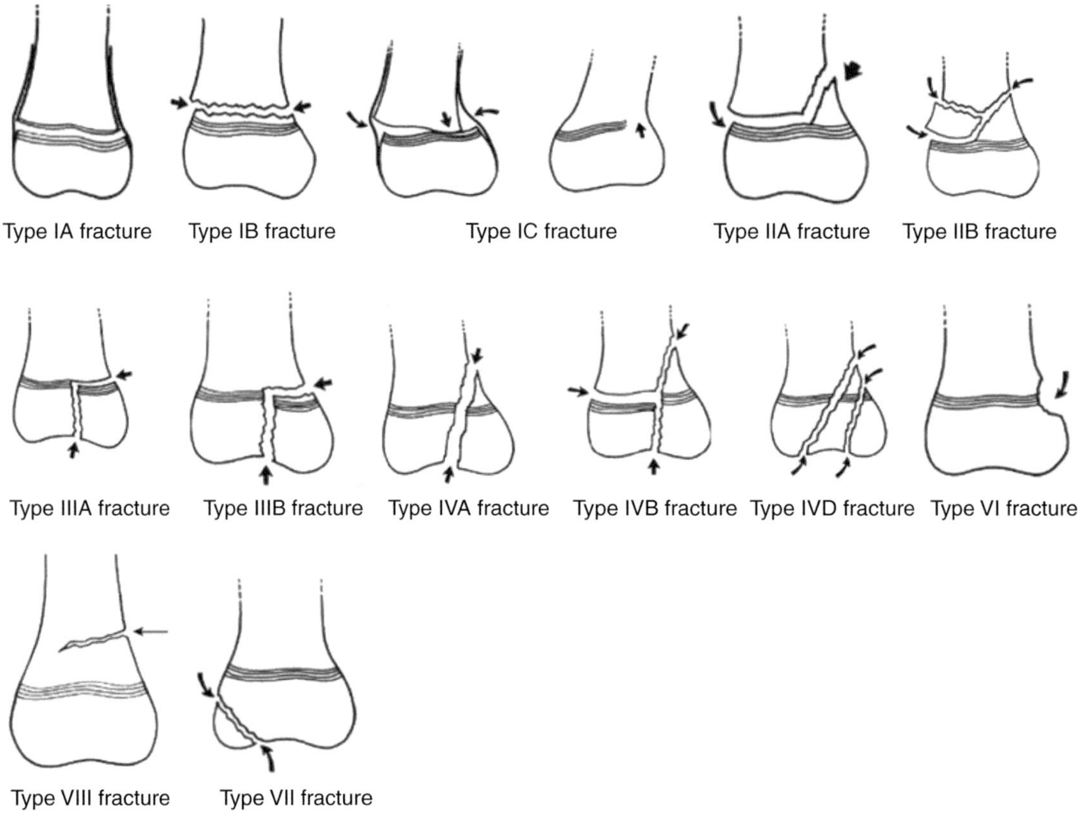

Physical Examination

Upon presentation it is important to evaluate the child for any neurovascular compromise. With open injuries vascular damage may be present along with sensory deficits. Likewise, areas of significant ecchymosis or severe swelling may influence screw placement. While compartment syndromes are rare with transitional pediatric ankle fractures, a good vascular exam and efficient closed reduction can reduce impending necrosis, wound development, or further complications. Both the dorsalis pedis and posterior tibial pulses should be palpable and documented. In the presence of significant edema, a Doppler may be utilized.

Malleoli tenderness is often present upon exam as compared to ligamentous injury alone. This should warrant completion of x-rays. Palpation should include above the ankle to the knee to evaluate for proximal fibula fractures. Fifth metatarsal base fractures are often associated with ankle fractures as well. With significant force, a child may present with concomitant foot fractures.

At times, excessive translation of fragments can compress the anterior aspect of the ankle. This may produce increased pain, hypoesthesia, numbness of the first interspace, and/or weakness of toe extensors [32, 33]. This requires efficient surgical release to minimize complications or functional deficits associated with extensor retinaculum syndrome [9]. Hence, time to closed reduction is important.

Conservative Management

Tillaux fractures as compared to triplane fractures can be less amenable to closed reduction as they are avulsion fractures of the anterior tibial-fibula ligament [34].

Plantarflexion, internal rotation followed by maximum ankle dorsiflexion, has been successful at reducing Tillaux fractures [35]. Closed reduction of triplane fractures generally requires internal rotation of the foot, followed by anterior translation and ankle dorsiflexion. With both fracture types, flexion of the knee at 90 degrees can relieve some tension and assist with reduction.

After closed reduction, often under conscious sedation, a splint or cast is applied. A CT scan confirms reduction. A gap distance greater than 2 mm warrants surgical intervention. If the gap distance is less than 2 mm, then conservative care is implemented and a long leg cast is applied for the first 3 weeks with serial images completed weekly to evaluate for any loss of reduction. Thereafter, the patient can be converted to a non-weight-bearing short leg cast to complete the 6-week course of immobilization. It is important to exclude any nonaccidental trauma and any atypical presentations that may present (Fig. 14.1).

Atypical Presentation

Pediatric patients are often healthy and present with strong bone. Particular care should be taken when children present without a history of trauma or one of vague trauma. An inability to ambulate may be associated with malignancy or hematogenous osteomyelitis. Pathologic fractures in the setting of malignant lesions, bone tumors, or osteogenesis imperfecta can take place. Likewise, metaphyseal corner fractures of the tibia are suspicious for nonaccidental trauma in very young patients [35]. Pain out of proportion following minor trauma or in association with fracture may be linked to complex regional pain syndrome. Early recognition of this pain syndrome as well as management with physical therapy and medications such as gabapentin and/or amitriptyline can be helpful in cessation of this condition.

Surgical Management of Displaced Ankle Fractures

Displacement of >2 mm in any plane is an indication for surgery for all transitional ankle fracture patterns [17]. With the use of CT scans, fracture mapping, and knowledge of fracture patterns, closed manipulation is complemented by percutaneous screw compression to stabilize. Arthroscopy can also be utilized to confirm appropriate reduction of the articular surfaces. Hardware is generally not associated with physeal arrest with transitional fractures as this population is close to physeal closure at the time of injury.

While alignment can be addressed with closed reduction and percutaneous fixation, physeal widening often requires an open approach due to invagination of tissue. A small incision overlying the affected physis provides good visualization for evacuation of the periosteum which blocks reduction of physeal widening.

Under general anesthesia, one uses a percutaneous technique with manual manipulation. Lag technique or lag by design is utilized for reduction of fragments in which there is pure distraction. If there is greater than 4 mm of distraction, one may utilize a periarticular reduction clamp for assistance [9]. With Tillaux fractures, one can use a guide wire from a 4.0 cannulated screw set from lateral to medial confined to the epiphysis [8]. The guide wire may be used to reduce the fracture fragments, or a clamp is applied prior to wire placement to assist with reduction [8]. The wire can be antegraded medially with intention of retrograde placement of screws if the fibula does not allow for seating of the intraepiphyseal screw heads [8]. Fluoroscopic images are used to assess reduction as well as transphyseal screw placement. Care is taken to avoid any further trauma to the physis or intra-articular surface. Arthroscopy can be utilized to assist with visualization of reduction.

For triplane fixation, one would implement the same percutaneous approach to transphyseal screw placement as discussed with respect to Tillaux fracture fixation. It is important to review the location of various fracture fragments via CT scans to determine exact position of screws and small incisions. Further, intrametaphyseal screws can be placed above the physis to complete triplane fixation. It is often helpful to fixate the intra-articular fragments prior to the metaphyseal fragments, so reduction is not blocked. Intraoperative imaging confirms less than 2 mm displacement following operative reduction. Fractures not amenable to this technique may require an open surgical approach (Fig. 14.2).

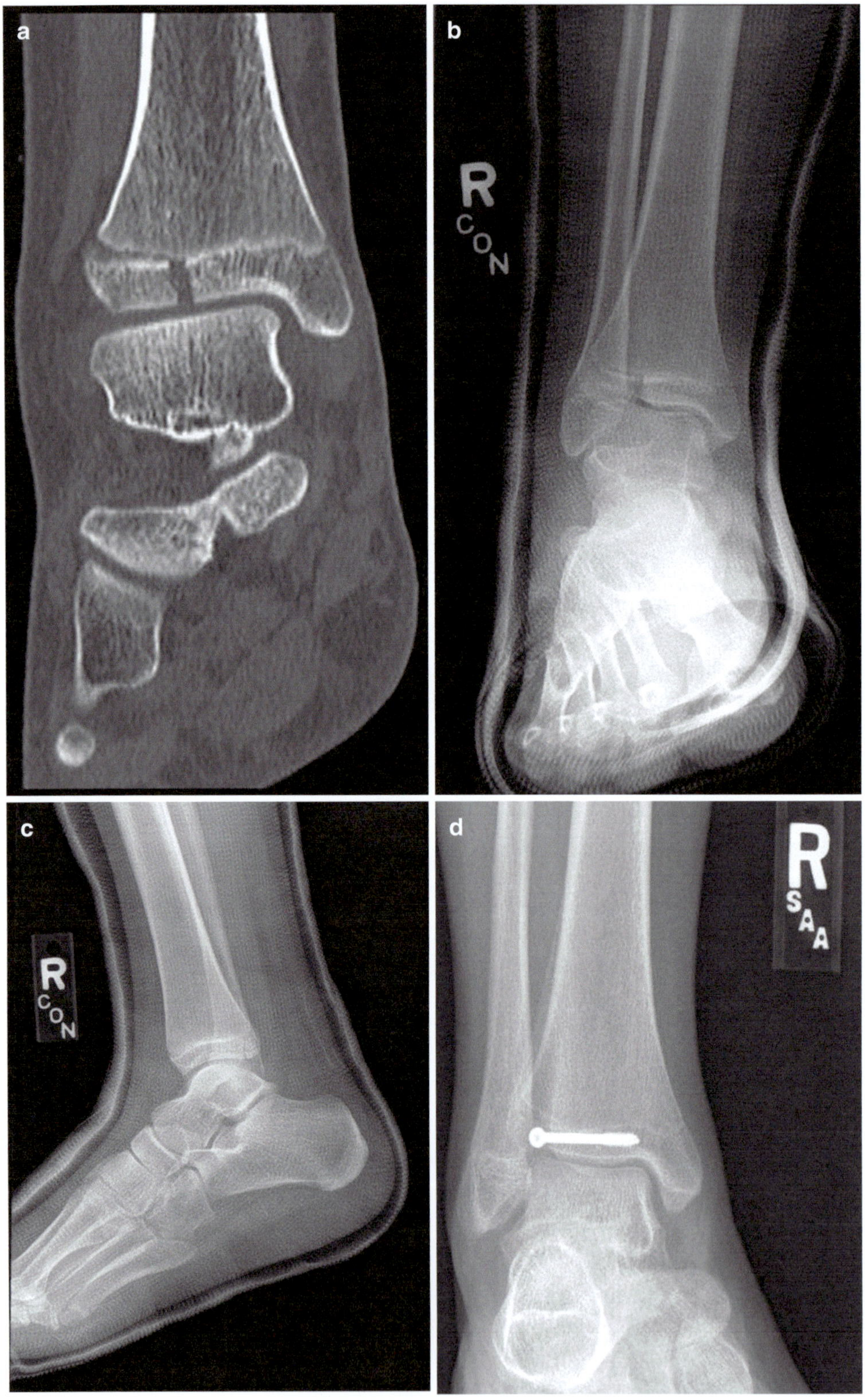

Fig. 14.1 Tillaux fracture: (**a**) CT scan, (**b**) AP x-ray post closed reduction, (**c**) lateral x-ray post closed reduction, (**d**) Tillaux intraepiphyseal fixation AP, (**e**) Tillaux intraepiphyseal fixation lateral

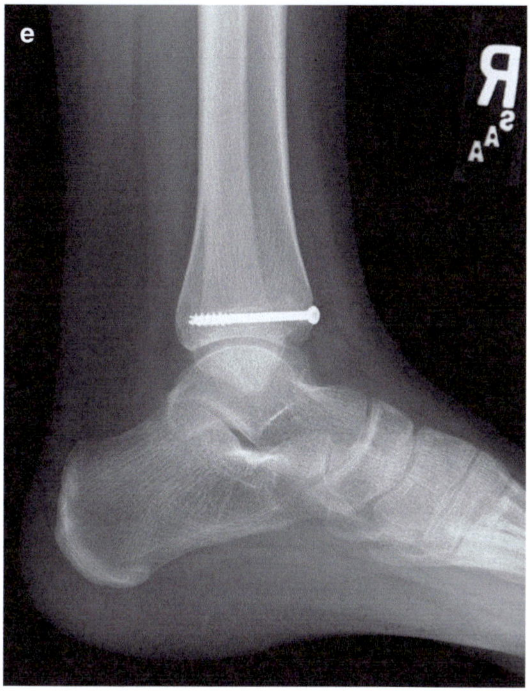

Fig. 14.1 (continued)

Fibular Fractures

Fibula fractures that are displaced or shortened greater than 2 mm should be reduced and then stabilized with plate fixation or intramedullary fixation in transitional fractures. As the tibia and fibula relationship is not static [36, 37], if the fibula deformity persists, it can drive the joint toward an angular deformity. The fibula normally moves more posteriorly with growth. In children where greater than 3 years of growth is expected, the fibular physis should be respected, and if fixation across it is necessary, smooth wires should be utilized [9]. Syndesmotic instability is rarely encountered (Fig. 14.3).

Complications

Limb Length Discrepancies/ Growth Disturbance

Growth arrest leading to angular deformities or limb length inequality is rare following treatment of transitional ankle fractures. Still, it is uncertain how much growth needs to be present for physeal arrest to cause a significant deformity. Given that these fractures occur in adolescence, the physis is in the process of closing already. Children who present with 3 years of growth or more should undergo preservation of the physis. To evaluate for growth arrest, one can visualize Park Harris lines (growth arrest lines) on x-rays. These lines represent the position of the physis at the time of injury and form on long bones due to growth arrest.

With evaluation of a limb length discrepancy, one must determine growth available. If a great deal of growth is available, then an epiphysiodesis of the elongated limb can be helpful. If little growth is available, then limb-lengthening procedures on the short limb may be utilized. The timing of epiphysiodesis should be identified carefully using one of the four accepted methods. These methods include the Anderson et al. [38] growth remaining charts, the White-Menelaus arithmetic method [39], the Moseley [40] straight line graph, and the Paley et al. [41] multiplier method.

Angular Deformities

While anatomic reduction, appropriate surgical technique, and minimizing attempts at closed reduction can certainly decrease further injury of the physis, it still appears that the mechanism of the injury [42, 43], initial displacement [44, 45], comminution [46] and post-reduction displacement [47] are most important in assessing growth plate injury and prognosis. In the presence of angular ankle deformities, a supramalleolar osteotomy may be required to restore alignment. One should evaluate for the center of rotation of angulation (CORA) with respect to deformity when determining osteotomy location.

Arthritis

In general, the type of Salter-Harris fracture, amount of initial displacement, and quality of reduction remain the main predictors of outcome.

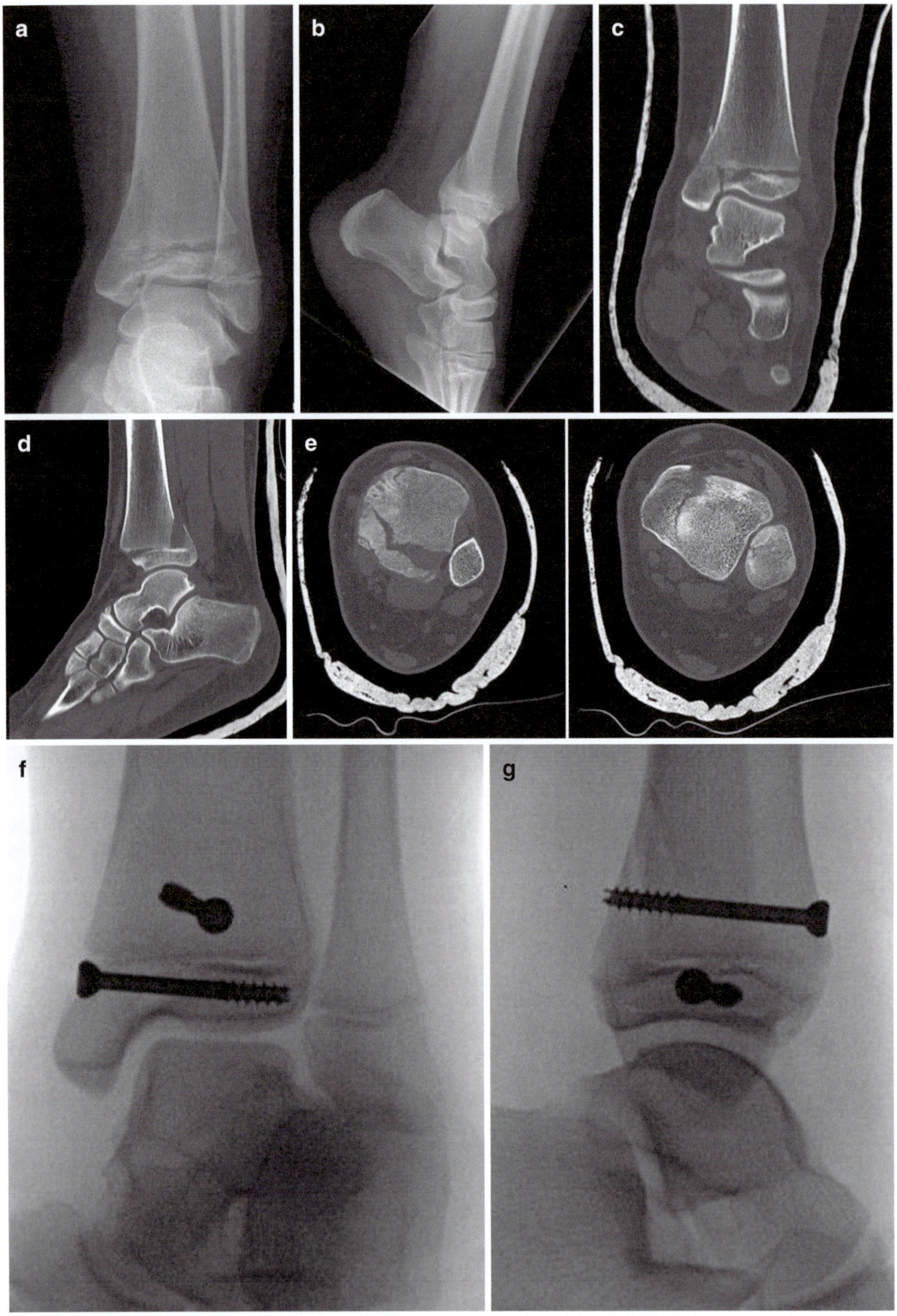

Fig. 14.2 Triplane ankle fracture: (**a**) AP x-ray of triplane fracture, (**b**) lateral x-ray of triplane fracture, (**c**) coronal CT scan triplane, (**d**) sagittal CT scan triplane, (**e**) axial CT scan triplane, (**f**) AP x-ray triplane ORIF, (**g**) lateral x-ray triplane ORIF

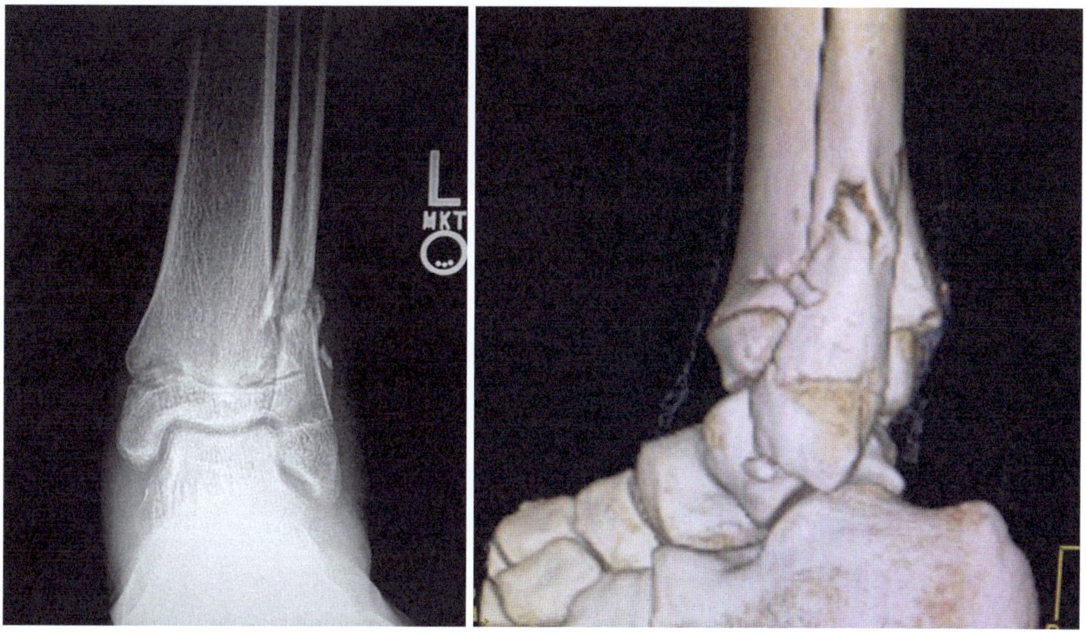

Fig. 14.3 Fibula fracture: angulation of the distal fibula is appreciated

Authors note that transitional fractures have good long-term outcomes provided the gap distance and step-off remains less than 2–2.5 mm [19, 48]. Any severe damage to cartilage may allow for progressive degeneration with growth over time. Surgical intervention is advised in SH-III and SH-IV medial malleolus fractures with more than 1 mm of displacement to minimize any delay in osseous healing. While non-unions are rare in this patient population, SH-III, SH-IV, and medial malleolus fractures have been associated with delayed healing (Figs. 14.4 and 14.5).

Infection

Timely closed reduction of ankle fractures reduces skin necrosis and pressure on anatomic structures and minimizes any vascular compromise. This in turn can minimize risks of infection and soft tissue complications. Children are at risk of infections throughout their life at the metal-tissue interface. The glycocalyx (glycoprotein and polysaccharide) forms fibers that extend from cell to metal surfaces [49]. Hence, implanted metals tend to potentiate bacteria. Often hematogenous spread is noted among patients where infection does not arise until years later. Acute surgical site infections tend to be rare in this patient population.

Metallic Implant Removal

In the second half of the twentieth century, improvements in metal quality reduced the initial concern of corrosion in the pediatric population [49–53]. Others were still concerned with risks of carcinogenicity with retained metallic implants. Now concerns over leaving hardware implanted indefinitely stem from stress shielding issues. Fractures associated with stress shielding of retained plates can be difficult to treat [54].

One of the greatest concerns of retained transphyseal screws is with respect to an increase in articular pressure that may cause premature degenerative joint disease. Charlton et al. demonstrated that transphyseal metallic implants in the distal tibia significantly change the articular pressure in the ankle joint with simulated weight bearing [55]. While this was a cadaveric study with a small sample size, the results remain concerning for increased peak contact pressures.

The authors recommend removal of transphyseal hardware upon osseous union for this reason. Likewise, any hardware that traverses the physis should be removed as soon as possible. When the risk of removal outweighs hardware retention, then it is prudent to leave the implant alone.

Key Points

- A gap distance of less than 2 mm is acceptable [8].
- X-rays underrepresent displacement.
- CT scans are advised following closed reduction.

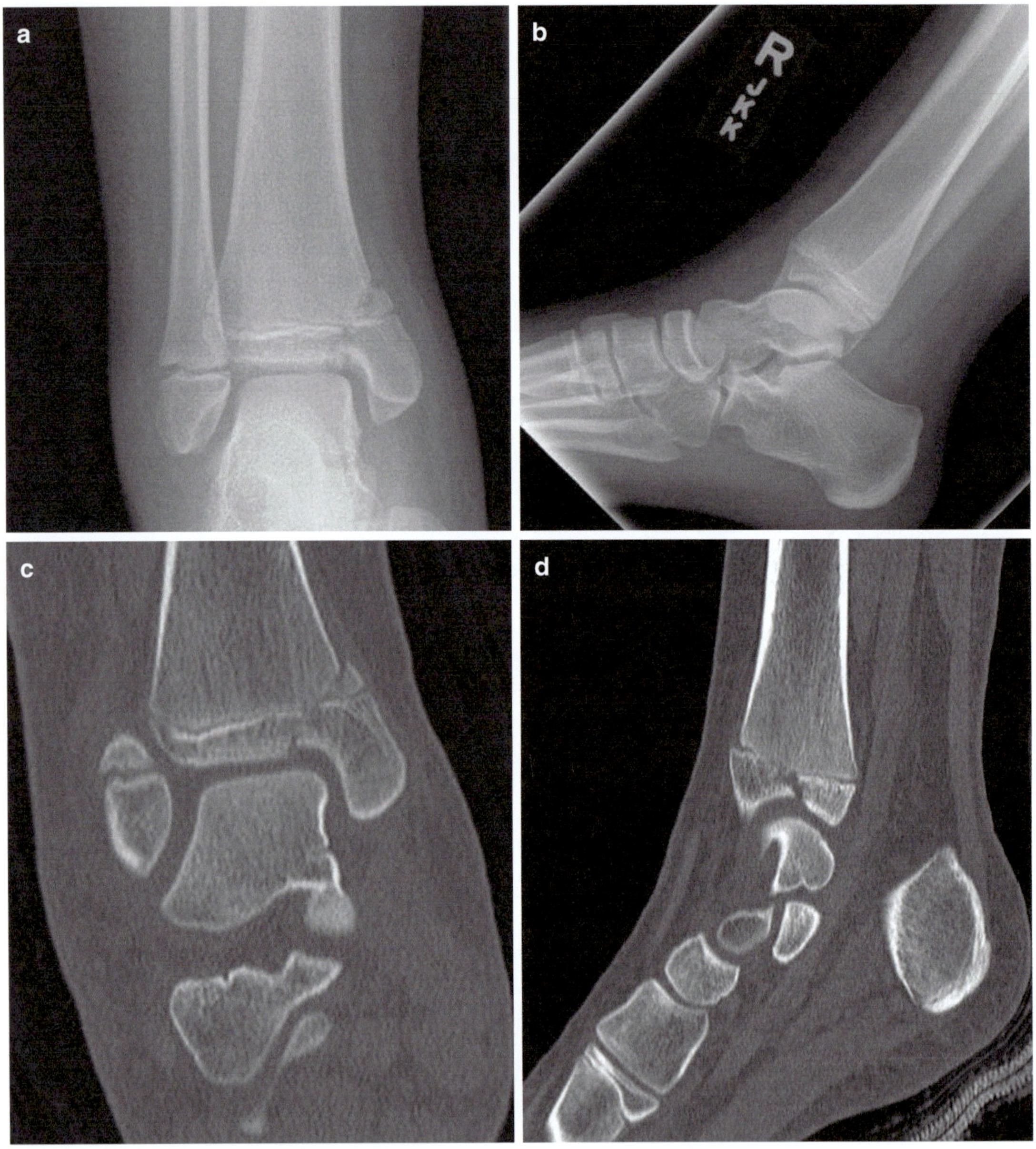

Fig. 14.4 Medial malleolus fracture SHIV: (**a**) AP x-ray, (**b**) lateral x-ray, (**c**) coronal CT scan, (**d**) sagittal CT scan, (**e**) CT 3D reconstructive view posterior ankle, (**f**) AP post ORIF, (**g**) lateral post ORIF

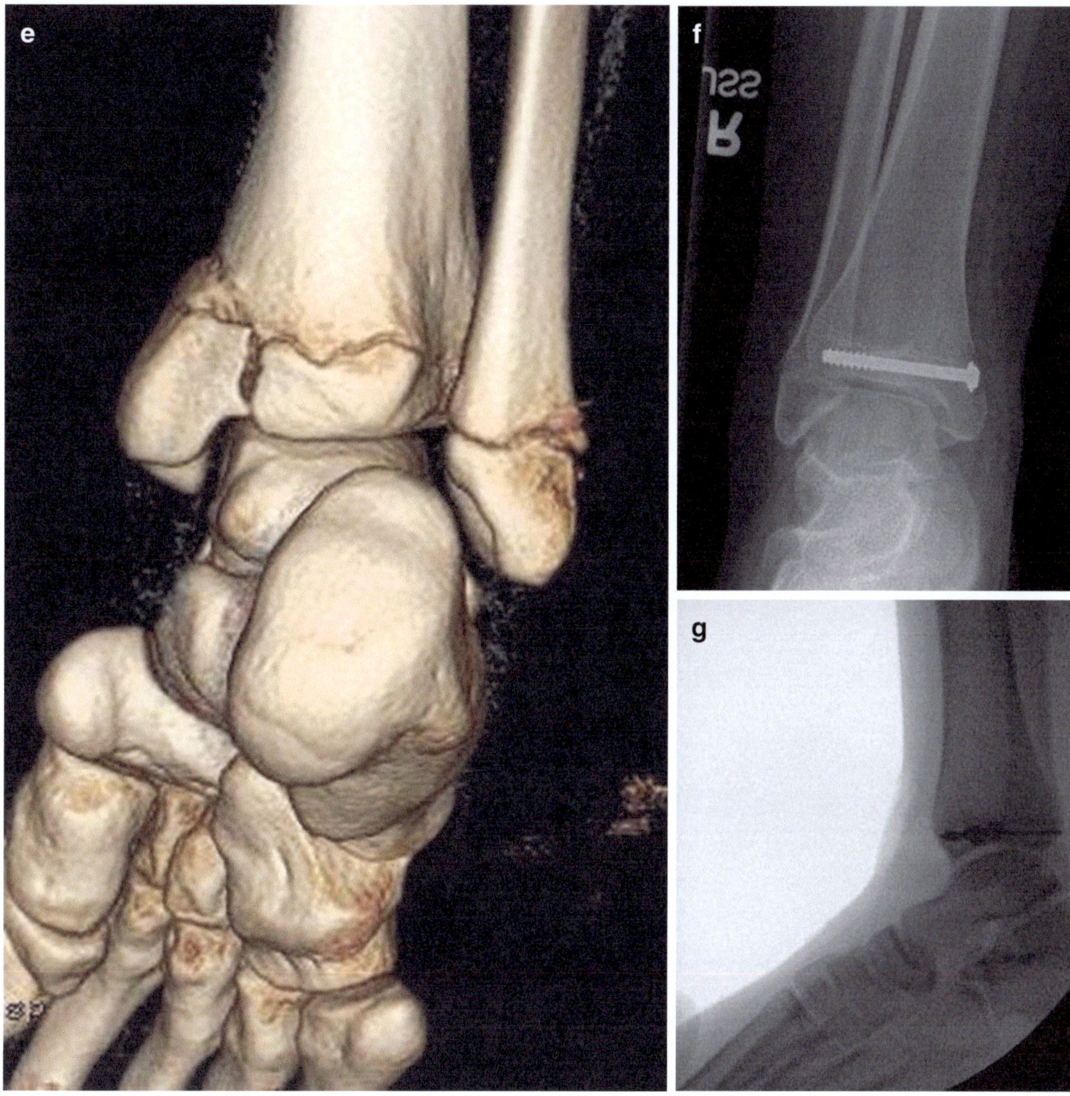

Fig. 14.4 (continued)

- In an ankle where >3 years of growth is expected, one should respect the physis.
- Percutaneous and/or arthroscopic approach is recommended for transitional ankle fractures in need of surgery. Intraepiphyseal and intrametaphyseal fixation should be utilized.
- The relationship between the tibia and fibula changes with growth.
- Intra-articular fractures should be reduced and fixed to less than 2 mm of displacement [19].
- Mechanism of the injury, initial displacement, comminution, and post-reduction displacement are most important in assessing growth plate injury and prognosis [45].
- Transphyseal metallic implants in the distal tibia significantly change the articular pressure in the ankle joint with simulated weight bearing. The authors recommend removal of hardware upon osseous healing if patient is stable for surgery [55].

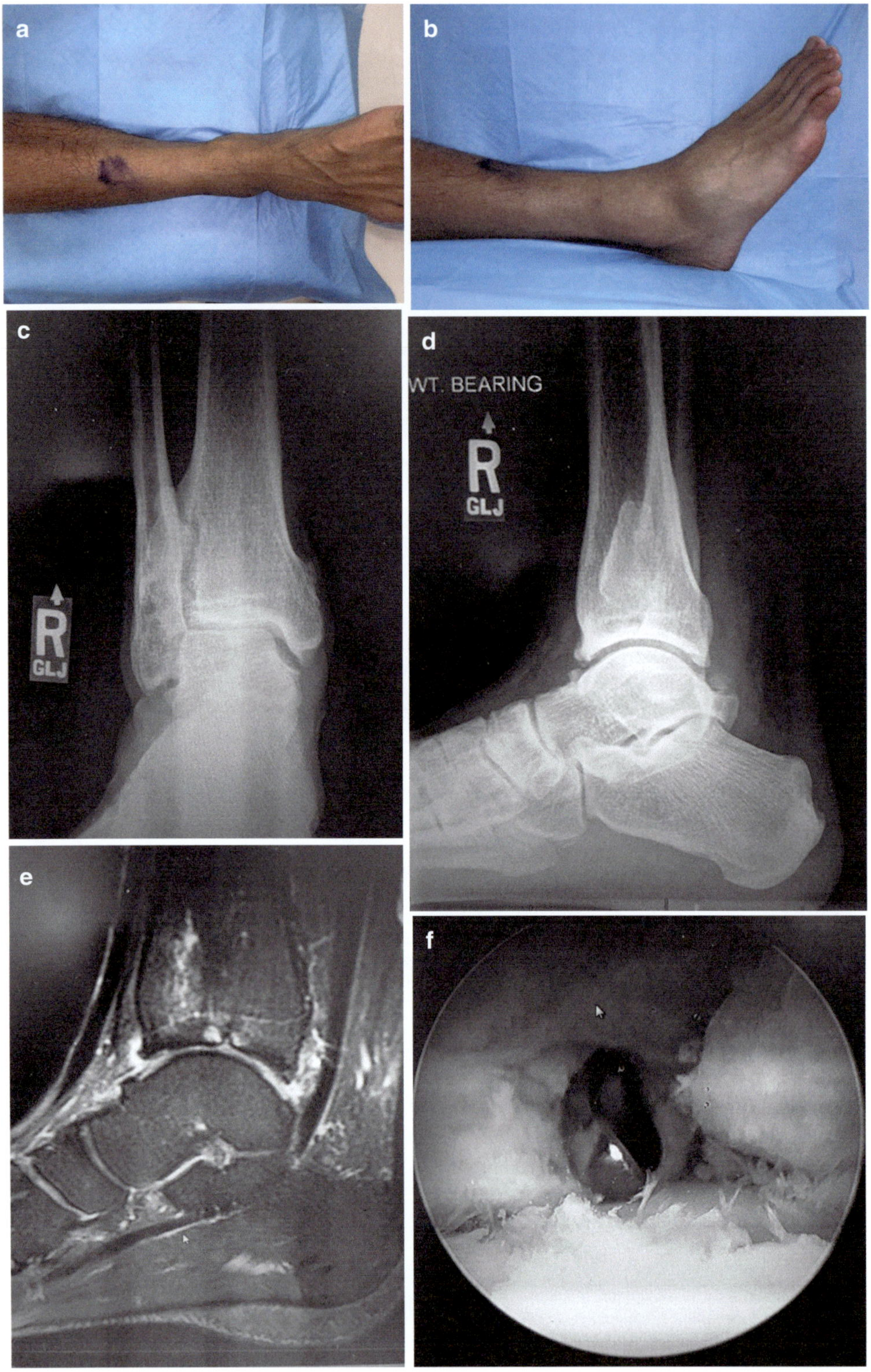

Fig. 14.5 Degeneration: patient status post-pediatric triplane ankle fracture 15 years prior to ankle arthroscopic images. (**a**) Clinical photo, (**b**) clinical photo, (**c**) AP x-ray, (**d**) lateral x-ray, (**e**) MRI, (**f**) arthroscopic evaluation

Foot Fractures

Anatomy

In the pediatric patient, there are relatively few fractures, but there are many anatomic variants that mimic fractures. Many children have accessory bones in which up to 20% have been reported in the literature. There are 24 different accessory ossicles in the foot which include accessory navicular bone, os peroneum, os trigonum, os intermetatarseum, os vesalianum, os subfibulare, os subtibiale, os calcaneus secundarius, os calcaneus accessorium, os supratalare, os sustentaculi, os talotibiale, os tali accessorium, talus secundarius, os subcalcis, os cuboideum secundarium, os supranaviculare, os infranaviculare, os paracuneiforme, os intercuneiforme, os cuneometatarsale I tibiale, os cuneometatarsale plantare, os cuneo-I metatarsale-II dorsale, and os aponeurosis plantaris [56]. Careful attention should be paid to these, as they are easily confused with fractures. If not sure as to whether it is a fracture or an accessory bone, do not hesitate to image the other foot for comparison. During the gait cycle, the foot performs many different tasks. It must be both flexible at foot strike and rigid at lift off to function appropriately, so careful attention must be paid to ensure that any fracture does not affect this normal function.

Talus Fractures

Fractures of the talus are rare in children, but when they do occur, careful attention must be paid to the anatomy and blood supply of the talus as these injuries have high rates of non-union, AVN, and osteoarthritis especially after a high-energy mechanism [57–59]. The posterior tibial artery has a branch to the tarsal canal. This artery then divides and provides multiple branches to the talar body. The dorsalis pedis artery has a lateral branch to the talar body. The dorsalis pedis also has a branch that communicates with the perforating peroneal artery. Arising from the peroneal artery are branches to the posterior talus tubercle region. Disruption of the blood supply to the talus puts a patient at high risk for avascular necrosis. Most fractures of the talus result from trauma such as a fall from a height in which there is forced dorsiflexion at the ankle. Although fractures through the pediatric talar neck are rare, they must be reduced as soon as possible if there is dislocation. There has been no specific classification system developed for pediatric talar neck fractures, but the classification developed by Hawkins has been adopted by most in the evaluation of pediatric talar neck fractures. The larger the type of fracture, the more risk of avascular necrosis occurs. Hawkins classification is as follows[60]:

- Type 1 – minimally displaced talar neck fracture
- Type 2 – talar neck fracture that also includes subluxation or dislocation of the subtalar joint
- Type 3 – includes type 2 with the addition of ankle dislocation
- Type 4 – Canale [61] added a type 4 to the classification, which includes type 3 with the addition of dislocation of the talar head from the navicular

Most of these fractures can be treated with closed reduction and casting. The technique for reduction is done by plantarflexing and everting the forefoot [62]. Once the reduction is obtained, it is best to treat with an above-the-knee cast holding the foot in a slight plantarflexed and everted position. Post-reduction radiographs must be taken to ensure that the reduction has not resulted in a varus alignment. If closed reduction cannot be obtained or you are dealing with a probable non-compliant patient, then surgical reduction and fixation is necessary. If reduced in the operating room, a large number of these fractures can be fixated with percutaneous screws from anterior to posterior. If closed reduction cannot be obtained, then a dorsomedial approach is utilized followed by two screws crossing the talar neck.

Whether treated conservatively or surgically, the pediatric patient should be kept non-weight bearing in a long leg cast for 6–8 weeks. All patients who suffer a talar neck fracture should

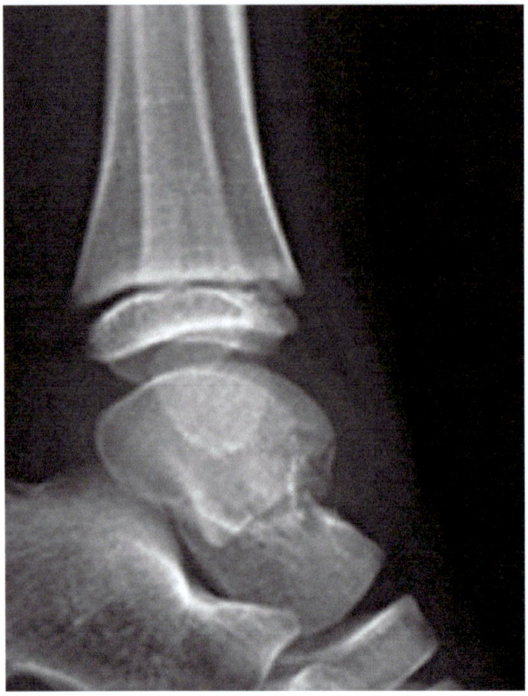

Fig. 14.6 Non-displaced Hawkins type I fracture

be followed up long term to insure that avascular necrosis does not develop [63] (Fig. 14.6).

Other Fractures of the Talus

Although fractures of the talar body and talar dome are extremely rare, they are intra-articular fractures and anatomic reduction must be obtained.

Calcaneal Fractures

Calcaneal fractures in the pediatric population are not common. When they do occur, the majority of these fractures are non-displaced [64]. It is reported in the literature that a high percentage of these fractures are extra-articular, which can be attributed to low trauma and the flexibility and resiliency of the cartilage, bone, and soft tissues [65]. The standard treatment protocol for all pediatric calcaneal fractures is nonoperative treatment [64]. The pediatric patient may have some loss of subtalar motion and joint arthrosis, but this is rare and has little effect on normal gait [64]. There have been some recent studies in treating the displaced fracture with the standard approaches used for surgical repair of adult calcaneal fractures with good clinical outcomes and few complications [65]. Intraoperative treatment of calcaneal fractures is rarely indicated even for displaced intra-articular fractures as the remodeling that occurs leads to satisfactory results [62]. When there is a depressed posterior facet, utilization of a small sinus tarsi incision and manipulation of the fracture fragment with direct visualization are utilized. These can be fixated with k-wires or screws, and in most cases the fixation is removed after fracture consolidation (Fig. 14.7).

Tarsometatarsal Injuries

Injuries to the tarsometatarsal joint are rare in children, but they are easily missed due to the incomplete ossification of the foot bones on radiographs. In the pediatric patient, the distance between the base of the first and second metatarsal is quite constant (below 3 mm), and the distance between the medial cuneiform and the base of the second metatarsal is larger before the age of 6. Both of these distances approach adult values (below 2 mm) at the age of 6 [66]. Tarsometatarsal joint injuries can be caused from direct or indirect mechanisms and may be either high- or low-energy trauma. High-energy injuries are usually the result of a fall from a height or motor vehicular accidents. Usually with these high-energy injuries, a fracture dislocation occurs at the tarsometatarsal joint. The low-energy fractures usually occur from landing on a foot in a tiptoe position after a jump or from a marked compression load to the heel while the patient is in a kneeling position which produces indirect dorsiflexion and plantarflexion forces [67, 68]. These low-energy injuries usually occur during athletic activities and are usually a purely ligamentous injury [69]. These injuries in the pediatric population can be treated nonsurgically with closed reduction and casting or

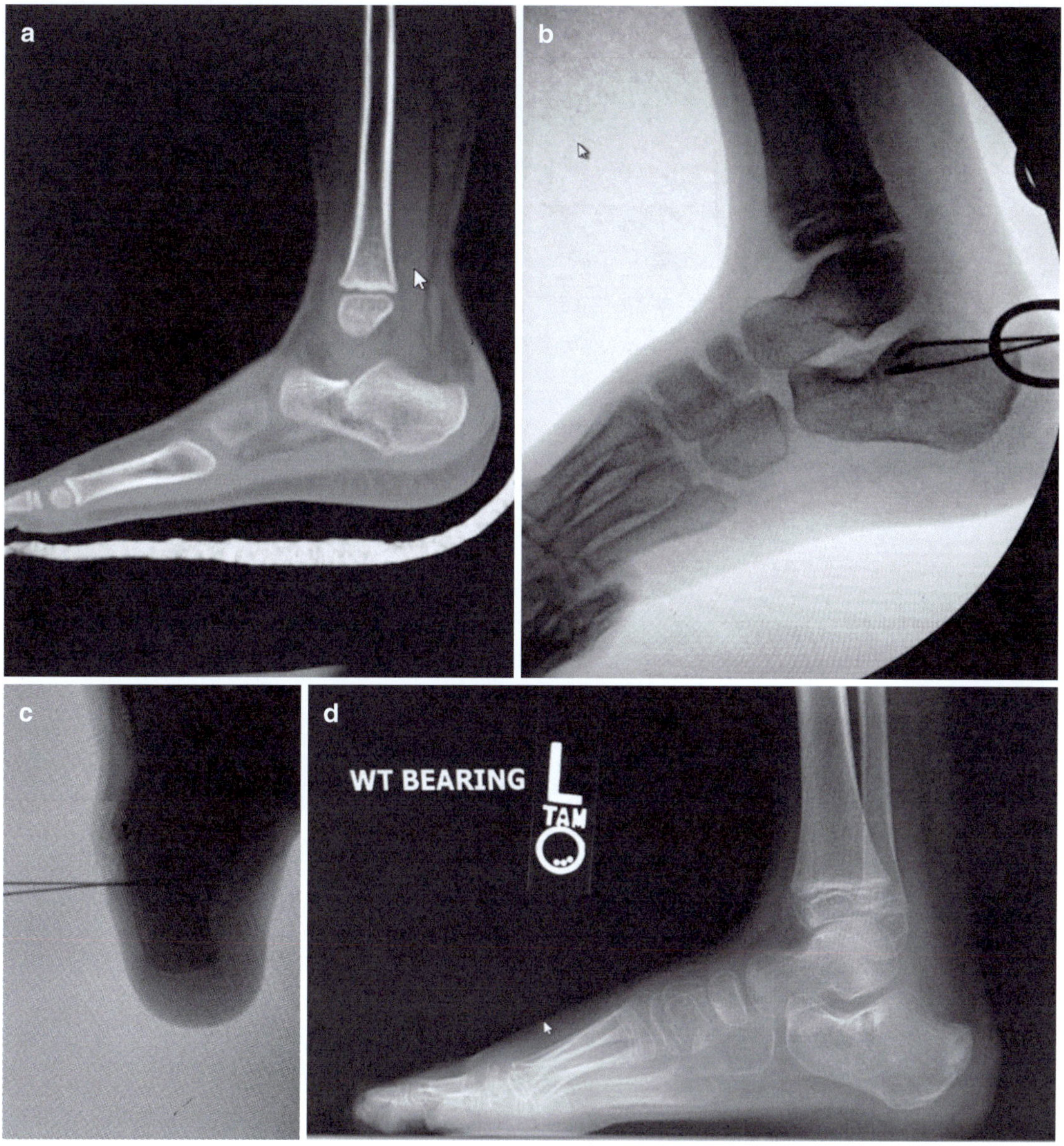

Fig. 14.7 Eight-year-old patient with intra-articular joint depression of posterior facet of calcaneus from fall from a high height. (Case shared by Jason Pollard D.P.M.) (**a**) Lateral x-ray injury film. (**b**) Intra-op lateral x-ray post joint reduction with k-wire fixation. (**c**) Intra-op calcaneal axial x-ray post-reduction with k-wire fixation. (**d**) Lateral x-ray post pin removal

with surgical intervention if reduction is unable to be obtained. The short-term outcomes have generally been favorable with patients having no limitations in athletic or everyday activities [68, 70]. Fixation for pediatric Lisfranc injuries is with a smooth k-wire in most cases. Bridge plating and screws can be used if needed but requires fixation to be removed after consolidation (Figs. 14.8 and 14.9). Even with anatomic reduction and immobilization, studies suggest that long-term outcomes may be similar to those of adults. In adults, degenerative arthritis in the tarsometatarsal joints is the most common complication.

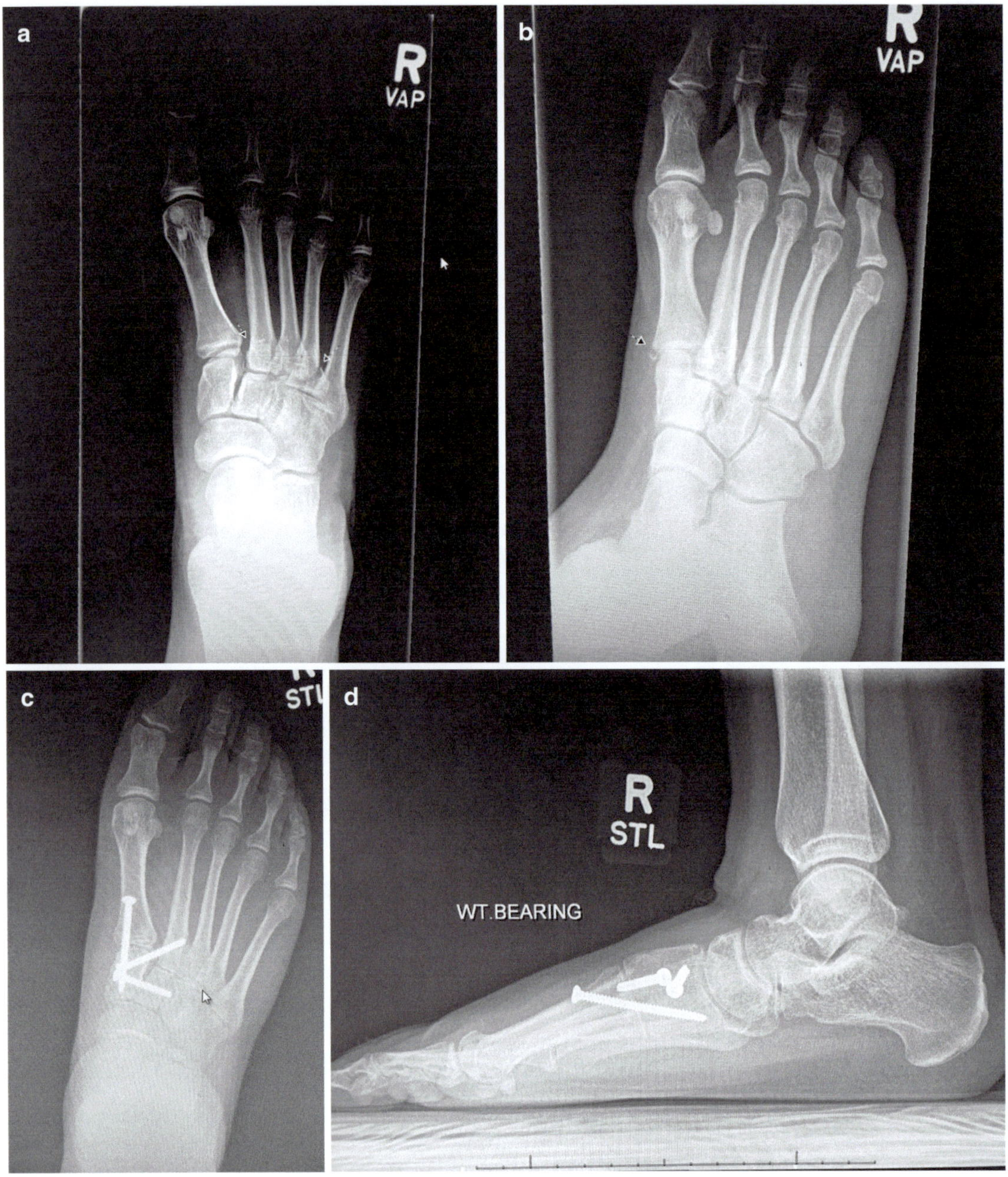

Fig. 14.8 Pediatric Lisfranc's injury with instability and fractures. (**a**) AP x-ray injury film. (**b**) Oblique x-ray injury film. (**c**) Postoperative AP x-ray with screw fixation. (**d**) Postoperative lateral x-ray with screw fixation

Metatarsal Fractures

Fractures of the metatarsals necks and shaft can be treated closed most of the time. They represent a large portion, 61%, of all pediatric foot fractures [71]. Minimally displaced fractures are treated with a walking cast for approximately 1 month. If there is significant displacement, then they need to be reduced under anesthesia. The most common reduction method utilizes distraction with Chinese finger trap device followed by percutaneous pinning with a Kirschner wire.

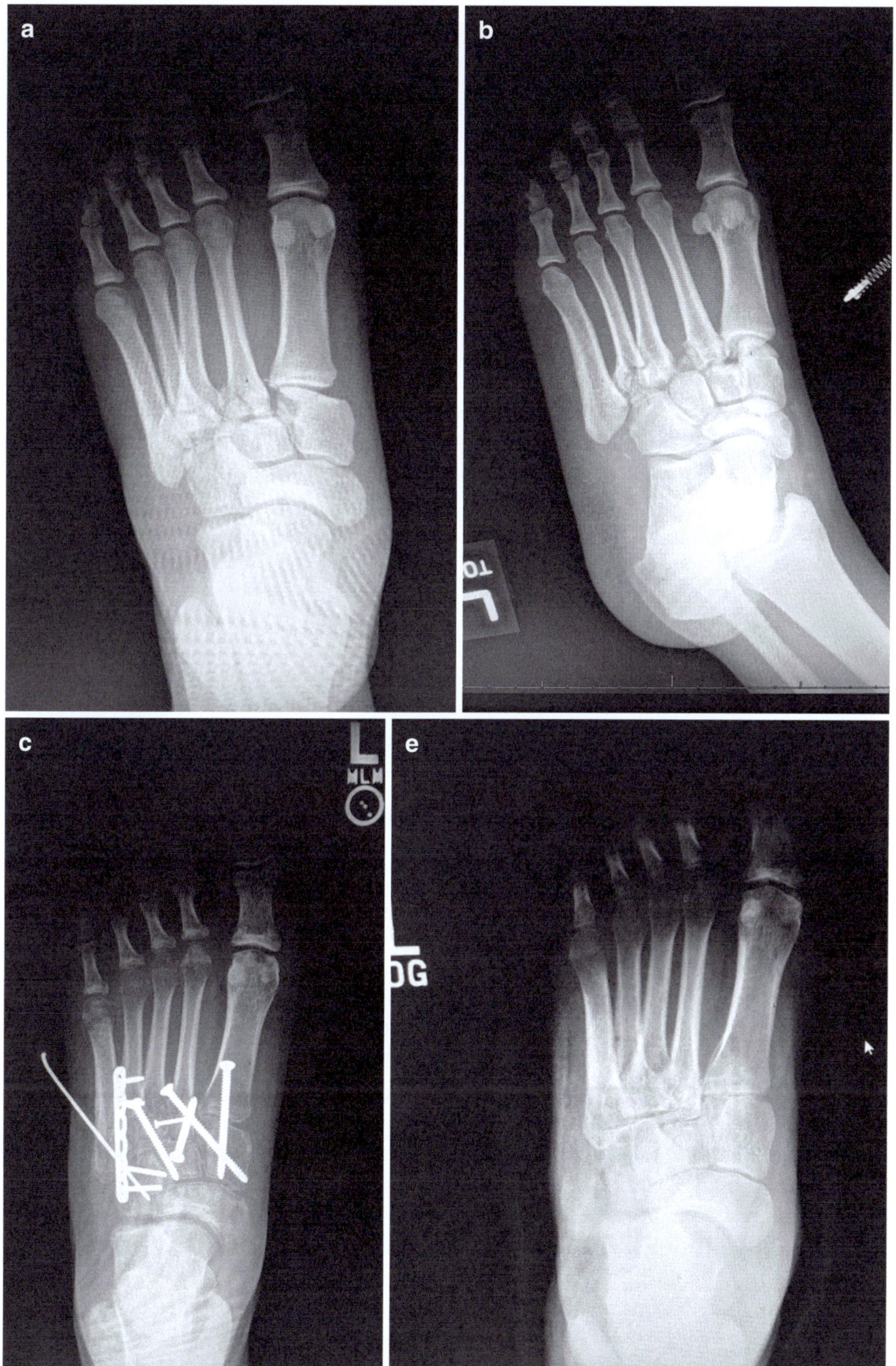

Fig. 14.9 Lisfranc's with comminuted intra-articular metatarsal base fractures. (**a**) AP x-ray injury film with comminuted metatarsal base fracture, angulation changes, and displaced medial cuneiform. (**b**) Oblique x-ray showing comminuted metatarsal bases with dislocation. (**c**) Post-reduction AP x-ray with k-wire, screws, and bridge plating. (**d**) Post-reduction lateral x-ray with k-wire, screws, and bridge plating. (**d**) Postoperative AP x-ray 1 year after hardware removal

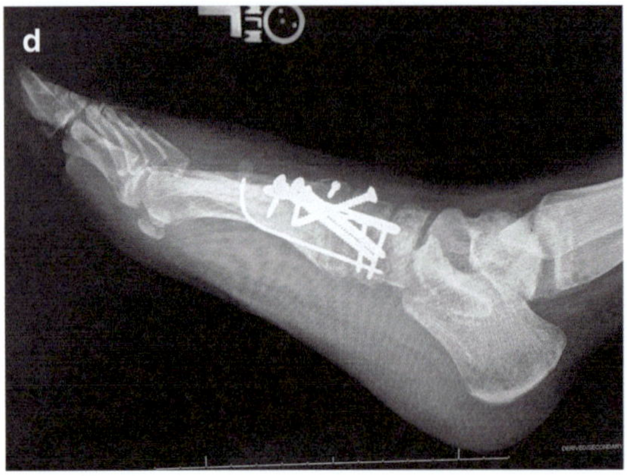

Fig. 14.9 (continued)

Rarely do these fractures need to be surgically opened; however, when necessary, it is done through a small incision with Kirschner wire insertion through the fracture site, which exits through the skin in the sulcus and is then advanced across the fracture site in a retrograde fashion. Avulsion fracture to the fifth metatarsal base is not uncommon in the pediatric patient. It results in pain with weight bearing and walking but usually has less edema than a typical metatarsal fracture. Treatment for these is weight bearing for 4–6 weeks in a short leg cast or fracture boot. Immobilization can be discontinued when the edema and tenderness have resolved. Stress fractures can occur in children, but they are a lot less common in adults (Fig. 14.10).

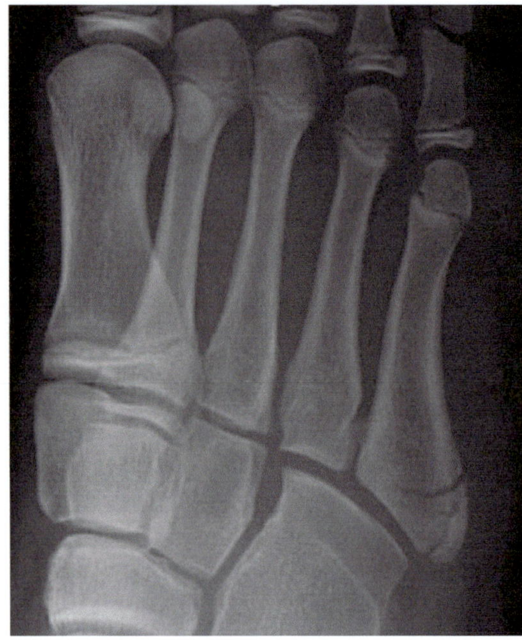

Fig. 14.10 Non-displaced fracture of the fifth metatarsal base with open physis. Treated conservatively with no complications

Pain Management

Managing pain after fractures in the pediatric population is often underappreciated. It is falsely believed that children do not experience pain or have much higher pain tolerance than the adult population. Other factors that play a role in the undertreatment of pediatric pain are lack of pain assessment and the fear of adverse effects such as respiratory depression from analgesic medications.

Understanding the common pharmacologic agents for the acute pain management can make the post-injury period more tolerable for both the patient and the parents. Acetaminophen is the most commonly used analgesic agent in the pediatric population secondary to minimal side effects and good safety profile. It is appropriate for mild to moderate pain and can be used in combination with narcotics for more severe pain. The medication is dosed at 10–15 mg/kg, with single dosing of 20 mg/kg noted to be well tolerated and safe. The daily maximum should not exceed 75 mg/kg for oral preparations.

Similar to acetaminophen, ibuprofen is a commonly used nonsteroidal anti-inflammatory drug for mild to moderate pain. It too comes in both a tablet and liquid form. Unlike in adults, the gastrointestinal and renal side effects are negligible [72]. Parenteral ketorolac can be administered postoperatively at a single dose of 0.8 mg/kg and has been shown to decrease opioid use by 30% after surgery [73]. Finally, opioids can be administered for more severe pain. In older children, and adolescents, Norco can be given at adult dosage in tablet form. In some circumstances, younger children can be given the liquid form. However, more commonly, younger children are given codeine in combination with acetaminophen.

Maltreatment

Although it is not likely to be encountered with isolated foot and ankle injuries, it is important to understand some of the features in identifying child abuse. Orthopedic injuries result in the care of 30–50% of abused children [74]. Fortunately, the large majority of fractures are related to a fall from heights, motor vehicular accidents, and other non-abusive trauma and metabolic conditions such as osteogenic imperfecta. However, it is important to recognize abuse since 25% of children suffer from further abuse, and 5% of children are at risk for death [75].

To identify child abuse as the cause of fractures, the physician must take into consideration the history, the age of the child, the location and type of fracture, the mechanism that causes the particular type of fracture, and the presence of other injuries while also considering other possible causes such as social circumstances of the child and family members.

Although there are not any significant predictors, there are certain patterns of injury that should raise potential awareness for child abuse. A systematic review demonstrated the cases of abuse most often occurring in infants and toddlers (< 3 years of age) and including multiple fractures [76].

A review of 32 studies demonstrated that once major trauma was excluded, rib fractures had the highest probability for abuse (0.71; 95% confidence interval, 0.42 to 0.91). The probability of abuse given a humeral fracture lies between 0.48 (0.06 to 0.94) and 0.54 (0.20 to 0.88), depending on the definition of abuse used. Analysis of fracture type showed that supracondylar humeral fractures were less likely to be inflicted. For femoral fractures, the probability was between 0.28 (0.15 to 0.44) and 0.43 (0.32 to 0.54), depending on the definition of abuse used, and the developmental stage of the child was an important discriminator. The probability for skull fractures was 0.30 (0.19 to 0.46); the most common fractures in abuse and non-abuse were linear fractures. Insufficient comparative studies were available to allow calculation of a probability of abuse for other fracture types.

References

1. Goldring MB. Chondrogenesis, chondrocyte differentiation, and articular cartilage metabolism in health and osteoarthritis. Ther Adv Musculoskelet Dis. 2012;4:269–85.
2. Löfgren M, Ekman S, Svala E, Lindahl A, Ley C, Skiöldebrand E. Cell and matrix modulation in prenatal and postnatal equine growth cartilage, zones of Ranvier and articular cartilage. J Anat. 2014;225(5):548–68. https://doi.org/10.1111/joa.12232.
3. Shapiro F, Holtrop ME, Glimcher MJ. Organization and cellular biology of the perichondrial ossification groove of Ranvier: a morphological study in rabbits. J Bone Joint Surg Am. 1977;59:703–23.
4. Makarov MR, Dunn SH, Singer DE, Rathjen KE, Ramo BA, Chukwunyerenwa CK, Birch JG. Complications associated with epiphysiodesis for management of leg length discrepancy. J Pediatr Orthop. 2018;38(7):370–4.
5. Candela ME, Yasuhara R, Iwamoto M, Enomoto-Iwamoto M. Resident mesenchymal progenitors of articular cartilage. Matrix Biol. 2014;39:44–9. https://doi.org/10.1016/j.matbio.2014.08.015.
6. Schneidmueller D, Bühren V. Verletzungen des Jugendlichen – die Übergangsfraktur Nomenklatur, Diagnostik und Therapie. Trauma Berufskrankh. 2016;18(Suppl 2):101–4.
7. Lavelle WH, Uhl R, Krieves M, Drvaric DM. Management of open fractures in pediatric patients: current teaching in Accreditation Council for Graduate Medical Education (ACGME) accredited residency programs. J Pediatr Orthop B. 2008;17(1):1–6.
8. Crawford AH. Triplane and Tillaux fractures: is a 2 mm residual gap acceptable? J Pediatr Orthop. 2012;32(Suppl 1):S69–73.
9. Olgun ZD, Maestre S. Management of pediatric ankle fractures. Curr Rev Musculoskeletal Med. 2018;11(3):475–84.
10. Landin LA, Danielsson LG. Children's ankle fractures. Classification and epidemiology. Acta Orthop Scand. 1983;54:634–40.
11. Peterson HA, Madhok R, Benson JT, et al. Physeal fractures: part 1. Epidemiology in Olmsted County, Minnesota, 1979–1988. J Pediatr Orthop. 1994;14:423–30.
12. Peterson CA, Peterson HA. Analysis of the incidence of injuries to the epiphyseal growth plate. J Trauma. 1972;12:275–81.
13. Mizuta T, Benson WM, Foster BK, et al. Statistical analysis of the incidence of physeal injuries. J Pediatr Orthop. 1987;7:518–23.
14. McHugh MP. Oversized young athletes: a weighty concern. Br J Sports Med. 2010;44:45–9.
15. Zonfrillo MR, Seiden JA, House EM, et al. The association of overweight and ankle injuries in children. Ambul Pediatr. 2008;8:66–9.

16. Mann DC, Rajmaira S. Distribution of physeal and nonphyseal fractures in 2,650 long-bone fractures in children aged 0–16 years. J Pediatr Orthop. 1990;10:713–6.
17. Ertyl JP, Barrack RL, Alexander AH, et al. Triplane fracture of the distal tibial epiphysis. Long term follow up. J Bone Joint Surg Am. 1988;70:967–76.
18. Eismann EA, Stephan ZA, Mehlman CT, Denning J, Mehlman T, Parikh SN, Tamai J, Zbojniewicz A. Pediatric triplane ankle fractures: impact of radiographs and computed tomography on fracture classification and treatment planning. J Bone Joint Surg Am. 2015;97:995–1002.
19. Rapariz JM, Ocete G, González-Herranz P, López-Mondejar JA, Domenech J, Burgos J, Amaya S. Distal triplane fractures: long term follow –up. J Pediatr Orthop. 1996;16(1):113–8.
20. Hadad MJ, Sullivan BT, Sponseller PD. Surgically relevant patterns in triplane fractures. J Bone Joint Surg Am. 2018;100:1039–46.
21. Cooperman DR, Spiegal PG, Laros GS. Tibial fractures involving the ankle in children. The so called triplane epiphyseal fractures. J Bone Joint Surg Am. 1978;60(8):1040–6.
22. Marmor L. An unusual fracture of the tibial epiphysis. Clin Orthop Relat Res. 1970;73:132–5.
23. Kärrhom J, Hansson LI, Laurin S. Computed tomography of intraarticular supination-eversion fractures of the ankle in adolescents. J Pediatr Orthop. 1981;1(2):181–7.
24. Smekal V, Kadletz R, Rangger C, Gföller P. A new type of triplane fracture in 19-year- old snowboarder. J Trauma. 2001;50(1):155–7.
25. von Laer L. Classification, diagnosis, and treatment of transitional fractures of the distal part of the tibia. J Bone Joint Surg Am. 1985;67(5):687–98.
26. Denton JR, Fischer SJ. The medial triplane fracture: report of an unusual injury. J Trauma. 1981;21(11):991–5.
27. El-Karef E, Sadek HI, Nairn DS, Aldam CH, Allen PW. Triplane fracture of the distal tibia. Injury. 2000;31(9):729–36.
28. Peiró A, Aracil J, Martos F, Mut T. Triplane distal tibial epiphyseal fracture. Clin Orthop Relat Res. 1981;(160):196–200.
29. van Laarhoven CJ, van der Werken C. 'Quadriplane' fracture of the distal tibia: a triplane fracture with a double metaphyseal fragment. Injury. 1992;23(7):497–9.
30. Salter R, Harris WR. Injuries involving the epiphyseal plate. J Bone Joint Surg Am. 1963;45(3):587–622.
31. Ogden JA. Skeletal growth mechanism injury patterns. J Pediatr Orthop. 1982;2(4):371–7.
32. Mubarak SJ. Extensor retinaculum syndrome of the ankle after injury to the distal tibial physis. J Bone Joint Surg Br. 2002;84:11–4.
33. Haumont T, Gauchard GC, Zabee L, Arnoux J-M, Journeau P, Lascombes P. Extensor retinaculum syndrome after distal tibial fractures: anatomical basis. Surg Radiol Anat. 2007;29:303–11.
34. Stefanich RJ, Lozman J. The juvenile fracture of Tillaux. Clin Orthop Relat Res. 1986;210:219–27.
35. Manderson EL, Ollivierre CO. Closed anatomic reduction of a juvenile Tillaux fracture by dorsiflexion of the ankle. A case report. Clin Orthop Relat Res. 1992;276:262–6.
36. Kärrhom J, Hansson LI, Selvik G. Changes in tibiofibular relationships due to growth disturbances after ankle fractures in children. J Bone Joint Surg Am. 1984;66:1198–210.
37. Chung T, Jaramillo D. Normal maturing distal tibia and fibula: changes with age at MR imaging. Radiology. 1995;194:227–32.
38. Anderson M, Green W, Messner M. Growth and predictions of growth in the lower extremities. J Bone Joint Surg. 1963;45A:1–14.
39. Menelaus MB. Correction of leg length discrepancy by epiphyseal arrest. J Bone Joint Surg. 1966;48-B:336–9.
40. Moseley CF. A straight- line graph for leg length discrepancies. J Bone Joint Surg. 1977;59-A:174–9.
41. Paley D, Bhave A, Herzenberg JE, et al. Multiplier method for predicting limb length discrepancy. J Bone Joint Surg. 2000;82-A:1432–46.
42. Kling TF, Bright RW, Hesinger RN. Distal tibial physeal fractures in children that may require open reduction. J Bone Joint Surg Am. 1984;66:647–57.
43. Luhmann SJ, Oda JE, O'Donnell J, Keeler KA, Schoenecker PL, Dobbs MB, et al. An analysis of suboptimal outcomes of medial malleolus fractures in skeletally immature children. Am J Orthop. 2012;41:113–6.
44. Caterini R, Farsetti P, Ippolito E. Long term follow up of physeal injury to the ankle. Foot Ankle. 1991;11:372–83.
45. Leary JT, Handling M, Talerico M, Yong L, Bowe JA. Physeal fractures if the distal tibia predictive factors of premature physeal closure and growth arrest. J Pediatr Orthop. 2009;29:356–61.
46. Spiegel PG, Cooperman DR, Laros GS. Epiphyseal fractures of the distal ends of the tibia and fibula. A retrospective study of the two hundred and thirty-seven cases in children. J Bone Joint Surg Am. 1978;60:1046–50.
47. Barmada A, Gaynor T, Mubarak SJ. Premature physeal closure following distal tibia physeal fractures: a new radiographic predictor. J Pediatr Orthop. 2003;23:733–9.
48. Choudhry IK, Wall EJ, Eismann EA, Crawford AH, Wilson L. Functional outcome analysis of triplane and Tilleaux fractures after closed reduction and percutaneous fixation. J Pediatr Orthop. 2014;34:139–43.
49. Peterson HA. Metallic implant removal in children. J Pediatr Orthop. 2005;25(1):107–15.
50. Bransby-Zachary MA, MacDonald DA, Singh I, et al. Late fracture associated with retained internal fixation. J Bone Joint Surg Br. 1989;71:539.
51. Kahle WK. The case against routine metal removal. J Pediatr Orthop. 1994;14:229–37.

52. Labosky DA, Cermak MB, Waggy CA. Forearm fracture plates: to remove or not to remove. J Hand Surg Am. 1990;15:294–301.
53. Müller ME, Allgöwer M, Schneider R, et al. Manual of internal fixation techniques recommended by the AO Group. 2nd ed. (English translation by J Schaatzker). Berlin: Springer; 1979. p. 148–53.
54. Rosson JW, Petley GW, Shearer JR. Bone structure after removal of internal fixation plates. J Bone Joint Surg Br. 1991;73:65–7.
55. Charlton M, Costello R, Mooney JF III, et al. Ankle joint biomechanics following transepiphyseal screw fixation of the distal tibia. J Pediatr Orthop. 2005;25(5):635–40.
56. Keles-Celik N, Kose O, Sekerci R, Aytac G, Turan A, Güler F. Accessory ossicles of the foot and ankle: disorders and a review of the literature. Cureus. 2017;9(11):e1881. Published 2017 Nov 26. https://doi.org/10.7759/cureus.1881.
57. Kruppa C, Snoap T, Sietsema DL, Schildhauer TA, Dudda M, Jones CB. Is the midterm Progress of pediatric and adolescent talus fractures stratified by age? J Foot Ankle Surg. 2018;57(3):471–7.
58. Smith JT, Curtis TA, Spencer S, Kasser JR, Mahan ST. Complications of Talus fractures in children. J Pediatr Orthop. 2010;30(8):779–84.
59. Meier R, et al. Fractures of the talus in the pediatric patient. Foot Ankle Surg, [s l]. 2005;11:5–10.
60. Hawkins LG. Fractures of the neck of the talus. J Bone Joint Surg Am. 1970;52(5):991–1002.
61. Canale ST, Kelly FB. Fractures of the neck of the talus. Long-term evaluation of seventy-one cases. J Bone Joint Surg Am. 1978;60(2):143–56.
62. Polyzois VD, Vasiliadis E, Zgonis T, Ayazi A, Gkiokas A, Beris AE. Pediatric fractures of the foot and ankle. Clin Podiatr Med Surg. 2006;23:241–55.
63. Metzger MJ, Levin JS, Clancy JT. Talar neck fractures and rates of avascular necrosis. J Foot Ankle Surg. 1999;38:154–62. https://doi.org/10.1016/S1067-2516(99)80030-1.
64. Mora S, Thordarson DB, Zionts LE, Reynolds RA. Pediatric calcaneal fractures. Foot Ankle Int. 2001;22(6):471–477.
65. Petit CJ, Lee BM, Kasser JR, Kocher MS. Operative treatment of intraarticular calcaneal fractures in the pediatric population. J Pediatr Orthop. 2007;27(8):856–62.
66. Knijnenberg LM, Dingemans SA, Schepers T, Terra MP, Struijs PAA, Schep NWL. Radiographic anatomy of the pediatric lisfranc joint. J Pediatr Orthop. 2018;38(10):510–3.
67. Wilson DW. Injuries of the Tarso-metatarsal joints. J Bone Joint Surg. 1972;54-B:677–86.
68. Buoncristiani AM, Manos RE, Mills WJ. Plantarflexion tarsometatarsal joint injuries in children. J Pediatr Orthop. 2001;21:324–7.
69. Bloome D, Clanton T. Treatment of Lisfranc injuries in the athlete. Tech Foot Ankle Surg. 2002;1:94–101.
70. Hill JF, Benton EH, Lierhaus A, Kocher MS, Mahan ST. Lisfranc injuries in children and adolescents. J Pediatr Orthop B. 2017;26:159–63.
71. Singer G, Cichocki M, Schalamon J, Eberl R, Höllwarth ME. J Bone Joint Surg A. 2008; 90(4):772–6.
72. Southey ER, Soares-Weiser K, Kleijnen J. Systematic review and meta-analysis of the clinical safety and tolerability of ibuprofen compared with paracetamol in pediatric pain and fever. Curr Med Res Opin. 2009;25(9):2207–22.
73. Vetter TR, Heiner EJ. Intravenous Ketorolac as an adjuvant to pediatric patient controlled analgesia with morphine. J Clin Anesth. 1994;6(2):110–3.
74. Akbarnia BA, Akbarnia NO. The role of orthopedist in child abuse and neglect. Orthop Clin North Am. 1976;7(3):733–42.
75. Schmitt BD. Current pediatric roles in child abuse and neglect. Am J Dis Child. 1979;133(7):691–6.
76. Kemp AM, Dunstan F, Harrison S, Morris S, Mann M, Rolfe K, Datta S, Thomas DP, Sibert JR, Maguire S. Patterns of skeletal fractures in child abuse: systematic review. BMJ. 2008;337:a1518.

Correction to: The Pediatric Foot and Ankle

Michelle L. Butterworth and John T. Marcoux

Correction to:
M. L. Butterworth, J. T. Marcoux (eds.), *The Pediatric Foot and Ankle*
https://doi.org/10.1007/978-3-030-29788-6

The following chapters were inadvertently published with incorrect chapter title:

Chapter 2: Radiology of the Normal Foot
Chapter 3: Neurological Abnormalities
Chapter 4: Pediatric Digital Deformities
Chapter 5: Brachymetatarsia: Correction Through Callus Distraction
Chapter 6: Metatarsus Adductus (Midfoot Adduction)
Chapter 8: Equinus in the Pediatric Patient
Chapter 10: Pediatric and Adolescent Pes Valgus Deformity
Chapter 11: Tarsal Coalition and Pes Planovalgus: Clinical Examination, Diagnostic Imaging, and Surgical Planning
Chapter 13: Pediatric Foot and Ankle
Chapter 14: Pediatric Fractures

The correct titles have been updated in the book, and the correct titles are as follows:

Chapter 2: Radiology of the Pediatric Foot and Ankle
Chapter 3: Neurological Abnormalities of the Pediatric Foot and Ankle
Chapter 4: Digital Deformities of the Pediatric Foot
Chapter 5: Pediatric Brachymetatarsia
Chapter 6: Pediatric Metatarsus Adductus
Chapter 8: Pediatric Equinus Deformity
Chapter 10: Pediatric Flexible Pes Valgus Deformity
Chapter 11: Pediatric Tarsal Coalition and Pes Planovalgus
Chapter 13: Sports Medicine of the Pediatric Foot and Ankle
Chapter 14: Fractures of the Pediatric Foot and Ankle

The updated online version of this book can be found at
https://doi.org/10.1007/978-3-030-29788-6

M. L. Butterworth, J. T. Marcoux (eds.), *The Pediatric Foot and Ankle*,
https://doi.org/10.1007/978-3-030-29788-6_15

Index

M. L. Butterworth, J. T. Marcoux (eds.), *The Pediatric Foot and Ankle*,
https://doi.org/10.1007/978-3-030-29788-6

MIX
Papier aus verantwortungsvollen Quellen
Paper from responsible sources
FSC® C105338

If you have any concerns about our products,
you can contact us on
ProductSafety@springernature.com

In case Publisher is established outside the EU,
the EU authorized representative is:
Springer Nature Customer Service Center GmbH
Europaplatz 3, 69115 Heidelberg, Germany

Printed by Libri Plureos GmbH
in Hamburg, Germany